Kenew Copy

Anaesthesia and Resuscitation: A Houseman's Guide

Anaesthesia and Resuscitation

A Houseman's Guide

Edited by

R. D. M. Jones MBBS, LLB (Hons), MD, FANZCA, FRCA, FHKCA

Professor and Director
Division of Anaesthesiology and Intensive Care
Royal Brisbane Hospital
The University of Queensland
Australia

and

R. B. Holland MBBS, FFARACS, FANZCA, FHKCA

Formerly, Professor and Chairman
Department of Anaesthesia and Intensive Care
The John Hunter Hospital
The University of Newcastle
Australia

BUTTERWORTH
HEINEMANN

Butterworth-Heinemann
Linacre House, Jordan Hill, Oxford OX2 8DP
A division of Reed Educational and Professional Publishing Ltd

A member of the Reed Elsevier plc group

OXFORD BOSTON JOHANNESBURG
MELBOURNE NEW DELHI SINGAPORE

First published 1997

British Library Cataloguing in Publication Data
A catalogue record for this book is available from the British Library

Library of Congress Cataloguing in Publication Data
A catalogue record for this book is available from the Library of Congress

ISBN 0 7506 2960 6

Typeset by Keyword Typesetting Services Ltd, Wallington, Surrey
Printed and bound in Great Britain by Hartnolls Limited, Bodmin, Cornwall

Contents

Contributors

Philip Allen	MB BCh(Dublin), FFARCSI	Visiting Specialist Anaesthetist The Royal Brisbane Hospital
Christopher Andrews	BE(Hons), MBBS, MEngSc, PhD, DipCompSc, EDIC	Anaesthetic Registrar The Royal Brisbane Hospital
Anthony Brown	MBChB, MRCP, FRCS(Ed), FACEM, FFAEM	Staff Specialist Department of Emergency Medicine The Royal Brisbane Hospital
Alan Brown	BSc, MB,ChB, FRCA	Consultant Anaesthetist Victoria Infirmary, Glasgow
Charles Cheung	BSc(Hons)	Equipment Scientist Division of Anaesthesiology & Intensive Care The Royal Brisbane Hospital
Tess Cramond, AO, OBE	MBBS, FFARCS, FFARACS, FFARCSI, FRCA, FANZCA	Professor Emeritus Division of Anaesthesiology & Intensive Care The University of Queensland Director of Chronic Pain Clinic Consultant in Palliative Medicine The Royal Brisbane Hospital
Philip Cumpston	MBBS, FFARACS, FFARACS (Intensive Care), FACEM, FANZCA, FFICANZCA	Senior Lecturer Division of Anaesthesiology & Intensive Care The University of Queensland The Royal Brisbane Hospital
Ross Holland	MBBS, FFARACS, FANZCA, FHKCA	Formerly Professor and Chairman Department of Anaesthesia & Intensive Care The John Hunter Hospital The University of Newcastle
Michael Irwin	FRCA	Honorary Clinical Lecturer The University of Hong Kong
Douglas Jones	MBBS, LLB(Hons), MD, FANZCA, FRCA, FHKCA	Professor and Director The University of Queensland The Royal Brisbane Hospital
Jon Kornberg	MB,ChB, FRCA, FHKCA, FHKAM (Anaes)	Formerly, Lecturer Department of Anaesthesiology University of Hong Kong
John Morgan	MBBS, FFARACS, FANZCA, FFICANZCA	Staff Intensivist Division of Anaesthesiology & Intensive Care The Royal Brisbane Hospital
Allan Palmer	BMedSci, FRCA, FANZCA	Lecturer Division of Anaesthesiology & Intensive Care The University of Queensland The Royal Brisbane Hospital
Brenda Roberts	MB,ChB, FFARCSI, FFARCS, FRCA, DA RCP & RCS	Staff Anaesthetist The Royal Brisbane Hospital
Jeremy Rushmer	MBBS, BSc, MRCP(Edin), FRCA	Senior Registrar in Anaesthetics Western General Hospital Edinburgh
Anil Visram	FRCA	Senior Registrar in Anaesthetics Royal Free Hospital, London

Foreword

Few experiences in a medical career can produce anxiety to compare with the abrupt transition from final year medical student to intern. Where 95% might once have seemed a fine examination result, 5% failure in the workplace represents embarrassing incompetence. Worse still, unless detected promptly, serious, even lethal results are possible from mistakes occurring at a rate of 1 in 20 decisions.

Students crave the knowledge and skills which they know they will need. Unfortunately, they often lack discriminatory processing of the mass of theoretical information which has accumulated in five or six years and the efferent limb of the knowledge/action loop is undeveloped.

Attachments to clinical units at the sharp end of acute hospital medicine can, if well organised, go some way to developing the problem-solving and executive skills which must be activated if the intern is to function effectively. To obtain maximum benefit from these attachments, the student must have a clear understanding of what the experience can offer, and a firm grasp of certain vital theoretical concepts which may not hitherto have been emphasised. For instance, the relationship between tissue oxygen delivery and its determining triad of cardiac output, haemoglobin concentration and oxygen saturation is often a revelation to final year students.

This book attempts to fill such gaps in understanding, and to help the new graduate to cross the bridge which spans the gulf between academic interest on the one side and clinical responsibility on the other. Authors have been chosen for their practical, as well as academic skills in the major acute disciplines: anaesthesia, emergency medicine and intensive care.

The focus is, without apology, on the hot spots, and pays little attention to more contemplative concerns. The latter are not only well covered in most undergraduate curricula, but more importantly, in the non-acute situation there is ample time to research the subject and/or seek more mature advice. It is not that the authors wish to encourage interns to exceed their responsibilities, but being paralysed by doubt and indecision in a crisis is just as bad as being cocksure.

The format chosen is intended to be user-friendly, in that elegant prose has been eschewed in favour of the bullet presentation. Students are inveterate summarisers of prolix texts, but unfortunately their summaries are frequently either inaccurate or miss the major points. It is our hope and intention to render summarisation redundant.

Those of us who have attempted similar, but much more modest productions in the past, have found student feedback to be especially positive. This publication takes the concept further, and we the co-defendants eagerly, if anxiously, await the jury's verdict.

Ross B. Holland
Formerly, Professor & Chairman, Department of Anaesthesia & Intensive Care
The John Hunter Hospital,
The University of Newcastle
Australia

Preface

AIMS

- To provide medical core knowledge on subjects in which anaesthesiologists have most expertise
- To use pattern recognition in evaluation of illness and risk assessment
- To provide safe programmes of response in critical incidents
- To integrate physiology and pharmacology applicable to anaesthesia
- To present new trends in data acquisition and interpretation

This is NOT intended to be a 'How to give an anaesthetic book'!!

Part I

Topics Related to Anaesthesia

Chapter 1

Preparation for anaesthesia

The pre-anaesthetic consultation

Anaesthesia is a means to an end. It is neither diagnostic nor therapeutic except in certain very limited applications, but almost always serves to make a procedure (such as an operation) or an experience (like having a baby) painless. It is never trivial; even in the best circumstances, with highly trained individuals delivering the service, there is a hazard which can never be totally eliminated, although risk reduction has made great progress, and the mortality from anaesthesia is steadily being reduced.

The more you know about anaesthesia, the more able you are to anticipate what might go wrong, and the better prepared for trouble you are, the less likely it is to get out of control. The most important single principle of anaesthesia is that it is

BETTER TO STAY OUT OF TROUBLE,

THAN TO GET OUT OF TROUBLE.

If risks are taken, the stakes are provided by the patient, not by the anaesthetist, and the penalty for indiscretion is the patient paying with his life. Therefore everything must be done which will minimise risk. Risk reduction relies upon a sound knowledge of the basic sciences and adequate patient preparation. This means a meticulous workup for the elective case and vigorous resuscitation of the emergency.

Consultation by an anaesthetist is essential for the medical assessment of a patient prior to any anaesthetic procedure. Its purpose is to ensure that the patient is in the optimal state for anaesthesia, surgery or a related procedure. This requires additional skills and judgement which differ from those that are used to administer an anaesthetic.

General principles

- all doctors need to appreciate any potential anaesthetic problems to provide informed advice on the risks of surgery, for their patients.
- the pre-anaesthetic consultation should be performed by the anaesthetist who is to administer the anaesthetic.
- this consultation should take place at the appropriate time prior to surgery and anaesthesia, so that any necessary therapeutic or investigatory measures can be performed.
- it is acknowledged that early consultation is not always possible (e.g. life-saving surgery), but assessment is still necessary prior to commencement of anaesthesia and surgery, even in these circumstances.

Specific objectives

- establish a doctor/patient relationship
- history and examination
- develop a management strategy

Pre-anaesthetic consultation recommendations

- identification of the patient
- confirmation of the nature of the procedure and where applicable, the side on which it is to be performed
- a medical history and clinical examination of the patient, including a review of any current medication and results of any special investigations
- arrangement of any further therapeutic or investigatory measures, consultation with colleagues in other medical or surgical disciplines where appropriate (physicians, intensivists etc.)
- an attempt to satisfy the psychological needs of the patient
- the ordering of appropriate pre-medication if considered necessary
- a written summary which becomes part of the medical record of the patient

The anaesthesiology outpatient clinic

Why?

- the incidence of concurrent medical disease is high in surgical patients
- improves detection of previously unknown conditions
- improves a patient's general condition for surgery

Which patients?

- major surgery
- specific anaesthetic techniques required
- older patients with multiple pathology
- requested opinion on risks associated with surgery
- calm environment allows discussion, explanation and social circumstances to be considered

Some typical unsuspected findings!

- shadows on X-rays
- cardiac dysrhythmias
- anaemia
- hypokalaemia
- glycosuria
- cardiac murmurs
- hypertension
- goitre
- breast lumps

Preoperative assessment

The medical student should be competent in history taking and performing a general examination. This next section provides the student with important perspectives rather than a list of symptoms and signs.

What specific information pertinent to the conduct of anaesthesia should be sought from a patient?

History

Past history

- any unusual response to anaesthesia by any relatives
- any allergies, particularly medication sensitivity
- previous admissions to hospital
- previous anaesthesia
- present medications (+ traditional therapies & recreational drugs)

Past complications associated with surgery or anaesthesia

- chest infection
- deep vein thrombosis
- nausea and vomiting
- awareness
- dental trauma

Leading questions

Cardiovascular system

- past history
- exercise tolerance (consider concurrent disease-limited mobility e.g. osteoarthritis)
- chest pain, palpitations
- dependent oedema
- hypertension

Chest

- difficulty breathing
- snoring
- asthma
- cough – effectiveness and sputum production
- tobacco consumption

Hiatus hernia

- 'heartburn' (gastro-oesophageal sphincter incompetence)

Central nervous system

- loss of consciousness, hearing or vision
- epilepsy
- numbness

Alcohol and drug abuse

Examination

Body weight

- drug doses, fluid and blood requirements, ventilation, urine output and many more parameters are calculated using the body weight and lean body mass is estimated.

Dentition

- dentures, crowns, caps and caries

Airway and intubation problems

- anterior larynx
- cervical spine fixation
- temporomandibular joint opening
- # nose, nasal blockage

Cardiovascular and pulmonary systems

Venous access

- relationship to proposed surgery

Regional anaesthesia

- examine the surface anatomy
- existing neural deficits

Psychological assessment

- a personal visit and interview by the anaesthetist is a more potent anxiolytic than administration of a pharmacological preparation alone

Preoperative patient optimisation

Chronic obstructive airways disease

- physiotherapy, bronchodilator therapy

Atrial fibrillation

- pharmacological conversion from a rapid to a controlled rate

Cardiac failure

- treat the cause ± diuretics, digoxin

Obesity

- a patient may lose up to 10 kg due to the incentive effect of facilitating their surgery

Allay preoperative anxiety which may be due to

- poor general health
- fear of the operation or of postoperative discomfort
- leaving the family
- uncertain future
- fear of death
- loss of consciousness or 'control'
- anaesthesia

Thyrotoxicosis

- beta blockade

Jaundice

- vitamin K

Steroid dependence

- medication timing and dosage adjustment

Classification of physical status

At the conclusion of the consultation the anaesthetist should classify the patient's risk status and record it on the anaesthetic assessment chart.

American Society of Anesthesiologists (ASA) Classification

Class **1** – a normal healthy patient
Class **2** – a patient with mild to moderate systemic disease caused by the condition to be treated surgically or by any other disease
Class **3** – severe systemic disease or disturbance from any cause
Class **4** – severe systemic disorders that are already life threatening
Class **5** – the moribund patient with little chance of survival for more than 24 hours
Emergency is denoted by the letter **E**

Mortality rate per 1000 surgical operations

ASA	**1**	0.06 – 0.8
	2	0.27 – 0.4
	3	1.8 – 4.3
	4	7.8 – 23
	5	9.4 – 51

An alternative method used to assess procedural risk is the

Cardiac Risk Index (CRI)

Patients are separated into one of four classes according to their total point score:

third heart sound or raised jugular venous pressure	11
acute myocardial infarction within six months	10
more than 5 ventricular extrasystoles per minute	7
rhythm other than sinus (incl. premature atrial contractions)	7
age more than 70 years	5
emergency operation	4
intraperitoneal, intrathoracic, aortic operation	3
significant aortic stenosis	3
poor general condition	3
	53

ASA	**CRI**	
1 or 2	1	0 – 5 points
3	2	6 – 12
4	3	13 – 25
5	4	> 26 points

Note the appropriately large weighting given to cardiac failure and a recent history of myocardial infarction. A patient with a score > 26 has < 50% chance of surviving the operation.

Special conditions and anaesthesia

Pregnancy

- avoid anaesthesia during the first and last trimesters

Physical and mental disabilities

- use a sympathetic and intelligent companion
- provide heavy sedation with premedication
- hydrocephalus – difficult intubation
- absent limbs – difficult venous access
- deafness and blindness – leave hearing aid and glasses in situ

Psychological considerations

- personality – people who feel loved and secure have lower anxiety with separation and anaesthesia
- discuss patient fears
- preoperative visit – be humane, confident and competent
- some aspects of anaesthesia require special consideration
  - ◊ cardiac surgery
  - ◊ changes in body configuration
  - ◊ pain
  - ◊ local anaesthesia
  - ◊ paediatric patients – tell the truth
  - ◊ psychiatric patients
  - ◊ monoamine oxidase inhibition and lithium

Nutritional considerations

- obesity
  - ◊ body weight exceeds 30% of ideal
  - ◊ respiratory function
    - work of breathing increased
    - functional residual capacity decreased
    - gas exchange decreased
  - ◊ cardiac output and blood volume increased
  - ◊ blood pressure measurement inaccurate
  - ◊ difficulty with venous access
  - ◊ difficulty with intubation
  - ◊ increased risk of gastro-oesophageal reflux
  - ◊ increased postoperative complications
- malnutrition
  - ◊ due to disease
  - ◊ preoperative nasogastric alimentation
  - ◊ fluid and electrolyte depletion
  - ◊ increased susceptibility to infection
- diabetes
  - ◊ diagnosis
    - fasting blood sugar (FBS) > 8 mmol/L
    - post-prandial blood sugar > 11 mmol/L
  - ◊ insulin dependent diabetic
    - preoperatively convert to soluble insulin
    - schedule operation early in the day
    - FBS > 13 ... postpone!!
    - K^+ 1–2 mmol/ kg/ day plus an insulin infusion 50u / 50ml @ 1–2 ml/hr 10% dextrose by syringe pump to maintain BSL 4–10 mmol/L
  - ◊ non insulin dependent diabetic
    - FBS < 8 mmol/L ... OK
    - chlorpropamide has a half life of 36 hours, therefore STOP the day BEFORE surgery
    - major surgery – use soluble insulin for smooth and safe control

Liver disease

- cirrhosis associated with portal hypertension and haemorrhage
- coagulation defects
- oedema secondary to low plasma albumin
- interference with detoxification of drugs
- cerebral effects of drugs produce increased depression
- obesity, chronic hypoxia and heredity predispose to hepatic halothane sensitivity
- liver enzyme induction alters drug disposition

Alcoholism

- require CXR, ECG, FBE, BGA, BSL, U & Es, LFTs as a **routine**
- cirrhosis
- cardiac myopathy
- electrolyte imbalance
- hypoglycaemia

Drug interactions

- current therapy should NOT be discontinued abruptly, especially digoxin, diuretics, insulin, beta blockers, anti-hypertensives, steroids, anticoagulants, antibiotics.
- contraceptive pill – oestrogen-containing pill should be discontinued four weeks preoperatively because of the increased risk of deep vein thrombosis. This risk increases with obesity, age, smoking, and high oestrogen, however the progesterone pill need not be stopped.
- the aspirin induced anti-platelet thrombotic effect lasts about 1 week and may precipitate serious bleeding (e.g. in transurethral prostatic resection)

Immediate preoperative preparation

- fasting requirements
    - ◊ adults – last intake of solids 6 hours prior to elective surgery to prevent pulmonary aspiration
    - ◊ infants – clear dextrose fluids up to 2 hours preoperatively
- cosmetics removed – except covering scars
- dentures and artificial limbs removed in theatre
- hearing aid should remain attached to patient
- empty bladder
- operation site marked and patient labelled
- consent form signed
- anticipation of postoperative care (ICU bed, nursing manpower)
- preparation of the appropriate monitoring apparatus, resuscitative equipment, cross-matched blood and other equipment essential for the performance of the chosen anaesthetic technique
- emergency anaesthesia requires rapid patient preparation but hypovolaemia, electrolyte disturbances and acid-base derangements MUST be corrected prior to surgery

Preoperative medication

Preoperative medication has been dominated by tradition. In the past it was used to minimise the effects of ether and cyclopropane, however the major present day indication is to attenuate patient anxiety.

Various drug combinations

- major tranquilliser
- anticholinergic
- sedative/hypnotic
- narcotic analgesic
- none

There is NO standard premedication

- a premedication regimen is designed to meet the specific needs of a particular patient in a specific surgical situation

Drug administration and timing

- drug and dosage depends on
    - ◊ age
    - ◊ weight
    - ◊ ASA status
    - ◊ current medication
    - ◊ type and duration of surgery
- timing of premedication administration varies from seconds (intravenous), up to 2 hours (oral administration) prior to induction.
    - ◊ shocked patients should receive drugs intravenously
    - ◊ vagal nerve block and antibiotic therapy are given with induction
    - ◊ antisialagogue is given 2 hours preoperatively
    - ◊ gastric antacid is given 20 minutes preoperatively
- routes of drug administration
    - ◊ oral, inhaled
    - ◊ intramuscular, intravenous
    - ◊ sublingual, transdermal, rectal

Responses to premedication

All or some of the following effects of premedication may be desirable

- anxiolytic
- amnesia
- analgesia
- sedation
- antisialagogue
- vagolytic
- antiemetic
- antihistamine (allergy prophylaxis)
- smoother induction procedure (dampen reflex responses to surgical stimuli)
- lowered induction drug dosage (± decreased intraoperative anaesthetic requirements)
- antacid (increased gastric pH and decreased gastric volume)

Other selective preoperative treatment regimens

- antithrombosis – subcutaneous low dose heparin
- antiplatelet – NSAIDS, aspirin
- fluid, acid-base and electrolyte balance
- blood transfusion
- haemodilution
- autologous transfusion
- antibiotic preparation
- preparation for specific disease problems

Chapter 2

Tracheal intubation

Introduction

- intubation of the trachea is performed as a routine part of many general anaesthetics but it also plays an important part of the management of patients during resuscitation, intensive care and in the emergency department
- you may need this skill during resuscitation during your internship year

Indications for tracheal intubation

- ventilation of the lungs
  - ◊ when paralysis of voluntary muscles is produced by drugs to facilitate surgery
  - ◊ to hyperventilate a patient with an injured brain to lower the $PaCO_2$ and reduce cranial blood volume
  - ◊ for respiratory support in patients with neurological, respiratory, cardiovascular, muscular or metabolic disease in the intensive care unit
  - ◊ when the type of surgery interferes with access to the airway for the anaesthesiologist, e.g. neurosurgery, head & neck, dental surgery or prone position
  - ◊ resuscitation following cardiac arrest
- prevention of pulmonary aspiration
  - ◊ an unconscious patient is at risk of regurgitation and aspiration (see below). This may occur in the ward, emergency department, recovery or operating room or by the road side
  - ◊ a conscious patient may also lose his protective reflexes, e.g. stroke, bulbar palsy, Guillain–Barré disease
- access to the lungs
  - ◊ suction of secretions, blood or pus from the lungs and major bronchi through the tracheal tube during anaesthesia or in intensive care
  - ◊ administration of drugs during advanced cardiopulmonary resuscitation
- bypass obstruction
  - ◊ anywhere in the airway above the carina due to trauma, oedema, cancer or, rarely, a foreign body.
  - ◊ the commonest and most important cause of obstruction of the airway is impaction of the base of the tongue in the laryngopharynx

Equipment

- the minimum equipment to intubate a patient is a working laryngoscope, an appropriate size tracheal tube and a syringe to inflate the cuff
- in addition one should also have the facility to ventilate the patient's lungs with a mask and self-inflating bag, anaesthetic circuit or a ventilator. If you are in a situation where these are not available (e.g. at the scene of a drowning) then you can blow down the tracheal tube to inflate the patient's lungs.
- in hospital there should also be a supply of oxygen, suction facilities and a full range of tube sizes
- a range of laryngoscope blade shapes is also useful and a stylet or bougie may aid difficult intubation
- a second back-up laryngoscope should always be available
- a competent assistant

Method

1. Position the patient

- to intubate under direct vision, the intubator has to convert what is normally a **right-angle** between the mouth and the laryngeal opening into a **straight line**.

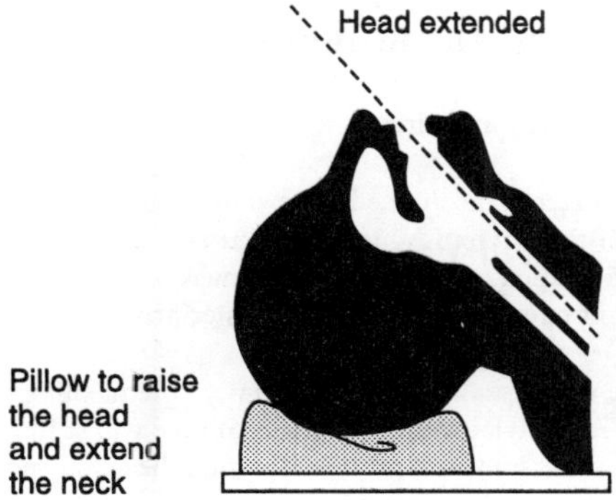

Head position for laryngoscopy

- use at least one pillow beneath the occiput to produce flexion of the neck, then gently tilt the head backwards to produce the classic 'sniffing the morning air' position by extension of the head on the neck.

2. take the handle of the laryngoscope in your **left** hand and carefully introduce the blade into the **right** side of the mouth and sweep the tongue away to the left. It may help if you have an assistant hold the mouth open.

3. orientate yourself to the midline by noting the position of the uvula. By gently lifting the tip of the laryngoscope blade you should try to view the tip of the epiglottis.

4. having identified the epiglottis, slide the tip of the laryngoscope blade anteriorly (i.e. on the upper surface of the epiglottis when the patient is supine) into the vallecula. *You should not lose sight of the epiglottis at any time during intubation as it is the major crucial landmark.*

5. holding the laryngoscope firmly by its handle, lift steadily up and forwards along the axis of the handle. DO NOT LEVER THE HANDLE BACK TOWARDS YOU. This will damage the patient's lips and teeth and will make intubation more difficult. *The laryngoscope should not be touching the upper teeth or lips if you are lifting in the correct direction.* The cords should now come into view posteriorly and below the epiglottis.

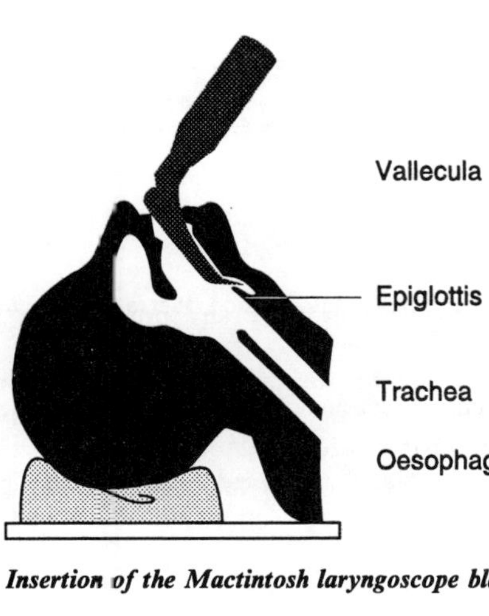

Insertion of the Mactintosh laryngoscope blade

6. hold the tracheal tube about 1/3 from the connector and introduce the tube at the angle of the lips into the side of the mouth so that the view of the larynx is NOT obscured by the tracheal tube.

- align the tip of the tube with the open cords, then pass it through and rotate the tube anticlockwise 90°. In the adult the tube should only be advanced so that the upper weld of the cuff lies 1 cm beyond the cords, thereby reducing the risk of endobronchial intubation. Check the length marking on the tracheal tube at the lips.

7. attach a self-inflating bag or anaesthetic breathing circuit and gently inflate the lungs with oxygen. There will be an audible leak around the tracheal tube until the cuff is inflated with sufficient air to stop the hissing sound of air-leak. If there is no leak the tracheal tube should be replaced by one of smaller size.

8. tie or tape the tube in place and check its position by listening in both axillae and over the epigastrium. If there is a capnograph available, attach it to the circuit and confirm expired carbon dioxide. This confirms that the tracheal tube is not in the oesophagus.

What to do if you fail to intubate

- ventilate the patient with oxygen using a mask, airway and circuit.
- send for help.
- *increase neck flexion.* Check that the head is correctly positioned. The most common reason for failure is not having a pillow under the head. If the larynx is anterior it is useful to place a second pillow under the occiput after reoxygenating the patient with the bag and mask.
- *laryngeal pressure.* Using the fingers of your right hand, press the larynx posteriorly. This will often bring the larynx into view.
- *intubating stylet.* Sometimes the vocal cords are well visualised but a prominent premaxilla prevents the tracheal tube aligning with the laryngeal inlet. A stylet within the tracheal tube will stiffen it and allow it to be curved into the desired shape. The stylet must not protrude beyond the distal end of the tracheal tube as it may damage the tracheal or laryngeal structures.
- if you still cannot intubate the patient, DO NOT PERSIST. Maintain the patient's ventilation with the bag, mask, airway and oxygen, and call for more experienced assistance.

Likely contributing factors to intubation difficulty

- neck
    - ◊ limitation of cervical spine movement – ankylosing spondylitis, rheumatoid arthritis, short muscular neck
    - ◊ burns scarring
- jaw
    - ◊ limitation of temporo-mandibular joint movement – arthritis
    - ◊ trismus associated with
        - dental abscess
        - trauma – # mandibular condyle
        - quinsy (rarely)
- lips and mouth
    - ◊ scleroderma, burns scarring
    - ◊ prominent premaxilla and receding mandible i.e. type II malocclusion, Pierre–Robin syndrome
    - ◊ tongue enlargement – Down's and Beckwith's syndromes
- pharynx, epiglottis and larynx
    - ◊ pharynx – # middle third of face, vascular tumours, caustic ingestion, angioneurotic oedema
    - ◊ epiglottis – infection, burns, smoke inhalation, cysts
    - ◊ larynx
        - anterior position
        - viral infection, oedema, tumour
        - sub-glottic stenosis

Predicting difficult intubation

Many of the factors contributing to difficult intubation are obvious but there is a need for a method of predicting a difficult intubation in patients who may appear normal.

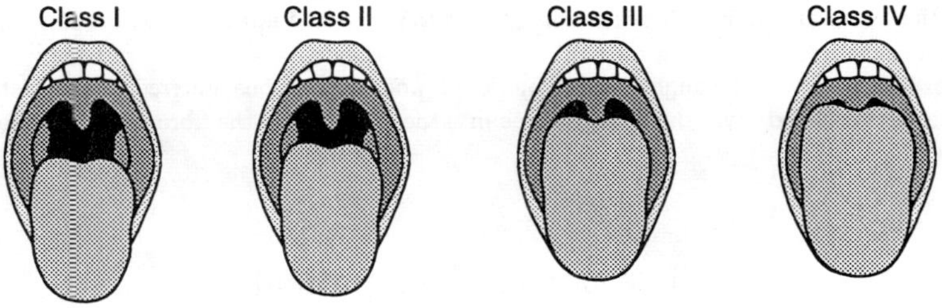

Mallampati assessment of the pharyngeal structures

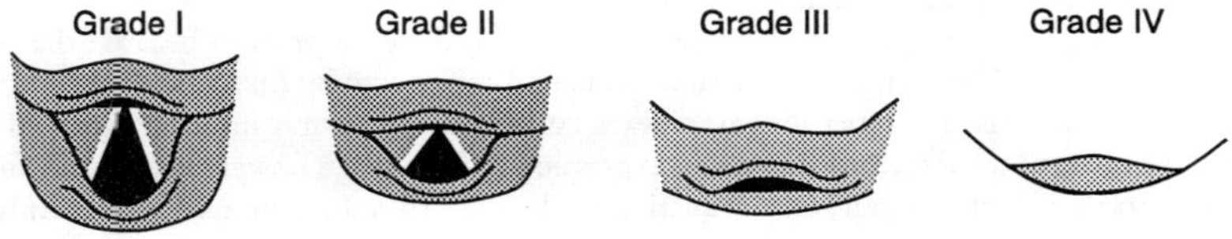

Corresponding laryngoscopic views (modified from Cormack & Lehane)

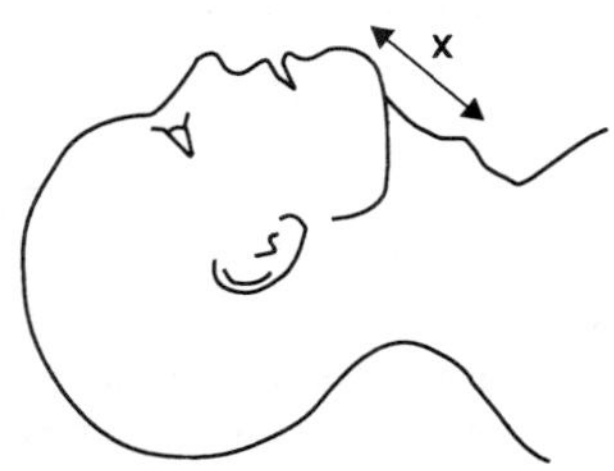

- Mallampati classified patients into four groups depending on the amount of pharyngeal soft tissue visualised when the patient opens the mouth while sitting opposite the examiner.
- this was correlated with the Cormack & Lehane classification of the laryngeal view seen at direct laryngoscopy, i.e. if the patient is assessed as class IV Mallampati preoperatively, the patient will most likely be Cormack & Lehane grade 3 or 4 during direct laryngoscopy and the intubator will be unable to intubate the patient by conventional means.
- **Thyromental distance:** with the neck fully extended, patients who have a distance of less than 7 cm between the prominence of the thyroid cartilage and the bony point of the chin are more likely to present difficulty in intubation, as the hyoid bone and its attached structures will be situated more anteriorly than normal.
- this assesses the capacity for the mouth and pharynx to accept the tongue sweep to the left and permit epiglottic exposure.

The patient who is unintubatable by direct laryngoscopy

- occasionally a patient may require intubation to facilitate surgery but be impossible to intubate using direct laryngoscopy.
- intubation is accomplished using a fibre-optic flexible laryngoscope through the nose.
- the patient is awake, although often sedated, and the nose and upper airway are anaesthetised with local anaesthetic.
- the cords are viewed through the laryngoscope and the trachea entered. The tracheal tube is advanced (railroaded) over the laryngoscope into the trachea and the fibre-optic laryngoscope withdrawn.

The unconscious patient

- to accept the passage of a tracheal tube the patient must have severely depressed or absent reflexes in the pharynx and larynx. These reflexes normally prevent liquids and solid material from entering the lungs through the laryngeal opening.
- in the operating room, the anaesthesiologist is able to intubate the trachea because the patient has been given a drug which depresses conscious state and reflex activity (induction agent). Use of this drug alone to depress the upper airway reflexes sufficiently to permit intubation would require a relative overdose of the induction agent and expression of the agent's unwanted effects. Combination with a muscle relaxant drug allows a reduction in the dose of induction agent and paralysis of the vocal cords.
- during induction there will be a period of time when the patient is unconscious and the lungs are unprotected by reflexes, before the tracheal tube has been placed through the larynx. During elective surgery in patients without a propensity to vomit, this is not a problem because the patients come to the operating room fasted. However certain groups of patients are at risk of regurgitating stomach contents and aspirating these into their lungs during periods of unconsciousness, such as during induction and recovery from anaesthesia.

Patients at risk of aspiration

- all unconscious patients have a compromised airway and are at risk of aspirating. Absence of 'gagging' after stimulation of the gag reflex by touching the back of the pharynx with a spatula implies a serious derangement of pharyngeal reflexes and it is correct to assume that laryngeal reflexes are similarly depressed
- any patient who has not been fasted for the normal period (4-6 hours) prior to surgery
- trauma patients in whom pain and shock combine to produce gastric stasis
- acute abdominal conditions which produce ileus and decrease abdominal compliance
- administration of opiates further decrease gastric emptying
- obstruction of the gastrointestinal tract
- hiatus hernia patients who regurgitate through an incompetent gastro-oesophageal sphincter: aspiration of stomach acid may still occur after fasting
- several factors combine to increase the risk in obstetric patients
    - ◊ the enlarged uterus causes an increase in intra-gastric pressure and a reduction in abdominal compliance
    - ◊ hormonal and mechanical changes cause relaxation and incompetence of the gastro-oesophageal sphincter
    - ◊ pain in labour results in gastric stasis, increased gastric secretion at a lower pH, decreased gastric emptying and an increase in gastric volume
    - ◊ opiate administration decreases gastric emptying and is associated with nausea

Prevention of aspiration during anaesthesia induction

- **guaranteed** emptying of the stomach **CANNOT** be achieved by insertion of a *nasogastric tube*, although this will decompress the stomach by providing a route for gas under pressure to escape to atmosphere
- a large bore *stomach tube* can be inserted for gastric lavage but is unpleasant and not completely effective
- *vomiting* (emesis) can be induced with intravenous apomorphine but is extremely unpleasant in an otherwise ill patient and may cause fluid, electrolyte and acid-base abnormalities.
- reduction in gastric acid volume and increase in pH with *H_2 receptor antagonists* such as ranitidine and cimetidine given several hours before surgery. These drugs are often used in patients at risk of regurgitation such as pregnancy and hiatus hernia
- 30 ml of 0.3 M sodium citrate can also be administered 20 minutes preoperatively to elevate gastric pH and thereby reduce the severity of the chemical pneumonitis which may result if accidental aspiration does occur.

Cricoid pressure

- regurgitation is *passive* and at low pressure (10–15 cm H_2O)
- vomiting is an *active* process and develops a high pressure within the upper gastrointestinal tract (40–60 cm H_2O)
- obstruction of the oesophagus using cricoid pressure can withstand a pressure of 100 cm H_2O
- posterior compression of the complete cartilaginous cricoid ring during induction of anaesthesia can prevent regurgitation from the stomach reaching the laryngeal inlet
- the patient is anaesthetised in the supine position. Prior to induction, an assistant familiar with Sellick's manoeuvre locates the patient's cricoid cartilage and positions his fingers in readiness to apply pressure. As consciousness is lost the assistant presses the cricoid cartilage with the middle finger and thumb, using the index finger to control the direction of pressure until the resistance of the cervical vertebral body is felt
- this produces compression of the oesophagus between the posterior aspect of the complete cricoid ring and the anterior aspect of the vertebral body

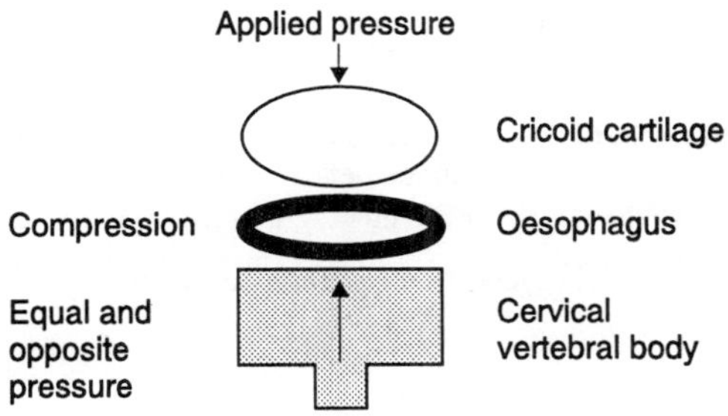

Cricoid pressure (Sellick's manoeuvre)

ALL doctors should be familiar with this procedure because anyone may be required to assist the anaesthetist during induction of anaesthesia.

Chapter 3

General anaesthesia and unconsciousness

General anaesthesia

Anaesthesia delivered to a patient may be general or regional. General anaesthesia is associated with unconsciousness whilst regional anaesthesia per se, is not. Regional anaesthesia may be employed either in combination with general anaesthesia or alone. It is appropriate for the student to acquire a broad appreciation of the type of anaesthesia being delivered to their patient. Regional anaesthesia is discussed in a later chapter.

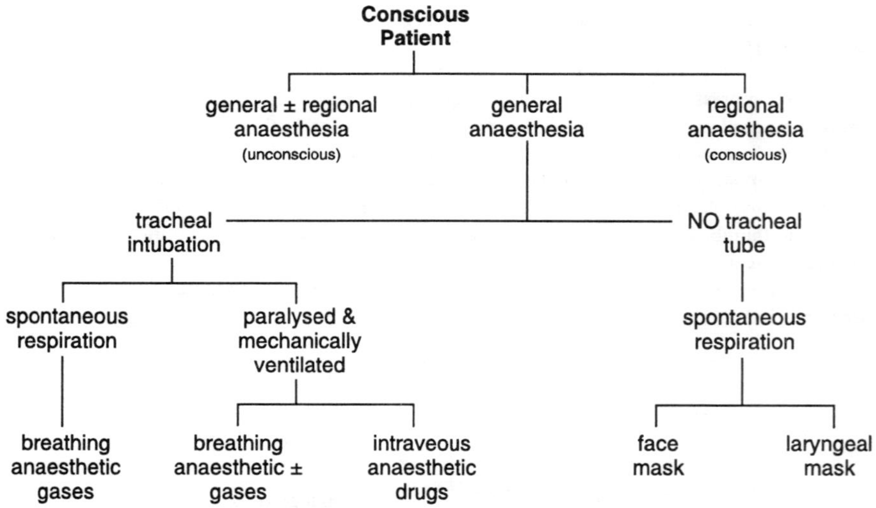

An overview of general anaesthesia

Anaesthesia involves the following phases

- preparation
- induction
- airway management
- maintenance
- reversal
- recovery
- postoperative care

Preparation

Preoperative planning and preparation is an essential part of limiting the hazards of anaesthesia. It commences with the preoperative consultation and continues until induction of anaesthesia. It requires a checklist analogous to that used by a pilot before takeoff –

- oxygen
- suction
- anaesthetic machine and gas delivery circuit
- intubation equipment
- drugs

Induction

This is the process of transforming the conscious patient to the unconscious state and may be accomplished intravenously by drugs like THIOPENTONE or PROPOFOL or by the patient inhaling anaesthetic agents such as ISOFLURANE or HALOTHANE. Intravenous induction is rapid (unconsciousness occurring in one arm–brain circulation time – approximately 15 seconds), pleasant and predictable. The blood level of the intravenous induction agent falls rapidly as the drug is redistributed throughout the body and consciousness is normally regained within 5 minutes of administration. Induction by inhalation of a volatile agent in oxygen may be used with those frightened of injections and in patients with threatened airway obstruction.

Airway management

Some surgical procedures require tracheal intubation. To facilitate placement of the tracheal tube through the larynx a muscle relaxant is administered. The muscle relaxant may be of the short acting type – lasting say 5 minutes (SUXAMETHONIUM) or longer acting – more than 15 minutes and lasting up to an hour (ATRACURIUM or VECURONIUM). It is possible to administer suxamethonium, intubate, allow the paralysis to 'wear off' so that the patient breathes spontaneously with the tracheal tube in situ, whilst anaesthesia is maintained. Usually when surgery requires tracheal intubation a longer acting muscle relaxant is administered; the patient remains paralysed and **must be mechanically ventilated** to maintain normal respiratory gas exchange. Patients having peripheral minor surgery may not require tracheal intubation and their oxygen-anaesthetic gas mixture is delivered via a face mask and Guedel airway or laryngeal mask.

Maintenance of anaesthesia

Anaesthesia can be maintained with intravenous drugs or inhalational agents. Narcotics, sedatives, muscle relaxants and induction agents may be administered intravenously in various combinations either as intermittent aliquots or as continuous infusions. These intravenous drugs may be supplemented by inhalational agents or alternatively, anaesthesia may be maintained by inhalation agents alone. Nitrous oxide together with oxygen is delivered to the patient from FLOW METERS situated on the anaesthetic machine. Nitrous oxide is a weak anaesthetic and by itself is insufficient to maintain a satisfactory depth of anaesthesia for major surgery. To deepen anaesthesia it is usual therefore to add a volatile agent which is dispensed from a VAPORISER attached to the flow meters.

Reversal

When the surgical procedure has concluded, the long acting muscle relaxant may be reversed by neostigmine or the blood levels allowed to decline due to spontaneous drug metabolism. Atropine is usually concurrently administered, although its vagolytic half life is of shorter duration than neostigmine and delayed bradycardia may result. The inhalational agents are excreted via the lungs to the atmosphere and as the concentration of anaesthetic drugs fall in the brain, so the patient gradually regains consciousness.

Recovery

The unconsciousness produced by general anaesthesia is associated with the same potential hazards which accompany coma, but because trained anaesthetic staff are present, steps can be taken to minimise these hazards. Recovery from anaesthesia is not immediate and requires supplemental oxygen administration to combat nitrous oxide induced diffusion hypoxia. Furthermore a period of intense monitoring is required to ensure there are no early untoward consequences of surgery.

When

the patient can maintain an airway without support
the upper airway protective reflexes have returned
the respiratory and cardiovascular systems are stable
the patient demonstrates a satisfactory elevation of conscious state

Only then can the patient be returned to the ward.

Hazards of acute unconsciousness

When consciousness is abolished, either deliberately by the anaesthetist, or as a consequence of trauma or disease, serious physiological aberrations occur which potentially threaten the patient's life. Some of these hazards are:

- Loss of ***muscle tone***. Of particular importance are the muscles supporting the upper airway, which in the supine position, allow obstruction of the laryngeal inlet when the tongue falls backward to the posterior pharyngeal wall, due to the force of gravity.
- Derangement or abolition of ***laryngeal reflexes***. Protection of the airways from contamination is either absent or inappropriate. In the latter case, the response is exaggerated so that laryngeal spasm may be so severe as to threaten asphyxia. In deeper states of unconsciousness, aspiration of liquids or solids may occur without impediment.
- Impairment of ***vasomotor control*** to a greater or lesser extent, depending on the depth of coma. In the head-up position, perfusion of the brain may fall to dangerously low levels.
- The patient is unable to respond to nociceptive stimuli, and will therefore be prone to injuries of various kinds, e.g. to the eyes, peripheral nerves and skin.

All of these hazards may be reduced by special techniques, but even in expert hands cannot be totally eliminated. These techniques are not unique to anaesthesia and have applications in the care of all unconscious patients.

The unconscious patient – acute care

All patients who are unconscious, no matter how briefly, run the risk of respiratory obstruction. When a head injury is associated with multiple trauma, there are additional risks of hypoxia, hypotension and hypoventilation which will harm the recently damaged brain. Unconscious patients must be afforded care appropriate to this state and attention to the head injury itself initially takes second place to ensuring that the body is well perfused with adequately oxygenated blood.

Respiratory system

Airway

- complete or partial airway obstruction is most commonly due to
  - ◊ the tongue falling backwards and obstructing the laryngeal inlet and/or
  - ◊ negative pressure causing collapse of toneless pharyngeal walls during attempted inspiration
- there may be vomitus, secretions, blood, CSF or a foreign body (e.g. dentures) in the mouth or pharynx
- rarely, there are direct injuries to the larynx or trachea.

All too often it is when the patient has reached hospital that insufficient attention is paid to the airway. **It is vital that the patient's airway is unobstructed:**
- clear the mouth and pharynx by finger sweep and suction the pharynx to remove blood, saliva and any regurgitated stomach contents
- place the patient in the left lateral position.
- insert an oral or nasopharyngeal airway ± jaw thrust
- tracheal intubation may be required

If the patient will tolerate an airway he needs one! However, inexpert attempts at intubation cause large rises in intracranial pressure and can only be harmful.

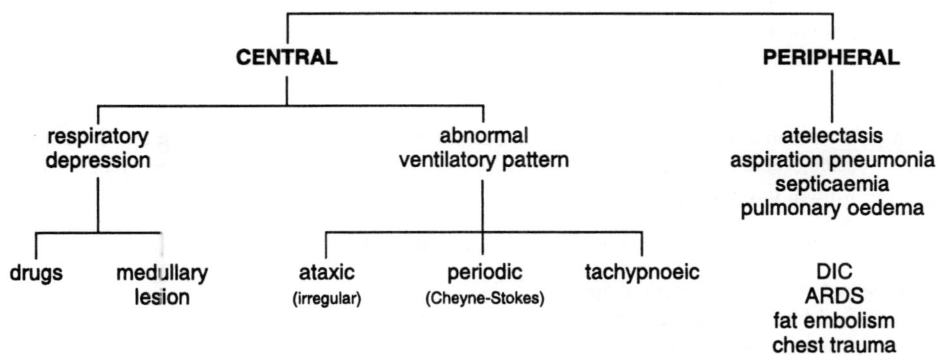

Causes of respiratory dysfunction in the unconscious head injured patient

Lungs

- pulmonary toilet (suctioning)
  - ◊ precede by analgesic or sedative administration
  - ◊ precede by hyperoxygenation (F_IO_2 1.0)
  - ◊ ensure a sterile, brief, intermittent and efficient procedure

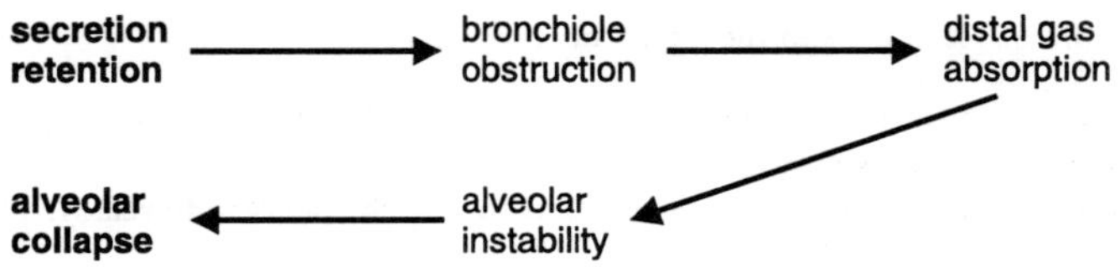

Aetiology of atelectasis in unconscious patients

- humidification of inspired gases
  - ◊ promotes mucociliary transport
  - ◊ prevents inspissation of secretions
  - ◊ saline instillation may be required
- chest physiotherapy
  - ◊ postural drainage
  - ◊ percussion and vibration
  - ◊ tracheal suction and artificial cough
- bronchoscopy
  - ◊ if humidification, physiotherapy and tracheal suction fail to prevent retention of secretions, flexible fibre-optic bronchoscopy may be used to aspirate the secretions under direct vision without interrupting ventilation

The most important physiological consequence of atelectasis is **hypoxia** which results from:

- increased ventilation/perfusion mismatch
- decreased functional residual capacity and pulmonary compliance
- increased work of breathing, respiratory rate and dead space

Patients suffering head and chest trauma have a high incidence of respiratory failure.
The following diagram illustrates some of the mechanisms:

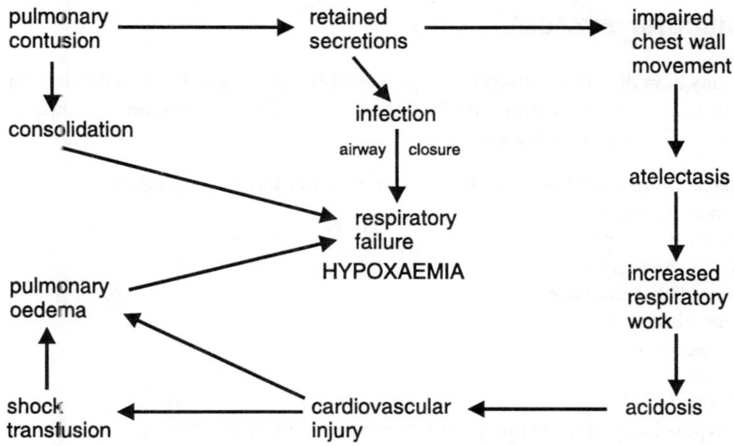

Respiratory failure following head and chest trauma

- **Pulmonary aspiration of gastric contents** is a constant threat to the unconscious patient because of
  - ◊ loss of gag and cough reflexes
  - ◊ a full stomach (trauma is often associated with alcohol consumption)
  - ◊ decreased rate of gastric emptying
  - ◊ gastric dilatation due to accidental insufflation during resuscitation
  - ◊ the passive, silent nature of regurgitation
- Aims of treatment of respiratory dysfunction associated with unconsciousness are:
  - ◊ maintain adequate pulmonary oxygen uptake
  - ◊ avoid carbon dioxide retention
  - ◊ provide a $PaO_2 > 75$ torr (10 kPa) and a $PaCO_2 = 30 - 35$ torr (4 – 4.5 kPa)
  - ◊ suction and physiotherapy preceded by sedation to prevent acute rises in intracranial pressure
  - ◊ intubation may be required to
    - maintain an airway by preventing upper respiratory tract obstruction
    - ensure adequate ventilation
    - ensure adequate oxygenation
    - control intracranial pressure
    - treat concomitant chest injuries or complications
    - reduce risk of aspiration

Cardiovascular system

Hypotension may have disastrous effects upon the recently injured brain, but hypotension per se is rarely a consequence of the injury to the brain itself. Hypotension and unconsciousness associated with trauma may arise in the following circumstances:

- hypovolaemia – loss of blood/fluid (overt bleeding or covert third space losses)
- associated chest injury
    - ◊ tension pneumothorax
    - ◊ direct cardiac injury
    - ◊ pericardial tamponade
    - ◊ aortic dissection
    - ◊ haemothorax
- spinal injury
- septic shock
- relative hypovolaemia exposed by positive pressure ventilation
- rarely, cranial causes
    - ◊ extensive scalp injury
    - ◊ extradural haematoma in a child
    - ◊ fracture involving a major venous sinus or artery

Chapter 4

Muscle relaxants

The neuromuscular junction

During your medical course it is unlikely that any other discipline will discuss the clinical pharmacology of the muscle relaxant group of drugs and therefore, contrary to the theme of this book, this chapter will provide some non-clinical background information.

Skeletal muscles are innervated by myelinated motor nerve fibres which arise in the anterior horn cells of the spinal cord, or in the brain stem. As the axon approaches the surface of the muscle fibre, it expands and divides into a number of motor endplates, each endplate contacting an individual muscle fibre. Where the membrane of neural origin comes into contact with the muscle fibre, a specialised area of the muscle membrane also develops, and the combination of the two forms the physiological unit via which a nerve impulse effects a contraction of the muscle fibre.

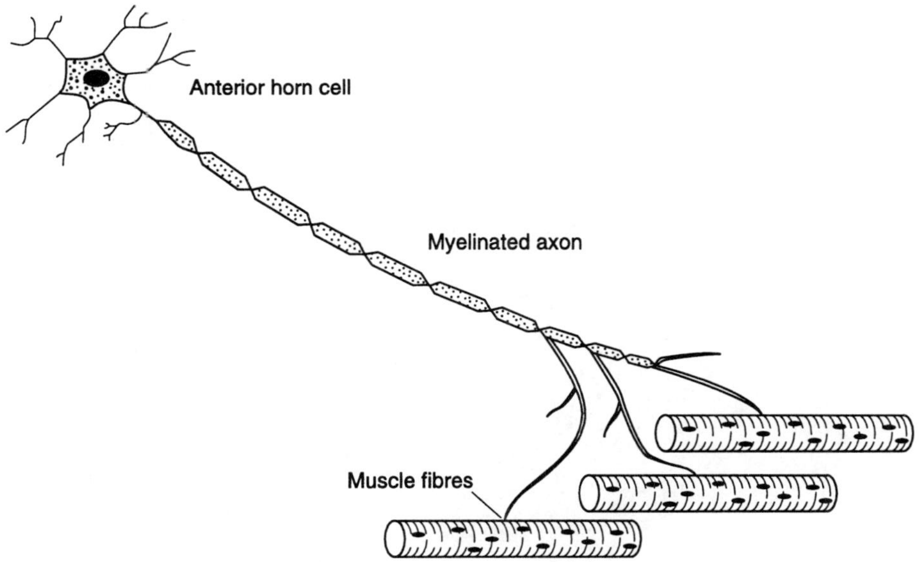

Neural innervation of skeletal muscle

Within the neural component (axon terminal), vesicles containing acetylcholine await the stimulus of a nerve impulse for their rupture and discharge into the cleft between the two components of the endplate. The muscle-derived component contains receptors which respond to acetylcholine, but they are not wholly specific, and can be occupied by the muscle relaxant class of drugs. Within the cleft itself, cholinesterase begins to hydrolyse acetylcholine as soon as it is discharged, ensuring that depolarisation is transient. The components are reabsorbed into the neural terminal where they are recycled. Drugs with anticholinesterase activity therefore allow the accumulation of acetylcholine in the cleft, prolonging and intensifying its action.

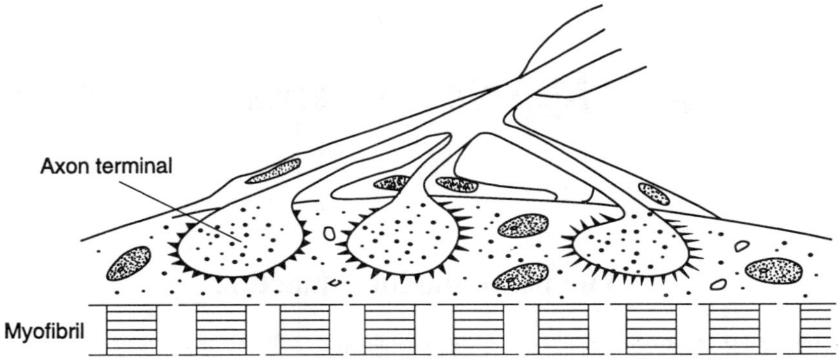

The neuromuscular junction

Once acetylcholine has occupied its receptor on the muscle component of the neuromuscular junction, a complex series of electrochemical events takes place culminating in the contraction of the muscle fibre. Channels in the membrane open, admitting sodium and calcium ions, whilst potassium ions escape into the extracellular space. A substantial shift in electrical charge depolarises the muscular component of the end-plate, and it is this electrical event which is then followed by muscle contraction. Return to the previous resting potential of −90 mV is necessary before another contraction can be initiated.

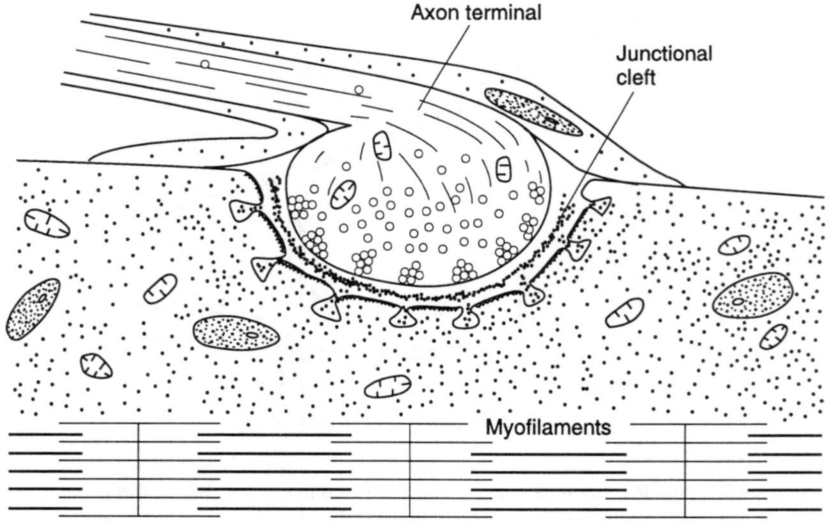

The muscular end-plate

The foregoing basic physiology is essential to an understanding of the action of muscle relaxants, of which there are two main types in clinical practice.

Non-depolarising muscle relaxants

The non-depolarisers, also sometimes called competitive blockers, occupy the acetylcholine receptors without activating them. When 70% of the receptors are so occupied, the onset of clinical paralysis ensues. Effective muscle relaxation for the performance of abdominal surgery requires 90% occupancy.

A **non-depolarising block** has the following characteristics:

- there is decreased reaction to a single impulse
- the response to a tetanic stimulus is not sustained, i.e. it fades
- at levels of occupancy of 70% and over, response to repeated stimuli at 1 Hz is characteristic. The 'train-of-four' stimuli can be used as a rough guide to percentage occupancy
- no fasciculation occurs prior to the onset of paralysis
- a single stimulus arriving after a period of tetany produces an enhanced response ('post-tetanic facilitation')
- it is antagonised by anticholinesterases.

There are many drugs in clinical practice which produce these effects:

Generic name	Proprietary name	Onset	Duration
d-tubocurarine (curare)	Tubarine	slow	long
alcuronium	Alloferin	medium-slow	medium
pancuronium	Pavulon	medium-slow	long
vecuronium	Norcuron	medium	short
atracurium	Tracrium	medium	short

Depolarising muscle relaxants

The other class of muscle relaxants, the depolarisers, is nowadays represented by a single drug, suxamethonium (succinylcholine). When this molecule occupies the receptor it triggers a depolarisation similar to that which follows acetylcholine occupancy, but the membrane does not recover as rapidly because the destruction of succinylcholine depends on pseudo-cholinesterase, and takes longer. Nevertheless, the onset of paralysis is very rapid (30 sec), and duration is ultra-short (< 5 min), making this agent ideal for certain purposes in which speed of onset and brevity of duration are important considerations.

The characteristics of **depolarising block** are:

- decreased response to a single impulse
- decreased amplitude, but sustained response to tetanic stimulation, i.e. there is no fade
- the train of four is not diagnostic of receptor occupancy
- muscle fasciculations occur prior to paralysis
- there is no post-tetanic facilitation
- anticholinesterases prolong the block

Choice of relaxant

The selection of a muscle relaxant is made according to the following considerations:

- duration of action
- cardiovascular effects
- class of relaxant and rate of onset

Duration

Pharmacokinetics

- suxamethonium is rapidly hydrolysed by plasma cholinesterase and plasma concentration falls exponentially
- most muscle relaxants are cleared from the plasma in a multiexponential manner with a rapid fall in plasma concentration due to redistribution and then a slower removal from the body via the kidneys or liver
  - ◊ gallamine is exclusively excreted by the kidney whereas atracurium is not renally excreted at all

Protein binding and receptor affinity affect duration

- suxamethonium – short
- vecuronium, atracurium – medium
- pancuronium, d-tubocurare, alcuronium – long

Age

- young and elderly – volume of drug distribution, lean body mass, renal function, hepatic blood flow

Electrolytes and pH

- acidosis and hypokalaemia prolong block

Drug interactions

- aminoglycosides, pseudocholinesterase inhibitors

Cardiovascular effects

- d-tubocurare produces hypotension secondary to ganglion blockade and histamine release
- pancuronium causes tachycardia due to vagolysis and some sympathetic stimulation
- vecuronium appears to have no cardiovascular effects

Pharmacological effects of each of the neuromuscular blocking drugs which produce cardiovascular changes:

Muscle relaxant	Ganglion blockade	Sympathetic stimulation	Vagolytic effect	Vagal stimulation	Histamine release
suxamethonium	-	-	-	+	+
vecuronium	-	-	-	-	-
atracurium	-	-	-	-	+
alcuronium	+	-	-	-	+
gallamine	+	+	+ + +	-	+
tubocurare	+ +	-	-	-	+ + +
pancuronium	-	+ +	+ +	-	-

These effects may be either useful or undesirable depending on individual situations.

Class of muscle relaxant

- intravenous suxamethonium provides excellent tracheal intubation conditions within 60 seconds of administration, lasting about 4–6 minutes. There are however several well known contraindications and side effects associated with its use
  - ◊ cardiac arrest due to hyperkalaemia
    - burns, trauma, renal failure, neural & neuromuscular disease
  - ◊ increases intraocular pressure
    - danger of vitreous extrusion
  - ◊ associated with muscle pains
    - especially in ambulatory women

Reversal of non-depolarising block

- reversal can be achieved with anticholinesterases provided that receptor occupancy is less than 90%
- the commonest reversal agent and the longest in duration is NEOSTIGMINE
- anticholinesterases produce powerful parasympathomimetic effects, such as bradycardia, bronchospasm, gut contraction and profuse upper airway secretions – these are blocked to some extent by ATROPINE or GLYCOPYRROLATE
- atropine and neostigmine are mixed in the same syringe and administered simultaneously intravenously
- the cardiac effects of atropine precede the muscarinic effects of neostigmine by 1–2 minutes and maximal reversal occurs within 5–10 minutes

Anticholinesterases must NOT be used in association with suxamethonium. Why do you think this is so?

Monitoring the neuromuscular block (NMB)

- ideally one should measure the force of muscle contraction during the operation but this is complicated and unsuitable for routine clinical practice
- the most practical way of monitoring muscle relaxation uses a peripheral nerve stimulator to deliver varying patterns of electrical stimuli such as single twitch, train-of-four (TOF) and tetanus and then the operator observes the response
- the table below correlates surgical conditions and ease of block reversibility with these assessments of the degree of block
- note that the patient can be reversed with neostigmine, even if twitch height is only 70% of untreated levels and the TOF ratio should be zero to provide adequate surgical relaxation
- visual and tactile monitoring can only differentiate recovery to a TOF ratio of 0.4 and therefore to be sure of complete recovery, tetanic stimulation should proceed without fade
- Double Burst Stimulation (DBS) has been recently introduced and this increases the sensitivity of tactile evaluation comparable to a TOF ratio of 0.7, enabling the use of a single nerve stimulation pattern right through to full recovery

Reversibility of block	Condition for surgery	Tetanic stimulus 50Hz/5sec	TOF ratio 0–1	TOF count 0–4	Twitch	Twitch height 0–100%
irreversible	intense NMB without response to twitch or TOF					0
possibly reversible 80µg/kg neostigmine wait 30 minutes	adequate surgical relaxation		0.00	1	-	10%
			0.00	2	-- -	20%
readily reversible 40µg/kg neostigmine < 15 min to reverse	'tight'		0.00	3	--- -- -	25%
			>0	4	---- --- -- -	neostigmine >25%
unable to lift head			0 0.4		-------- ------- ------ -----	75%
sustain head lift for 3 sec but decreased vital capacity and inspiratory force		fade	0.6		---------- --------- -------- -------	90%
responds to command, opens eyes widely, protrude tongue, effective cough, sustain head lift >5 sec, VC >15–30 ml/kg inspiratory force >25 cm H_2O negative pressure		no fade	0.75		------------ ------------ ----------- -----------	100%
			1		------------ ------------ ------------ ------------	100%

Chapter 5

Mechanical pulmonary ventilation

The mechanical ventilator

The modern mechanical ventilator delivers a tidal volume to the patient using positive pressure and is connected to the patient's airways either by a tracheal or a tracheostomy tube. The ventilator must overcome two forces, the resistance of the lungs and chest wall, and the airways resistance.

- The inverse of the resistance of the lungs and chest wall is the total compliance and is about 0.05 l/cm H_2O in a healthy, anaesthetised adult, but may fall dramatically with disease.
- Airway resistance of an intubated adult is approximately 6 cm H_2O/litre/sec which may rise to 20 cm H_2O/litre/sec with pulmonary disease.

Safe ventilation will depend on the level of supervision, the mode of function of the ventilator and its electromechanical reliability.

Mechanical ventilator requirements

Power source

- pressurised gas and/or
- electromechanical motor

Many ventilators which are powered by compressed gas also utilise a separate electrical supply to operate the displays, alarms, sensors and controls which determine how much and in what manner the patient is being ventilated. Conversely, ventilators which are electrically powered still need a supply of oxygen at least, so as to be able to enrich the inspired gases; many require a compressed air supply as well. Unless the power source(s) and/or gas supplies are connected and switched on, either nothing will happen, or an alarm system on the machine will tell you that something needs to be done.

Patient circuit

- this will incorporate some form of one-way valve system which will prevent rebreathing of expired gases and therefore the accumulation of carbon dioxide.

Intermittent gas flow

Ventilation mimics breathing and therefore there are four events which take place in each ventilatory cycle:

- inspiratory phase
- change over from inspiration to expiration
- expiratory phase
- change over from expiration back to inspiration

Inspiratory phase

There are two distinct methods of mechanical lung inflation which have different and important implications for patient care. Quite simply,

- a pressure generator has a pressure knob as its major control, which if not activated, will prevent the ventilator from working,
- a flow generator requires the setting of a gas flow or minute volume in order for the ventilator to work.

◊ **A pressure generator** exposes the patient to a constant pressure. This results in a flow waveform which is an exponential and therefore the rate of completion of tidal volume delivery depends upon the time constant of the ventilation and pulmonary systems (one time constant T = compliance x resistance). After one time constant 65% of the change is complete and after 3 time constants, changes are 95% complete.

- therefore if compliance is halved, the flow commences at the same rate but declines more rapidly. The time constant is halved and ventilation achieved in finite time is halved. To restore ventilation to the original amount, the generating pressure would need to be doubled
- if the airway resistance is doubled and the compliance remains unaltered, the initial flow declines to half and the time constant is doubled, and it now requires double the time to deliver the same tidal volume

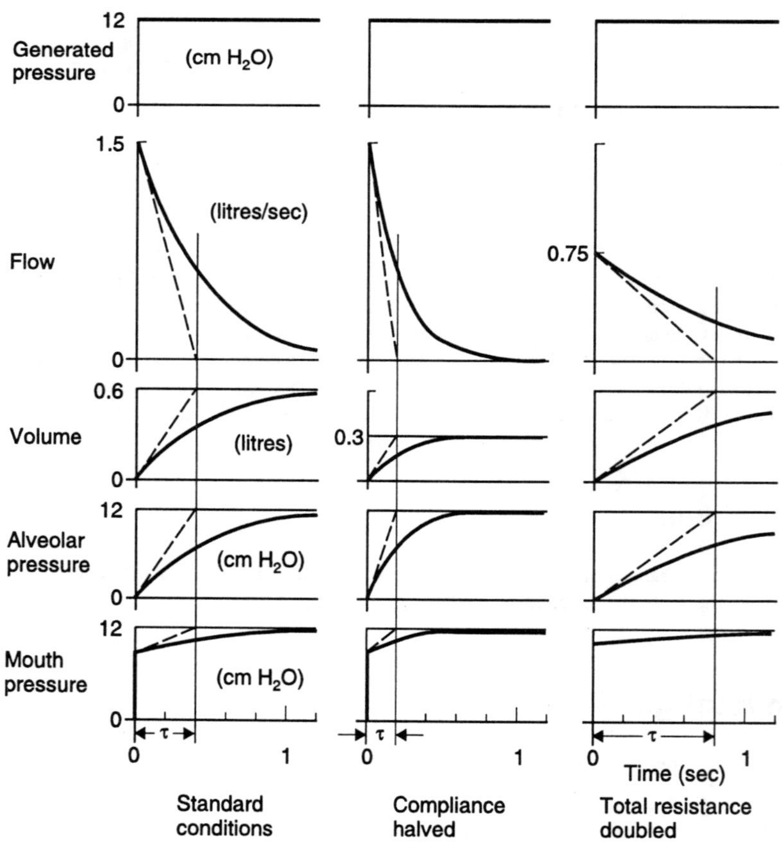

5. Mechanical pulmonary ventilation

◊ **A flow generator** is a ventilator which delivers gas at a constant flow rate throughout inspiration
- if the compliance is halved, flow is unaffected since the generated pressure is so high, BUT the alveolar pressure is doubled
- if the airway resistance is doubled, no change in the flow or alveolar pressure occurs

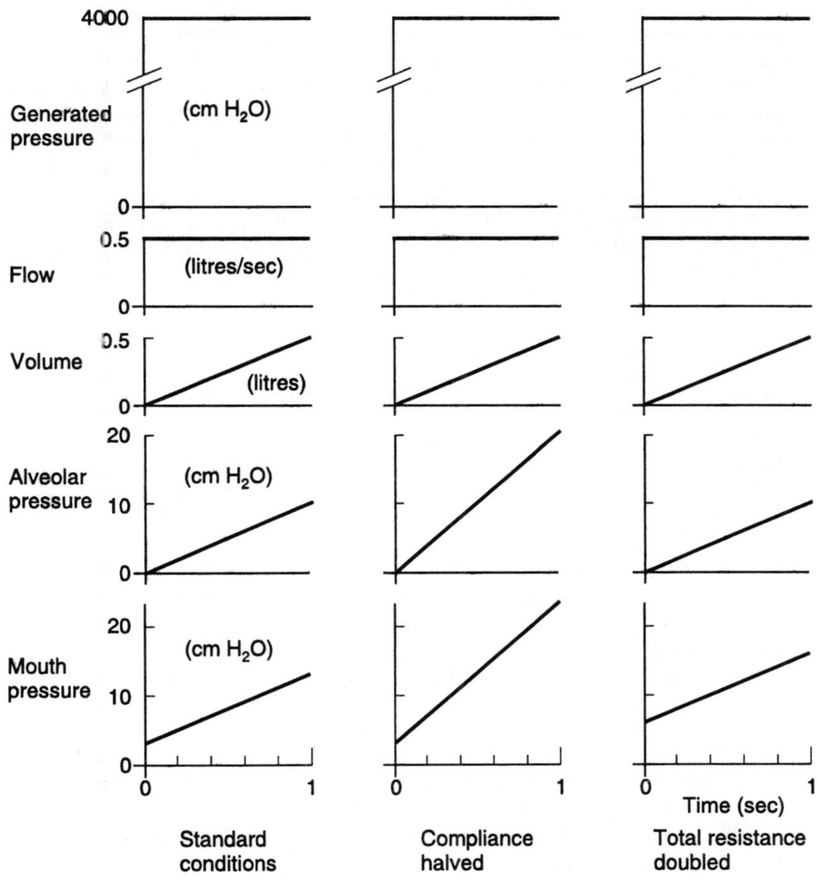

Inflation is active, in the sense that this is when the machine is actually performing the work which the patient's respiratory muscles normally do.

Clinical application of pressure and flow generators

- a pressure generator produces an exponential response whereas a flow generator is linear. Therefore the mean **alveolar pressure** during inspiration is higher with a pressure generator for a given tidal volume. This higher pressure improves the ventilation of parts of the lung supplied by narrow airways and increases the distension of relatively non-compliant areas, and so results in a more even distribution of gases. On the other hand, the higher mean alveolar pressure may have a compression effect, impeding the flow of blood through the pulmonary circulation.
- a flow generator delivers the same total volume of gas regardless of changes in compliance or airways resistance. With a pressure generator, a fall in **pulmonary compliance** will result in a fall in delivered tidal volume, unless the ventilator is manually reset to compensate for the compliance change.
- a pressure generator will tend to compensate for **leaks** which may develop in the circuit. The alveolar ventilation will only fall if the leak is so large that the maximum flow rate of gases from the machine is exceeded. Tracheal intubation in children requires that a gas leak be present around the tracheal tube, to prevent injury to a vulnerable tracheal mucosa.
- an inherent danger with a flow generator is that excessive pressure may develop within the pulmonary system resulting in **barotrauma** and therefore a pre-set pressure relief valve is mandatory. The pressure relief valve may be used to produce an inspiratory plateau prior to the opening of the expiratory valve to enable more even pulmonary gas distribution.

Change over from inspiration to expiration

The ventilator must cycle from inspiration to expiration. This may be achieved by

- pressure
- volume (flow)
- time

Pressure

◊ pressure cycled ventilators switch from inflation to deflation as soon as a preset pressure in the airways has been reached, irrespective of the time taken or the volume delivered.

◊ these machines therefore are very inefficient in the presence of stiff lungs or obstructed airways, since in these conditions, the cycling pressure will be reached early, before an adequate tidal volume has been delivered to the alveoli.

Time

◊ time cycling simply means that the changeover from inflation to expiration occurs after a preset time, usually 1–2 seconds, irrespective of the amount of gas which has entered the patient's lungs, or the pressure which has been generated.

◊ this could be dangerous if the pressure is too high, so time-cycled ventilators are almost always fitted with pressure-limiting devices which will not allow pressure inside the breathing circuit to rise above a certain level.

◊ they are unlikely to produce pressure injury to the lungs, and since they will not cycle unless their preset pressure has been reached, they give visual and usually audible evidence of disconnection.

Volume

◊ the disadvantages of time and pressure cycling have led to the development of the VOLUME VENTILATOR, i.e. one which is set to deliver a preset volume to the patient's lungs.

◊ in these machines the airway pressure which results is a function of

- delivered volume
- rate of inflation (i.e. inspiratory flow rate)
- lung compliance (normal = 0.05 litres/cm H_2O)
- airway resistance (normal = 6 cm H_2O/litre/sec)

◊ if an attempt is made to force the volume of gas into the lungs more rapidly than they can comfortably expand to receive it, then the peak pressure reached will be high.

- sometimes setting the cycling method is obvious. There will be a tidal volume knob or an inspiratory time knob, but many machines cycle by means of a rate knob which sets the number of cycles per minute and another control which alters the time ratio between inflation and deflation, usually called the I:E RATIO.
- some volume ventilators may make use of a flow control, which adjusts the speed with which gas is delivered to the patient. A fast flow delivers the same volume at a higher pressure in a shorter time, and a slower flow will take longer to get the gas in, but the pressure will not be so high.
- if there are settings for all components of the respiratory cycle, it will be possible to set a ventilator an impossible task, and some kind of fault signal will normally be generated to alert the operator in these circumstances.

Expiratory phase

Expiration is passive, and the machine simply allows the patient's respiratory tract to decompress, so that gas can escape to atmosphere.

- the generating pressure is the alveolar pressure and the lungs empty in an exponential fashion, with a declining flow rate which is at first rapid and then slows.
- expiration is complete when alveolar pressure equals atmospheric pressure
- it may be desirable to maintain the lungs in a partially inflated state. To do this, a small positive pressure is applied to the lungs at the end of expiration (Positive End Expiratory Pressure or PEEP).

Change over from expiration to inspiration

Two methods are used

- time cycling
- patient cycling
    - ◊ most ventilators used in Intensive Care (but usually not those in anaesthesia) have mechanisms which allow the patient to 'trigger' the ventilator. That is, if the patient takes a breath, the ventilator will switch to an inflating cycle, even if one was not due to occur at that precise time had the machine been left to do its own thing.
    - ◊ this 'assist' mode may be deliberately used in the 'weaning' of patients from mechanical ventilation, and can also be useful in acclimatising a conscious patient to artificial ventilation.

Ventilatory modes

IMV (intermittent mandatory ventilation)

- 'Smart' ventilators can also be fitted with intermittent mandatory ventilation (IMV) modes, which allow the patient to breathe spontaneously, but intervene with a positive pressure inflation at intervals, in order to maintain ventilation at a certain (mandatory) minute volume. Again, the purpose of this arrangement is to give the patient a chance to breathe on his own, but not to allow hypoventilation to occur.

PEEP (positive end expiratory pressure)

- It has been found that intermittent positive pressure ventilation (IPPV) results in 'shunting' within the lungs, resulting from the closure of small airways, and failure of some alveoli to ventilate. Blood flowing to these areas is not oxygenated, and PaO_2 falls. Correction is possible by increasing the FiO_2 (the percentage of oxygen in the inspired gases), but only up to a point, and the longer that IPPV goes on, the higher the FiO_2 has to be. Eventually, especially in patients who have poor lung function to begin with, or pulmonary damage due to septic or traumatic causes, even 100% oxygen cannot produce a satisfactory PaO_2. This is, of course, a critical situation.
- If the pressure in the lungs at the end of expiration is not allowed to fall to zero (i.e. atmospheric pressure), but maintained by a positive end expiratory pressure (PEEP) of 5–15 cm H2O, this problem can be overcome, and FiO_2 can be reduced, whilst PaO_2 can be maintained at a satisfactory level. In intensive care, most patients on prolonged ventilator care are on some degree of PEEP to help keep the FiO_2 of their inspired gases down to below 0.5.

Other ventilatory modes such as **pressure support,** synchronised intermittent mandatory ventilation **(SIMV),** and bilevel continuous positive airway pressure **(BIPAP)** are also used during ventilatory weaning but are beyond the scope of this book. Continuous positive airway pressure **(CPAP)** (pressure applied during both inspiration and expiration) may be applied in spontaneously breathing patients

Breathing systems

The gases which leave the ventilator do so via a breathing system which is connected to the patient's airway via a laryngeal mask airway, tracheal or tracheostomy tube. Breathing systems are made (usually) of corrugated wide-bore plastic tubing, and incorporate a number of components, as follows:

Breathing hoses

These are designed to resist kinking (hence the corrugations) and are of a diameter similar to that of the adult trachea, viz 2–2.5 cm. Their length is such as to enable the ventilator to be conveniently positioned, and is usually approximately 1 metre.

Connectors

These are rigid components which join hoses to each other (Y-piece), join a hose to a ventilator, or connect a tracheal tube to the breathing circuit. They have standard tapers by international convention, viz 22mm male and female and 15mm male or female. A 22mm male connector often has a 15mm female co-axial taper. These connectors may incorporate a leur-lock port which permits attachment of an aspirant gas composition or airway pressure monitoring line (F_{IO_2}, $E_{T}CO_2$, anaesthetic agent concentration, and respiratory rate).

Valves

Whilst many ventilators incorporate valves in their main mechanism, some make use of valves which form part of the breathing circuit. The commonest of these is the pressurised expiratory valve which is closed as the inspiratory cycle begins and opens as soon as the ventilator switches to the expiratory mode.

Moisture traps

Heated, humidified gases may produce sufficient condensation ('rain-out') in some breathing circuits to require inclusion of a receptacle for excess water.

Filters

The need to prevent bacterial and viral transmission (AIDS, hepatitis C) has led to the use of filters in the breathing circuit. These may include condenser humidification properties and are unidirectional, protecting the ventilator from contamination.

Thermometers

The breathing circuit incorporates a port near the patient end at which a thermometer may be mounted in order to monitor the temperature of inspired gases.

Spirometers

Most breathing circuits vent the expired gases from the patient into a device which indicates their volume – i.e. a spirometer or a pneumotachygraph. This is attached to an alarm which will signal failure to reach a preset volume.

Humidification

The need for humidification complicates all long-term IPPV, since the gases as delivered by the machine, having come from cylinders or a liquid oxygen reservoir, are absolutely dry, and the patient's own humidification system has been by-passed by the tracheal or tracheostomy tube. Failure to humidify has no short-term consequences – i.e. for up to an hour, but as time goes on, secretions will begin to dry, cilia function decreases, and the vulnerability of the respiratory tract to infections will increase. Humidification may be provided by:

Heater humidifiers

- most ventilators do not have their own built-in humidifier and rely on a separate device which is heated, since not enough water vapour can be obtained from water at room temperature.
- despite heating of the inspiratory arm of the breathing circuit, the warmed gases leaving the humidifier will cool during the journey to the patient resulting in some moisture condensation. The gas delivered to the patient should be saturated to 100% humidity at 37°C.

Condenser humidifier

- these devices are moisture/heat exchangers, saturating the inspired dry gas with expired moisture and raising its temperature towards 37°C by conserving heat loss from the respiratory tract, and are placed in the circuit close to the tracheal tube.

Ventilator alarms

Disruption of the patient–ventilator interface will result in inadequate pulmonary gas exchange, even if the ventilator is otherwise working perfectly. An alarm system will warn of this breach in the integrity, as may occur with accidental patient disconnection or ineffective pulmonary ventilation.

Alarms are fitted to all new ventilators to warn of

- disconnection
- the development of pressures outside a range which has been set by the operator
  - ◊ leakage
  - ◊ decreasing compliance
  - ◊ partial airway obstruction
  - ◊ alarms must be visual as well as audible, since it can be extremely difficult to determine which of a number of ventilators in a room is emitting an audible signal.
  - ◊ alarms also indicate failure of the gas supply, reduction of $F_{I}O_2$, and even power failure – such as might result from accidentally switching off the power outlet.

Practical ventilator management

- Non-activation of these alarms is always possible and the machine will still work. Hence it pays to concentrate on the basics of setting the volume, rate and I:E ratio controls, then the high and low pressure alarms, and making sure that all the connections fit. Other monitoring can be activated later if needed.
- If you are likely to have responsibility for a ventilated patient, you must at the earliest opportunity read the operator's manual for the machine which you will have to operate. Obtain a 'test lung' (a closed bag which is attached to the patient end of the breathing circuit) and experiment with the machine in this manner until you feel that you understand it.
- Always make sure that a self-inflating resuscitator is available and in working order, in case anything goes wrong.
- **Remember that if a patient 'fights' the ventilator, it may be because the ventilator is trying to kill him!** Until you have made quite sure that the machine is working properly, take the patient off it, check the airway, and use the manual resuscitator on 100% oxygen.

The ideal ventilator

would be one which most closely meets the following criteria:

- simple operation with minimal direct controls
- visual readout of
  - ◊ circuit pressure
  - ◊ volume expired
  - ◊ frequency
  - ◊ inspiratory time
  - ◊ inspiratory waveform
- direct control of inspired oxygen concentration ($F_{I}O_2$)
- capable of providing measurable PEEP
- small, portable, dual power source
- reliable, suitable for ICU, theatre and transport
- suitable for all patients with multiple ventilatory mode selection
- circuit easily sterilised
  - ◊ minimal dead space
  - ◊ low internal compliance
  - ◊ minimal resistance and minimal connections
- provision for humidification
- audible and visual safety alarms
- quiet, cheap, good service back-up with easy access for repairs

Adverse effects of IPPV

Cardiovascular system

- decrease in venous return producing decreased cardiac output
- pulmonary and systemic vascular pressures altered
- increased impedance to right ventricular ejection: increased intraluminal pressure, increased ventricular wall tension, myocardial ischaemia and ventricular dysfunction
- sympathetic nervous system stimulation with intubation

Respiratory system

- increased intra pulmonary shunt – V/Q, altered pulmonary vascular resistance
- increased dead space with high inflating pressures

Renal system

- inappropriate ADH secretion: fluid retention, particularly associated with a fall in cardiac output, decreased renal blood flow and excessive IV fluid administration
- increase aldosterone secretion – Na^+ retention
- decreased cortical blood flow – decreased urine flow and increased diuretic usage

Complications of IPPV

Disconnection, extubation and other machine or human failure — may result in patient death

- infection of upper airways and tracheostomy sites due to bacterial invasion especially in the presence of moisture. Pseudomonas, klebsiella and staphylococci are especially troublesome
- worsening hypotension in hypovolaemic states due to intrapulmonary positive pressure inhibiting venous return to the heart
- barotrauma, due to high inflation pressures which may be necessary to overcome poor compliance
- nasal, laryngeal and tracheal trauma, ulceration and stenosis as a consequence of prolonged indwelling tubes, especially if size is poorly chosen or cuffs over-inflated
- rise in intracranial pressure during suction of upper airways, manipulation of tubes or inadvertent hypoventilation
- alkalosis and arrhythmia due to inadvertent hyperventilation
- acidosis and cardiac depression secondary to hypoventilation

Chapter 6

Fluids, electrolytes and blood therapy

Perioperative fluid management

To make rational fluid therapy decisions, a knowledge of the normal physiological fluid distribution, composition and turnover is essential.

Distribution

The primary determinant of fluid and electrolyte therapy is the current clinical state of the patient. During anaesthesia and surgery the patient's well being is threatened by shifts in intravascular volume and cardiovascular performance caused by haemorrhage, unwise fluid management, pharmacological or mechanical effects on the heart and vessels, or aggravation of pre-existing cardiovascular disease.

Distribution of body water
(50 kg man lean weight)

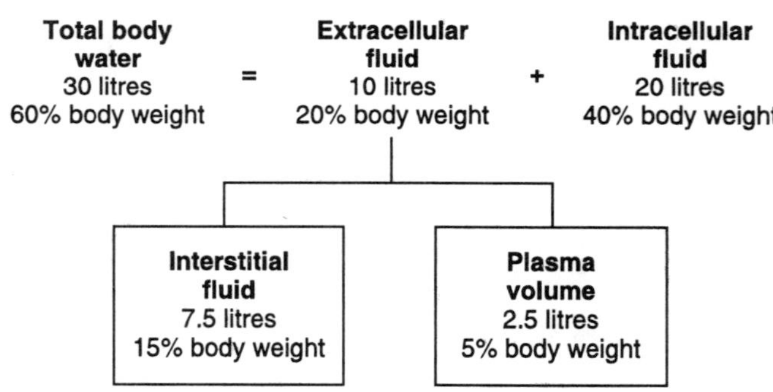

Composition

The intracellular fluid (ICF) is markedly different from the extracellular fluid (ECF). In the ICF the principal cation is potassium (K^+) and the principal anion is phosphate and with the exception of erythrocytes, it contains little sodium (Na^+) and almost no chloride (Cl^-). It has a high protein content which acts as an anion.

6. Fluids, electrolytes and blood therapy

The composition of some body fluids is shown in the following table:

Fluid	Na mmol/l	K mmol/l	Cl mmol/l	HCO_3 mmol/l	Comments
gastric	20–80	10–20	100–150	0.00	H^+ 20–120
bile	140–160	3–15	80–120	15–30	
pancreatic fluid	120–160	5–15	10–45	75–135	basal state
jejunal fluid	130–150	5–15	100–130	10–20	
ileal fluid	50–150	3–15	20–130	30–50	
diarrhoeal fluid	10–90	10–80	10–110	20–70	
sweat – normal	10–30	3–10	10–35	0	
–cystic fibrosis	50–130	5–25	50–110	0	
burn exudate	140.00	5.00	110.00	20.00	protein 30-50 g/l
saliva	10–25	20–35	10–30	2-10	unstimulated

The cell membrane is **selectively** permeable to ions and osmotic pressure equalisation is achieved by movement of water or ions, to which the cell is permeable. When the cell ceases to respire, its membrane loses its selectivity. The total concentration of intracellular ions exceeds that of the extracellular compartment, however the osmotically active particles in these compartments are equal (290–310 mOsm). The kidney is responsible for balancing the body water content, excreting more or less water, as intake varies. Antidiuretic hormone (ADH) assists in conserving water when intake decreases and in response to trauma. A healthy adult with **normal** kidneys can excrete the daily solute load in 0.5ml/kg/hour urine volume. Replacement intravenous therapy should be considered as a dose–response relationship; the dose is the amount and type of fluid administered and the response is the physiological interaction between the body fluids, the intravascular compartment and the kidneys. The response is assessed by clinical signs, urine output and biochemical estimations. Alterations to the dose may be necessary during replacement therapy.

Turnover

Normal fluid balance in a 65 kg adult

WATER GAIN			
	Ingested fluid	1,350 ml	
	Solid food	800 ml	
	Product of oxidative metabolism	350 ml	
		TOTAL WATER GAIN	**2,500** ml/day
WATER LOSS			
Alimentary tract	Saliva	1,500 ml	
	Gastric juice	1,500 ml	
	Bile	800 ml	
	Intestinal juice	1,500 ml	
		5,300 ml	
	Less reabsorbed	5,200 ml,	net loss 100 ml
Kidneys	Filtration	150,000 ml	
	Less reabsorption	148,500 ml,	net loss 1,500 ml
Skin	Transudation	500 ml	
	Sweating	0	
			net loss 500 ml
Lungs	Evaporation	400 ml,	
			net loss 400 ml
		TOTAL WATER LOSS	**2,500** ml/day

Fluid replacement

There are three components to perioperative fluid management
- provide **maintenance** fluid
- replace the **deficit**
- account for **on-going** losses

Maintenance

Water

Body weight (kg)	Water requirements
0–10	4 ml/kg/hr
11–20	40 ml/hr + 2 ml/kg/hr for each kg > 10
> 20	60 ml/hr + 1 ml/kg/hr for each kg > 20

Electrolytes

Na^+ : 2–6 mmol/kg/day
K^+ : 1–2 mmol/kg/day

Calories

1 calorie per ml of calculated maintenance water required

Deficit

Assessment

There are four components
- history
- clinical examination
- biochemical examination
- physiological examination

10% DEHYDRATED = 10% LOSS OF BODY WEIGHT

History

The composition and volume of fluid to be given will depend upon
- the **type,**
- **amount** and
- **rate** of loss of fluid from the patient.

Clinical examination

The state of hydration is assessed by skin turgor, urine output, pulse rate, central venous pressure, arterial blood pressure, haematocrit, serum osmolality, serum sodium and urine osmolality. None of these are accurate predictors by themselves and even collectively do not provide accurate information about fluid needs.

The most useful clinical signs of moderate dehydration are skin turgor and a low urine output. Dry mucous membranes depend on whether the patient is mouth breathing and acidotic, rather than being a specific sign of dehydration.

	Mild	Moderate	Severe
Body weight	5% loss	10% loss	15% loss
Skin turgor	↓	↓↓	↓↓↓
Mucous membrane	dry	dry	very dry
Skin colour	pale	grey	mottled
Urine	± oliguria	± oliguria	azotaemia ↓
Blood pressure Pulse	normal ±↑	normal ↑	decreased ↑↑

Overhydration is manifested as oedema. The factors which cause oedema are excess fluid administration, high levels of ADH, 'leaky' capillary syndrome, heart failure, renal failure and hypoalbuminaemia. In the intensive care setting there are often a number of these causes contributing at one time.

Modifications of fluid intake

Decrease	Adjustment required
humidified inspired air	x 0.75
base state (e.g. paralysed)	x 0.7
high ADH (IPPV, asthma, head injury)	x 0.7
hypothermia	- 12% per °C below 37°C
high room humidity	x 0.7
renal failure	x 0.3 (+ urine output)
Increase	
full activity + oral feeds	x 1.5
fever	+ 12% per °C above 37°C
room temperature > 31°C	+ 30% per °C above 31°C
hyperventilation	x 1.2
neonate – preterm radiant heater phototherapy	x 1.2 x 1.5 x 1.5
burns – first subsequently	+4% per 1% area burnt +2% per 1% area burnt

Biochemical examination
- haematocrit
- serum and urine electrolytes
- serum and urine osmolality
- urea and creatinine
- blood gases, pH and base deficit

Physiological examination
- clinical assessment
- non-invasive blood pressure (moderate dehydration, intra-arterial BP)
- ECG, E_TCO_2, S_PO_2
- urine output
- CVP ± (PCWP, cardiac output – in concomitant cardiac disease)

The signs of hypovolaemia are:

- ◊ narrow pulse pressure
- ◊ decreased systolic pressure
- ◊ increasing heart rate
- ◊ pale mucous membrane (conjunctivae, tongue, lips)
- ◊ flattening of neck veins
- ◊ retarded capillary refill after blanching
- ◊ cycling of systolic blood pressure with the positive phase of IPPV
- ◊ decreased peripheral venous pressure flash back in IV infusion on lowering the infusion bag.

The significance of central venous pressure readings is blurred in the presence of myocardial disease, and in any event a single observation is of much less value than a series of measurements taken at intervals.

On-going losses

MEASURE THE PREVIOUS HOUR'S LOSS AND REPLACE IN THE FOLLOWING HOUR

The questions to be answered now are

- which fluid?
- what volume?
- how fast should it be given?

Fluid

Simplistically, the fluid given should mimic the fluid lost. Vomiting and diarrhoea will result in loss of extracellular fluid and should be replaced with 0.9% saline. Loss of water would be replaced with 5% dextrose and loss of protein with 5% human albumin solution.

Some advantages of Polygeline ('Haemaccel')

- ◊ long shelf life (5 years), sterile & synthetic
- ◊ packaged in an unbreakable, collapsible plastic flask which does not require an air inlet
- ◊ similar to plasma and 50% remains in the intravascular space
- ◊ isotonic
- ◊ $T_{1/2}$ 4–5 hours, renal excretion
- ◊ does not interfere with cross-matching of blood
- ◊ no limit to the volume that can be infused
- ◊ very few side-effects (rare hypersensitivity reaction)

Commonly used intravenous fluids

Fluid	Na^+ mmol/l	K^+ mmol/l	Cl^- mmol/l	lact. mmol/l	gluc. g/l	Cals cals/l	Ca^{2+} mmol/l	Alb. g/l	Osm. mosm/l
Crystalloids									
0.9% NaCl	154	–	154	–	–	–	–	–	308
0.45% NaCl	75	–	75	–	–	–	–	–	150
0.45% NaCl + 2.5% dextrose	75	–	75	–	25 g	95	–	–	293
0.18% NaCl + 4% dextrose +2 g KCl	30	27	58	–	40 g	150	–	–	337
Hartmann's	131	5	111	29	–	–	2	–	272
5% dextrose	–	–	–	–	50 g	190	–	–	278
Colloids									
5% Albumin	130–160	4-6	130–160	–	–	–	–	50	
Concentrated albumin	85–13	–	85–130	–	–	–	–	250	
Haemaccel	145	5	145	–	–	–	6	–	

Volume

This will include the maintenance, deficit and on-going losses.

Rate of repair

The rate of fluid administration will depend on the ability of the cardiovascular system to accommodate a fluid load. The greater the degree of organ compromise, the slower the fluid should be given and the more intense the degree of patient monitoring required. A young, 'healthy' cardiopulmonary system will accept half the estimated fluid deficit volume in 8 hours and the remainder in the following 16 hours. An aged patient with bowel obstruction, left ventricular failure due to coronary artery disease and myocardial ischaemia may require 24 hours to administer half the deficit with pulmonary artery catheter monitoring, and a further 48 hours for administration of the remaining fluid deficit.

An example:

A 10 kg child is 10% dehydrated following 12 hours of severe diarrhoea.

Maintenance:

water – 4ml/kg/hr = 40 ml/hr = 1 litre/day
potassium – 2 mmol/kg/day = 20 mmol/day
sodium – 2–4 mmol/kg/day (see below)
calories – give water as 10% dextrose = 400 calories/litre i.e. 40% basal requirements

Deficit:

10% of 10 kg = 1 litre of fluid lost. Is there shock? Probably in a child losing this amount in a relatively short period.
shock – 20 ml/kg colloid over 1 to 2 hours = 200 ml, deficit = 800 ml
rate – half in 8 hours and remainder in 16 hours (no cardiac disease) 0.9% saline at 50 ml/hr for 8 hours, then 25 ml/hr for 16 hours = 150 mmol Na^+ = 15 mmol/kg/24 hours (see above)

On-going:

weigh nappies soiled in the previous hour
give weight as volume during the following hour
give as half normal saline 0.45%, to limit the sodium load (75 mmol Na^+ /litre), at say 50 ml/hr.

Practical considerations

- one or more large bore (14G in an adult) cannulae in situ **plus** the facility for measuring CVP
- formulae are imprecise and are only a guide because they may not be based on accurate data and various assumptions are made which may not necessarily apply
- Different fluids have different fates
  - ◊ 5% dextrose distributes to the total body water (TBW) and only 1/3 remains in the extracellular fluid (ECF) and 5% in plasma
  - ◊ 0.9% saline distributes to the ECF and only 25% remains in plasma
  - ◊ colloid distributes primarily to the plasma space
- iatrogenic administration of large volumes of 5% dextrose will result in hyponatraemia (water intoxication), especially in children
- K^+, Ca^{++} and lactate$^-$ (Hartmann's solution) are not always appropriate
- whole blood resuscitation should aim for a haematocrit (HCT) 30% in order to maximise O_2 transport
- dextrans should NOT be given more than 20ml/kg/day
- an abnormal laboratory result should always be viewed with caution and checked, especially if it is unexpected or inconsistent
- do not take blood samples from the limb attached to the intravenous infusion
- concomitant problems must be treated, particularly:
  - ◊ hypoxia
  - ◊ acidosis
  - ◊ sepsis
  - ◊ major disturbances of K^+, Ca^{++}, Mg^{++} and glucose
- therapy other than fluid administration may also be helpful during resuscitation, such as oxygen, steroids, inotropes, antibiotics and anti-arrhythmics
- always try to assess fluid volume requirements in terms of each body compartment – intravascular, interstitial, intracellular and third space losses

Haemorrhage and blood transfusion

- Bleeding as a cause of acute illness should be considered in a number of groups of patients:
  - ◊ trauma victims
  - ◊ recent surgery or invasive procedures
  - ◊ altered coagulation states
  - ◊ acute abdomen
  - ◊ gynaecological problems
  - ◊ history of upper gastrointestinal symptoms
- Postural hypotension (i.e. significant fall in systolic BP > 10 mmHg when patient moves from supine to erect position) is only certain to be present after more than 15% of blood volume (70 ml/kg) is lost.
- There are several causes of postural hypotension other than hypovolaemia, viz:
  - ◊ drugs – narcotics, vasodilators
  - ◊ autonomic neuropathies (diabetes)
  - ◊ increasing age
  - ◊ prolonged bed rest
  - ◊ spinal cord injuries

Typical blood loss associated with fractures (adult)

Type of fracture	Associated blood loss
Forearm	400–800 ml
Humerus	500–1,000 ml
Tibia and fibula	750–1,200 ml
Femur	1,000–1,500 ml
Pelvis	1,500–2,500 ml + +
Lumbar or thoracic spine	500–1,000 ml

Symptoms and signs of acute blood loss

Blood loss (% of blood volume)	Systolic blood pressure (mmHg)	Symptoms and signs
10–15	normal	postural hypotension mild tachycardia
15–30	slight fall	tachycardia thirst weakness
30–40	60–80	pallor oliguria confusion restlessness
>40	40–60	anuria air hunger coma death

The urgency of volume replacement and the rate of resuscitation are both functions of the **amount and rate** of loss. The initial assessment will suggest how much replacement is needed. If after this replacement is given the patient is still not stable, then it should be assumed that there is on-going, unrecognised bleeding.

Management of blood loss

In the initial phase of resuscitation in the emergency department cross-matched blood is usually not available. It is appropriate to use a colloid initially and then to use a mixture of packed red cells and clotting factors later as they become available. Since the patient usually has no oral intake in this situation it is important to consider maintenance fluid requirements as well.

Guidelines

- attend to the priorities of intravascular volume and tissue perfusion. Don't wait for blood to be available – start volume replacement with colloid.
- determine the required rate of replacement (slow onset of haemorrhage allows some compensation)
- titrate to an appropriate patient end-point
- correct 1/2 the abnormality and then re-evaluate
- replace deficits
- cover continuing losses
- provide maintenance

Massive blood loss

When 50% of the circulating blood volume has been lost in a short period, the **optimal** fluid for replacement is fresh whole blood, but volume replacement with colloid must commence while determining the patient's blood group. Blood cross-matching takes time and group-specific uncross-matched blood is very safe serologically, and if available can be given until fresh cross matched blood is procurable.

A review of the priorities in management of massive bleeding

- Cardiopulmonary resuscitation (CPR)
- First-aid control of haemorrhage
- Restitution of circulating volume
- Restitution of oxygen carrying capacity
- Medical and surgical haemostasis
- Management of specific injuries

Available blood components

- Stored whole blood
- Fresh whole blood (< 5 days old)
- Ultra fresh whole blood (uncooled)
- Red cell concentrates
- 5% normal serum albumin
- Concentrated albumin 20%
- Fresh frozen plasma
- Supernatant plasma (Factor VIII depleted plasma)
- Cryoprecipitate (Factors VIII, VWF, fibronectin, fibrinogen)
- Platelet concentrates
- Fibrinogen concentrates

6. Fluids, electrolytes and blood therapy

With increasing expertise and decreasing volumes of whole blood, more use is made of blood components. The acutely haemorrhaging patient who continues to bleed or has established shock is likely to require many of the components of blood.

Blood is a complex fluid which rapidly deteriorates outside its normal intravascular milieu. Complicated procedures are undertaken to prolong the life of its various components. These manoeuvres, together with the deterioration that occurs in blood in vitro, cause problems when the blood is returned to the cardiovascular system of the patient being transfused.

Potential hazards of massive and rapid blood transfusion

Hazard	Aetiology
Impaired oxygen transport	microaggregates* fluid overload defective red cell function* impaired haemoglobin function* ARDS*
Haemostatic failure	dilution of clotting factors depletion of platelets decreased clotting factor production
Electrolyte and metabolic disturbances	hyperkalaemia* sodium overload* acid-base disturbances* citrate toxicity* hypothermia*
Vasoactive reactions	kinin activation* damaged platelets and granulocytes*
Serological incompatibility	
Plasticiser toxicity	
Impaired reticuloendothelial function* Infection	 non A – non B hepatitis cytomegalovirus toxoplasmosis potentially AIDS

* = complications arising from changes which occur during storage.

Changes in stored whole blood

- 1 litre of cold blood removes 25 calories of heat energy from the patient.
- after transfusion the red blood cell level of 2,3 DPG returns to normal in four days.

The patient requiring massive blood transfusion is of course critically ill. If the patient survives, complications invariably occur in which blood transfusion therapy may be contributory – for example:

- Respiratory failure
- Sepsis – usually associated with cannulation and rarely transfusion per se
- Renal failure
- Pyrexia
- Multisystem failure
- Haemostatic failure
- Hyperbilirubinaemia
- Thrombophlebitis

Changes in stored blood over time

Component	Fresh	ACD	7/7	14/7	21/7	28/7
rbc survival	< 5% lysed	10%	10%	20%		30% lysed
rbc activity	10% normal @ 24 hr		flexible ovoid	rigid spherocytes		70% survive
wbc^s (%)	100% to 0 in 24 hr		0	0	0	0
platelets	3.5×10^5 0 in 24 hr		0	0	0	0
plasma free Hb						200 mg%
VII					70%	
VIII	50% @ 24 hr		50%			
V	50% in 10 days					
Fibrinogen	decreased					
Temp (°C)	37	4–37	4	4	4	4
pH	7.40	7.10	6.80	6.70	6.60	6.50
pCO_2 mmHg	46	46	60	150	200	300
pO_2 mmHg	40–100	40		40	20	5–15
HCO^-_3	24	15		7–10	2–5	2–5
Na^+	140	150–170	160	150		140
K^+	4–5	4-5	12	20	25	30
Lactic acid (mg%)	20	20		120	140	150
Glucose (mg%)	80-100	700		500	400	400
Ammonium (g%)	50	50		500		700
Ca^{++} (mmol/l)	4-5	0.50	0.50	0.50	0.25	
Citrate		500		500		
P_{50}	25.2			19.5 ± 1.5		
2,3 DPG activity	100%	**ACD** **CPD**	20% 60%	15% 50%	10%	5–10%
2,3 DPG level (ACD) (mmol/mole Hb)	0.76			0.24 ± 0.13		
Micro-aggregates	few	15×10^6	35×10^6	35×10^6	70×10^6	

Chapter 7

Physiological states – paediatrics, pregnancy, geriatrics

The practise of anaesthesia requires an understanding of human physiology and the changes that result from normal human development and are distinct from changes that occur as a result of the disease processes. This chapter describes the important differences from normal adult human physiology in pregnancy, infants and the elderly. Despite the emphasis on *differences* it is in fact the *similarities* that are most important. The fundamental physiological principles and anaesthetic 'rules' covered elsewhere remain the same.

Pregnancy

Physiological function has been extensively measured in pregnancy and most of the differences reflect the requirements of the developing foetus for:

- oxygen delivery
- nutritional support
- protection from environmental harm

These requirements increase as the foetus grows and so the physiological demands increase as pregnancy progresses.

The pregnant mother develops a utero-placental unit that strains maternal physiological resources (maternal blood being the source of oxygen and nutrition). In pregnancy the maternal circulation becomes hyperdynamic to supply the foetus with its increasing needs. If demand exceeds supply in early pregnancy the foetus suffers poor development but later, particularly during labour, the foetus may show the effects of hypoxia, recorded on a foetal heart rate monitor as foetal distress. During the last trimester, the physical presence of a large mass alters maternal vital organ function. When supply approaches demand, it is time for delivery.

BEWARE ! THIS IS WHEN THE ANAESTHETIST IS USUALLY REQUIRED

To fuel the oxygen demand of the foeto-placental unit, oxygen delivery must increase throughout pregnancy and consequently maternal oxygen uptake increases by 20%, as does carbon dioxide production.

Respiratory system changes

- measured lung *sizes* do not alter
- minute ventilation increases by 50% at term mostly accounted for by changes in tidal volume V_T
- functional residual capacity (FRC) is reduced by 20% (but vital capacity is unchanged)
- hyperventilation causes a *chronic compensated respiratory alkalosis* (normal pH, reduced bicarbonate and $PaCO_2$) and a rise in PaO_2 (by up to10 mm Hg)
- even at term the diaphragm is not completely splinted (it is still able to move) but the pregnant mother increasingly relies on thoracic breathing and when supine, one third of parturients have airway closure during normal tidal respiration. Consequently atelectasis occurs more commonly, predisposing to ventilation / perfusion mismatch and an
- increased alveolar–arterial O_2 gradient ($A–aDO_2$)

- intubation conditions are often worsened in pregnancy:
  - ◊ breast enlargement can make insertion of the usual Macintosh laryngoscope blade very difficult (have an open angled, short handled, obstetric blade available)
  - ◊ capillary engorgement of the mucosa of the upper respiratory tract makes passage of a normally sized tube difficult and / or hazardous (use a size 7 or 6.5)

At full-term the reduced FRC, increased V_T and high oxygen flux result in *rapid preoxygenation* (but less benefit due to a reduced oxygen reserve), *rapid gaseous induction* but equally ***rapid desaturation during apnoea.***

Labour

During contractions hyperventilation occurs due to pain:

- PCO_2 falls causing a metabolic alkalosis
- the raised pH and low PCO_2 may *inhibit* respiration after contractions causing a period of prolonged apnoea: this may cause hypoxia especially after the use of *Entonox* or opiates.
- Oxygen consumption is greater in labour aggravating the rapid fall in PaO_2 that occurs with apnoea.

Cardiovascular system changes

- cardiac output (CO) increases 30–40% by the end of the 2nd trimester. In the 3rd trimester *aortocaval compression* occurs in the supine position causing a dramatic reduction in venous return and CO
- since venous return is under threat from the gravid uterus, anything that causes a reduction in IVC flow will cause a sudden fall in blood pressure – dehydration, excessive vasodilatation due to anaesthetic drugs or sympathetic blockade
- at 40 weeks blood volume has increased about 1000ml (35–40%) but blood pressure does not normally rise because of a fall in systemic vascular resistance
- the apex beat is usually displaced to the left, and flow murmurs are common. ECG axis may change and the cardiothoracic ratio on chest X-ray may increase.
- during labour, *maternal* cardiovascular compromise may present as foetal distress due to inadequate uterine blood flow despite 'adequate' maternal pulse and blood pressure

Labour

- during a contraction circulating blood volume and cardiac output increase 10–25%
- on average 400–600 ml is lost during a normal vaginal delivery; up to 1000 ml is lost at caesarean sections or with twins.

Haematopoietic system changes

- the total oxygen carrying capacity of the blood increases by 20% as red blood cell mass increases from 25 to 30 ml/kg at term, but the rise lags behind the increase in total blood volume resulting in a dilutional anaemia with a decrease in haemoglobin concentration of 1.5 g/dl
- oxygen delivery becomes more efficient because:
  - ◊ maternal plasma viscosity is reduced due to the fall in haemoglobin
  - ◊ the maternal oxyhaemoglobin dissociation curve shifts to the right enabling oxygen to be more easily unloaded at the tissues. The P_{50} increases from 26.7 to 30.4 mm Hg
- increases in coagulation factors and fibrinogen result in a *hypercoagulable* state which in combination with poor venous drainage from the lower limbs (due to the pressure effect of the gravid uterus) predisposes to deep venous thrombosis.

Gastrointestinal changes

- gastric acid secretion increases (due to placental gastrin production)
- gastro-oesophageal reflux becomes more common due to the combined influence of progesterone causing reduced upper oesophageal sphincter pressure and the pressure effect of the gravid uterus, ***increasing susceptibility to aspiration.***

Labour

- once the pain of labour has started the stomach rarely empties adequately (it never empties if opiate pain relief has been given)

Paediatrics

In contrast to pregnancy, the physiological differences between children and adults become progressively less significant with time. Management of infants, except in the direst emergencies, should be by those skilled in their care.

Respiratory system

- anatomical airway differences:
  - ◊ the head is relatively large and the neck is short – place a thin head ring under the occiput to stabilise the head during intubation.
  - ◊ the tongue is large and may obstruct the airway.
  - ◊ the epiglottis is long, U shaped and projects posteriorly over the glottic opening and is commonly pushed postero-inferiorly by laryngeal mask insertion, resulting in airway obstruction. A straight blade laryngoscope lifts the larynx anteriorly during laryngoscopy.
  - ◊ the larynx is situated high and anterior in the neck. The arytenoid cartilages are large in comparison to the cords.
  - ◊ the narrowest portion of the infant airway is the cricoid cartilage. An overtight tube will cause sub-glottic stenosis. ***Always use an uncuffed tube and ensure an audible leak.***
  - ◊ the ribs are horizontal and relatively inefficient and breathing is mainly diaphragmatic. Gastric distension severely hampers respiration and must be deflated by a nasogastric tube.
  - ◊ airway reflexes are more sensitive and inappropriate airway manipulations when anaesthesia is inadequate result in laryngospasm.
- respiratory physiology differs from the adult:
  - ◊ the infant has a high metabolic rate (a high proportion of which is needed by an inefficient, easily fatigued respiratory system).
  - ◊ FRC is small relative to TLC.
  - ◊ preoxygenation and gaseous induction occur rapidly but upon apnoea rapid desaturation occurs. Apnoea accompanied by *hypoxia and bradycardia* may occur spontaneously in preterm infants, especially following anaesthesia.
  - ◊ efficient alveolar ventilation is achieved at higher respiratory rates and lower tidal volumes (newborn RR is 35–40/min).
  - ◊ all lung volumes are reduced proportionately compared to adults. Avoid increasing dead space and respiratory work by using low volume, low resistance anaesthetic equipment.
  - ◊ premature infants have uncompliant lungs due to a lack of surfactant causing *infant respiratory distress syndrome* (IRDS). Postmature infants may have residual lung damage.

Cardiovascular system

- the foetus has a right ventricular dominated cardiovascular system. As the patent ductus and foramen ovale close, the left ventricle predominates and the ECG axis approaches that of the adult at about 8–12 months.
- the low glomerular flow and immature tubular mechanisms of the infant requires care in fluid and electrolyte administration.

Vital signs change with age and are somewhat different from adult values:

Age	Heart Rate bpm	Blood pressure Systolic mm Hg	Diastolic	Respiratory rate min^{-1}
Newborn	120	60	35	45
2 months	120	95	45	40
4 years	100	98	60	30
8 years	90	112	60	20
12 years	80	115	65	20

Haematopoietic system

- haemoglobin F, with its high oxygen affinity (and consequent poor delivery), predominates (80% total) at birth and to deliver sufficient oxygen to the tissues, blood volume and haemoglobin concentration (13–19 g/dl) are high. Over 6 months HbF is replaced by adult HbA and a physiological anaemia (Hb 9–11 g/dl) is common at 3 months.

Homeostatic function

- Temperature: the large surface area to weight ratio results in rapid heat loss in infants and warming devices and a high ambient temperature is necessary to prevent 'cold' stress.
- Glucose: preterm and newborn infants have limited glycogen stores and hypoglycaemia rapidly develops with stress. Blood glucose levels should be measured in all sick, fasting infants and during surgery.

Central nervous system

- the immature retina of the preterm infant is susceptible to hyperoxia resulting in *retrolental fibroplasia*. Maintain SpO_2 90–95% .
- myelination of nerve fibres and muscle tone develop as the child grows and reflexes are immature but infants *respond to **pain.***
- children are also emotionally immature. With adequate explanation (usually from parents and nursing staff) the operating room need not be threatening.

Geriatrics

The ageing process represents a steady depletion of resources that will place limits upon the possible and the tolerable.

- age itself gives a poor indication of the degree of physiological limitation
- it may be impossible, or futile, to separate the reduction in physiological reserve solely due to aging from that due to disease

Although this decline in physiological function is a significant consideration when anaesthetising the elderly, they may gain considerable benefit from appropriately indicated surgery. ***Age in itself, is no bar to surgery.***

Cardiovascular system

- coronary heart disease is common and often asymptomatic.
- ventricular thickening with myocardial fibrosis, valve calcification and a decreased arterial elasticity result in an increased impedance to ejection. Cardiac index is well maintained but pulse pressure becomes wider and cardiovascular stability is dependent on volume loading.
- the elderly patient has sufficient cardiovascular resources to meet mild to moderate demand but failure of another organ system or major external stresses are likely to precipitate collapse.

Respiratory system

- progressive loss of elastin and replacement by fibrotic tissue; calcification of the chest wall results in rigidity with increased work of breathing.
- fibrotic alveoli result in inefficient gas exchange.
- residual volume increases, vital capacity decreases, airways closure occurs in tidal breathing.
- respiratory control centres have an attenuated response to hypoxia and increased sensitivity to the effects of narcotic analgesics.

Nervous system

- progressive increase in the stimulus thresholds for all forms of perception. This process of deafferentation contributes to the loss of hearing and visual acuity associated with degenerative disease in the elderly.
- the requirement for anaesthetic agents decreases with age. Both the ED_{50} (IV drugs) and the MAC (anaesthetic vapours) reduce by up to 30% in the elderly.
- reduced levels of neurotransmitters within the CNS result in impaired autonomic homeostasis affecting respiration, temperature and blood pressure control.
- despite deafferentation, the elderly do *not* have raised thresholds for pain, requiring adequate analgesia to promote early mobilisation.

Metabolic changes

- diabetes (usually non insulin dependent) becomes more common and is associated with a reduction in the ability to tolerate carbohydrate loads. Blood sugar should be checked routinely preoperatively.
- temperature regulation is impaired due to depleted thermoreception.
- autonomic regulation, poor peripheral tissue perfusion and impaired behavioural compensatory mechanisms.

Other systems

Organ system	Anatomical changes	Functional changes
Body composition	increased lipid fraction loss of skeletal mass	prolonged half life for lipid-soluble drugs ↓ O_2 consumption, heat production and cardiac output
Renal system	reduced vascularity tissue atrophy	↓ plasma flow and GFR ↓ drug clearance and ability to handle Na and H_2O ↑ plasma urea and creatinine
Hepatic system	↓ tissue mass	↓ hepatic blood flow and drug clearance

General anaesthesia

The 30 day perioperative mortality for appropriately prepared patients over 65 years is 5 to 10%. (One year mortality for *all* inpatients over 65 is 20%.)
Three factors have been identified that significantly increase peri-operative mortality in the elderly:

Operative site

Operative mortality after procedures that enter a body cavity is 10 to 20 times greater than that associated with surface surgery. In the elderly intra-abdominal surgery has a mortality equivalent to thoracic or major vascular procedures.

Patient condition

The preoperative physical status of the patient is a far more important predictor of morbidity and mortality than age itself. The presence of cardio-respiratory disease requires preventative measures to diminish the likelihood of perioperative deterioration.

Emergency

The risk of peri-operative death is 3 to 10 times greater with emergency surgery, often due to inadequate preoperative preparation and inappropriate timing of surgery.

No single technique has been proven advantageous. The following points should be remembered when selecting the mode of anaesthesia for the elderly:

- *adequate preoperative investigation and preparation*: occult illness and secondary injury are common in the elderly and time spent in their evaluation and treatment will be rewarded.
- *increased vigilance*: a reduced capacity to maintain physiological function requires extensive monitoring and early response to any deterioration of function, particularly in the early post-operative period.
- *prevention of cardiorespiratory stress*: the reduced capacity to compensate and the increased risk of tissue injury from destabilised physiology requires adequate analgesia and maintenance of tissue oxygenation by an ample supply of warm, well oxygenated blood to the cells.

Local anaesthesia in the elderly

Carefully executed conduction blockade provides long-lasting analgesia, excellent suppression of the stress response to surgery with relatively little sedation, cardiorespiratory compromise or motor impairment. This compares favourably with the low therapeutic index of sedative drugs and narcotic analgesics in the elderly.
Despite the appeal of these techniques there may however be problems in execution:

- poor patient communication (deafness, blindness, confusional states) makes procedure performance difficult without sedation.
- central conduction blockade may be technically difficult due to degenerative disease of the spine.
- spread of local anaesthetics is slower and more unpredictable.
- unwanted effects are more common and more threatening, especially a high central block with diminished cardiopulmonary reserve.
- both absolute and relative contraindications to conduction anaesthesia occur more frequently in the elderly.

Chapter 8

Monitoring the cardiovascular system

Principles

- ensure the adequacy of perfusion to essential organs
  - ◊ central nervous system
  - ◊ heart
  - ◊ kidneys
  - ◊ liver

- pressure versus flow
  - ◊ Pressure: easily measured but gives limited information
  - ◊ Flow: difficult to measure directly so look for effects of low flow

CARDIAC OUTPUT (CO) = HEART RATE (HR) × STROKE VOLUME (SV)

BLOOD PRESSURE (BP) = CO × TOTAL PERIPHERAL RESISTANCE (TPR)

- cardiac output depends firstly on preload
- blood pressure is a measure of afterload.
- indirect indicators of adequate organ perfusion
  - ◊ skin colour, temperature and venous filling
  - ◊ conscious level
  - ◊ urine output

- direct indicators of cardiovascular function
  - ◊ pulse rate
  - ◊ blood pressure
  - ◊ central venous pressure (CVP)
  - ◊ measured cardiac output
  - ◊

Indirect measures of cardiovascular function

Skin temperature

Blood from the body 'core' is warm but cools whilst flowing to the periphery.

- measure core–peripheral temperature difference (foot versus oesophageal)
- rate of cooling depends on
  - ◊ time blood spends in transit (cardiac output).
  - ◊ peripheral blood flow relative to environmental temperature – low flow in cool environment results in maximum cooling; high flow in warm environment results in minimum cooling.

- chart both core and peripheral temperatures, in different colours and look for trends:
  - ◊ converging lines indicate
    - improved tissue perfusion
    - improving cardiac output
    - improved vascular filling
  - ◊ Diverging lines indicate deterioration
    - falling cardiac output
    - increasing vascular resistance

Skin colour

Peripheral cyanosis in the absence of central cyanosis indicates a severe deficiency in peripheral blood flow.

- local tissue oxygen consumption depends primarily on temperature
- at low flow rates, blood spends a greater length of time in contact with the tissues so a greater quantity of oxygen is removed
- venous blood is desaturated and looks blue = peripheral cyanosis
- peripheral cyanosis indicates poor peripheral perfusion

Capillary return

- the rate at which pink coloration returns to an area of tissue which has been rendered ischaemic (white) by the application of pressure
- the rate of return of colour depends on the flow of blood to the blanched area and is an indirect indicator of cardiac output

Conscious level

- falling level of consciousness indicates critical cerebral hypoxia requiring urgent treatment. Hypoxia in this context means failure to deliver an adequate quantity of oxygen

OXYGEN QUANTITY = BLOOD OXYGEN CONTENT × BLOOD FLOW

- cerebral hypoxia frequently results from low cerebral blood flow (low cardiac output) even with a normal blood content (blood gas analysis)
- signs of hypoxia are
  - ◊ confusion
  - ◊ aggressiveness
  - ◊ vagueness, especially in the elderly
- the changes may be subtle and it is prudent to ask the relatives whether they notice any acute changes in mental state

Urine output

The kidney is a blood filter. A reduced flow of blood into the kidney results in decreased filtration which results in oliguria. Causes include:

- reduced cardiac output
- hypovolaemia
  - ◊ relative – vasodilatation secondary to septicaemia
  - ◊ absolute – haemorrhage
- decreased cardiac performance
  - ◊ ischaemia
  - ◊ arrhythmia
  - ◊ negatively inotropic drugs

- urinary tract obstruction
  - ◊ tumour
  - ◊ embolus
  - ◊ intra-abdominal pressure
  - ◊ surgical misadventure – ligated ureter

In all patients at risk of low cardiac output states:

- measure urine output hourly
- aim for minimum urine output of 0.5 ml/kg/hour
- never treat oliguria with diuretics
- fluid load until either a diuresis occurs, or there is evidence of imminent fluid overload
- consider inotropic support

Direct measures of cardiovascular function

Pulse rate

The radial pulse is traditional but not the most reliable – use carotid or femoral in low cardiac output states.

Assess:

- rate
- rhythm
- regularity
- volume

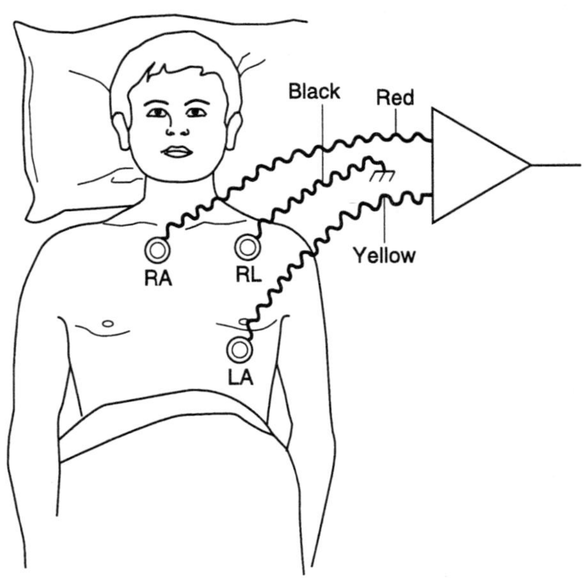

Electrocardiograph attachment to the chest – CM_5 configuration

ECG monitoring is readily available but beware its limitations:

- ECG indicates electrical activity, NOT cardiac output
- the rate counter expects a 'normal' QRS complex and therefore the ECG rate may be erroneous if waveform abnormal – peaked T waves, diathermy interference
- three lead ECG monitoring will detect arrhythmias and some ischaemic episodes. Lead II is often used for arrhythmia detection but is a poor monitor of the ST changes associated with ischaemia

CM_5 configuration for both arrhythmias AND major ischaemic events:

- red lead second intercostal space to the right of the manubrium sternum
- yellow lead in V_5 position
- earth or black lead can be anywhere but is usually placed in the infraclavicular region on the left
- set ECG monitor lead switch to lead I
- atrial fibrillation – monitor both ECG and a peripheral pulse rate to determine an effective pulse generation

Learn to recognise common arrhythmias and their precipitating causes:

- sinus tachycardia
  - ◊ pain, anxiety, hypovolaemia, infection
- atrial fibrillation
  - ◊ ischaemic heart disease
  - ◊ mitral valve disease
  - ◊ thyrotoxicosis
  - ◊ sepsis, especially chest infection in COAD
  - ◊ electrolyte imbalance
- ventricular ectopics
  - ◊ 'normal'
  - ◊ pain
  - ◊ electrolyte abnormalities (especially hypokalaemia)
  - ◊ ischaemia
  - ◊ drug toxicity
  - ◊ acid base disturbance
- ventricular tachycardia
  - ◊ severe electrolyte abnormalities especially K^+ and Mg^+
  - ◊ ischaemia
  - ◊ drug toxicity
  - ◊ acid base disturbance.

All need URGENT treatment of the underlying cause

Blood pressure

The manual sphygmomanometer is the gold standard.

- cuff should cover 2/3 length of the upper arm and the bladder should enclose half the arm circumference.
- chart measurements frequently and look for trends.
- assess pulse pressure
  - ◊ large volume pulse pressure may indicate low systemic vascular resistance (vasodilated circulation e.g. sepsis)
  - ◊ small volume pulse pressure may indicate high systemic vascular resistance (vasoconstricted e.g. dehydration)
  - ◊ postural hypotension is an excellent sign of hypovolaemia.

Non-invasive blood pressure monitoring

- convenient
- uses a technique of oscillometry which detects small pressure fluctuations as the cuff deflates
- false readings
  - ◊ irregular heart beat (atrial fibrillation)
  - ◊ patient movement
  - ◊ rapidly changing blood pressure e.g. haemorrhage
- complications
  - ◊ limb ischaemia if continuous readings
  - ◊ nerve entrapment leading to palsy

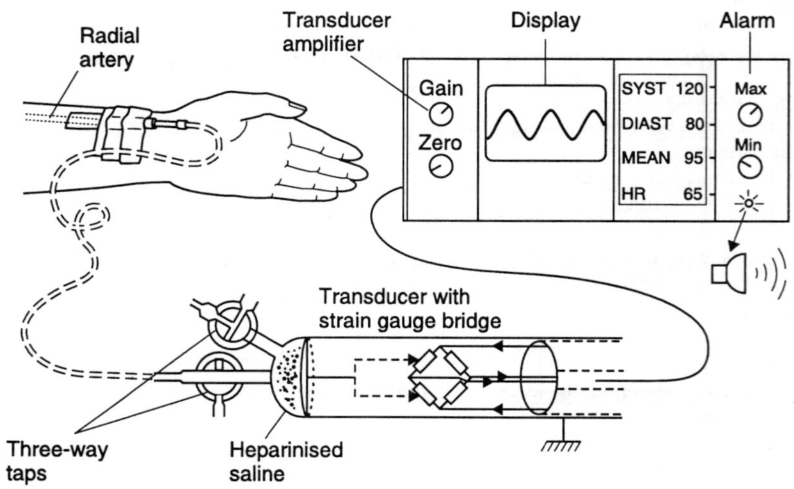

Pressure transducer, bridge amplifier, display and alarm

Intra-arterial blood pressure monitoring

- only used within high dependency areas because of risk of exsanguination
- requires specialised equipment
- provides continuous, beat by beat blood pressure, but is subject to artefact
- provides access for frequent blood sampling for blood gas analysis

A small cannula (22g) is inserted into a peripheral artery (radial, dorsalis pedis) and connected to an electronic pressure transducer. The monitor continuously displays the pulse waveform, systolic, mean and diastolic pressures. The waveform curves should be sharp with a clear upstroke and visible dichrotic notch. A rounded peak may indicate damping due to an air bubble, blood clot or a damaged cannula. Data from a damped waveform will be inaccurate.

- Modified Allen's test: this is used to exclude radial arterial dominance and confirm an adequate collateral arterial supply (ulnar artery) to the hand prior to cannula insertion.
  - ◊ the hand is placed in a neutral, supinated position and a tight fist made
  - ◊ both radial and ulnar arteries are compressed by the assessor and the patient asked to open his hand
  - ◊ the assessor releases pressure on the ulnar artery, while continuing compression of the radial artery, and looks for flushing of the blanched palm of the patient, and then releases the radial artery and looks for any further flushing to determine any tissue perfusion that is radial artery dependent
  - ◊ a rapid pink flush to all the hand confirms adequate collateral blood supply to the fingers if the radial artery becomes occluded following cannulation
- Hazards of arterial cannulation
  - ◊ haemorrhage – accidental disconnection
  - ◊ arterial damage – occlusion, aneurysm, arteriovenous fistula
  - ◊ embolus – distal ischaemia
  - ◊ infection – insertion site, emboli, systemic
  - ◊ accidental injection – thiopentone will cause severe arterial spasm followed by ischaemia and gangrene of supplied tissues

In the critically ill patient, the benefit of arterial monitoring far outweighs the risks but nevertheless the cannula should be inspected regularly and removed at the earliest opportunity.

Central venous pressure

Think of the heart as a bucket:

- The rate water flows out depends on
  - ◊ the rate water is poured INTO the bucket (preload)
  - ◊ the height of water in the bucket (contractility)
  - ◊ the size of the outflow pipe (total peripheral resistance)

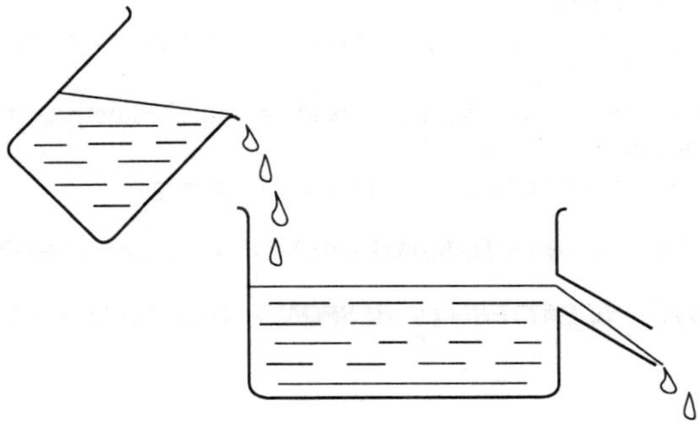

To some extent preload determines contractility (the rate water is poured in determines the height of water in the bucket) unless cardiac failure develops (bucket overflows) – STARLING

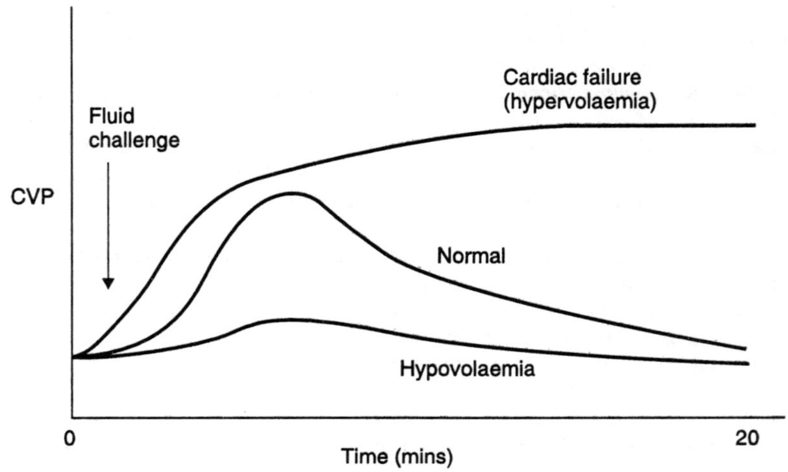

Central venous pressure gives an indication of the right heart preload which will determine right ventricular contractility, which will determine right heart output, which will in turn determine left heart filling pressure which will determine cardiac output.

- CVP is not a direct measure of cardiac performance or volume status.
- CVP indicates right heart filling pressure.
- cardiac output is determined primarily by the left ventricular performance which is a function of ventricular filling and contractility.
- requires insertion of a venous cannula into great veins of the thorax which is associated with certain risks
  - ◊ misplacement, dysrhythmias
  - ◊ pneumothorax, haemothorax
  - ◊ air embolus, catheter embolus
  - ◊ infection and septicaemia
- interpretation of CVP measurements requires prior confirmation of the position of the catheter tip in the superior vena cava by X-ray
- a single CVP reading is of little use. A series of readings must be interpreted in the context of the rest of a patient's cardiovascular physiology.
- CVP can be used to estimate volume status by a fluid challenge

A TECHNIQUE USED FOR OPTIMISING CARDIOVASCULAR PERFORMANCE IS TO OBSERVE THE PATTERN OF RESPONSE TO A FLUID CHALLENGE

- measure CVP using a pressure transducer at end-expiration
- infuse 250 ml 0.9% saline over 10 mins
- read CVP immediately after infusion
- re-read CVP at 5 min intervals for 20 mins

Optimisation of the CVS

It is often difficult to assess the state of a patient's cardiovascular system at the first meeting. This flow chart provides a series of actions which permit diagnosis and treatment to be combined into a logical sequence of events:

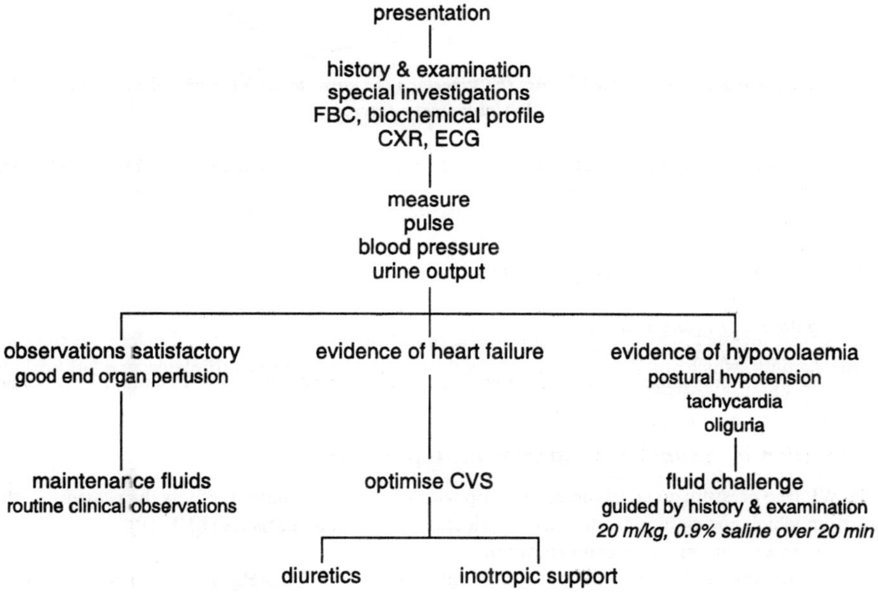

Pulmonary capillary wedge pressure (PCWP)

The Swan-Ganz catheter is an extension of central venous pressure measurement and is used to provide an indicator of left heart performance, particularly when there is concomitant right heart failure.

- the central venous circulation is catheterised (internal jugular, subclavian) with a pulmonary artery floatation catheter
- a balloon at the tip of the catheter is inflated with air and the catheter advanced into the heart
- the natural action of ventricular filling and emptying directs the catheter through the right heart and into the pulmonary artery, where the balloon lodges (wedges)
- catheter placement is guided by observation of the pressure and waveform in the catheter tip as it traverses the chambers of the heart and is confirmed by a CXR or using an image intensifier

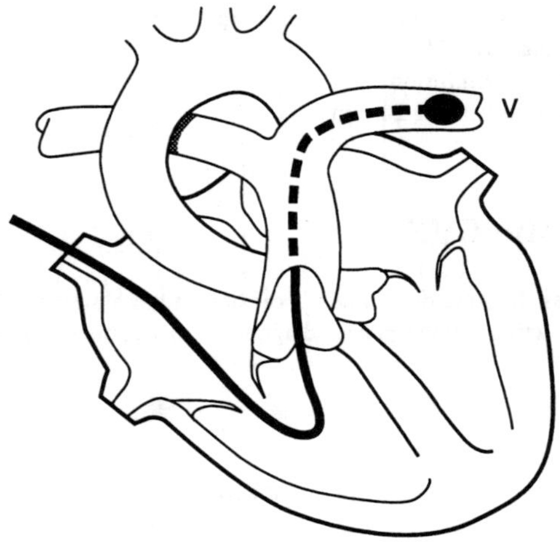

Passage of a pulmonary artery catheter from the superior vena cava through the chambers of the heart to the left pulmonary artery

- pulmonary artery catheter insertion carries risks over and above those associated with CVP insertion
  - ◊ misinterpretation, mesmerism
  - ◊ dysrhythmias
  - ◊ catheter knotting
  - ◊ tricuspid and pulmonary valve injury
  - ◊ cardiac perforation
  - ◊ pulmonary artery rupture
  - ◊ pulmonary infarction
    - ⊖ when the balloon is inflated, lung tissue distal to the obstruction is vulnerable to ischaemia.

Interpretation of Swan–Ganz catheter measurements

- PCWP (the pressure distal to the catheter tip with the balloon inflated) reflects the pressure in the left atrium which correlates with the left ventricular end diastolic pressure (LVEDP)
- measurements are made at end-expiration
- trends are more useful than single readings but a PCWP > 25 mmHg is likely to be associated with pulmonary oedema
- incorporation of thermistors in the right atrial and pulmonary artery components of the catheter permit measurement of temperature change in these regions. Injection of a bolus of cold fluid via the atrial (proximal) port and integration of the temperature change against time at the distal pulmonary artery port permits thermodilution measurement of cardiac output.
  - ◊ measuring the cardiac output directly, albeit intermittently, provides more precise manipulation of the cardiovascular system to achieve therapeutic goals
  - ◊ other clinical methods of CO measurement used by the anaesthetist are: dye dilution, transoesophageal echocardiography and Doppler

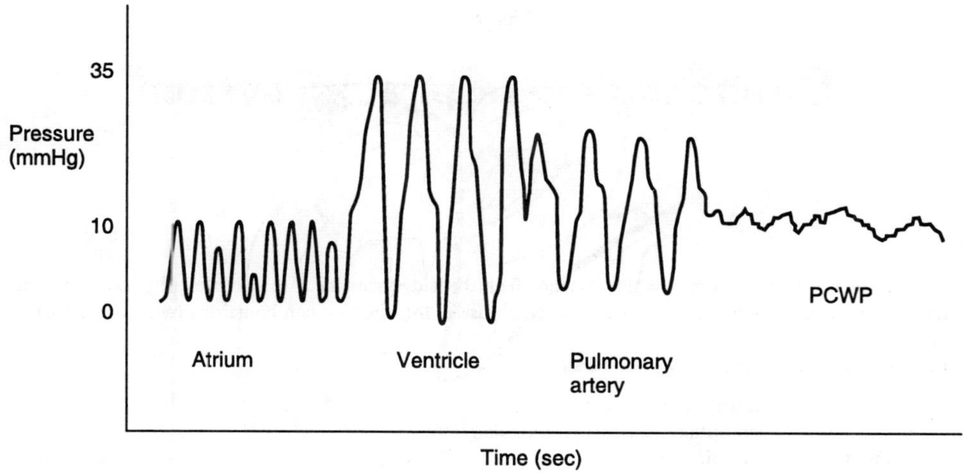

Waveform and pressure changes observed as the pulmonary artery catheter passes through the heart chambers

Chapter 9

Monitoring the respiratory system

The assessment of respiratory function extends from bedside assessment to complex physiological measurements requiring sophisticated apparatus. Much useful information can be gained by clinical observation.

The functions of the respiratory system include:

- ventilation (physical movement of gases)
- respiration (oxygen uptake and carbon dioxide removal)
- humidification of inspired gases
- non-respiratory functions of the lung (enzyme conversion)

The following discussion is limited to monitoring the acute ventilatory and gas exchange functions of the lung.

Functional classification of respiratory system monitoring

Monitors of gas exchange

- physical examination
- pulse oximetry
- arterial blood gases and acid/base
- trans-cutaneous blood gas measurements

Monitors of pulmonary mechanics

- physical examination
- end-tidal CO_2 monitoring
- airway resistance
- compliance of lung and thorax
- airway pressure measurements
  - ◊ PEEP
  - ◊ plateau
  - ◊ peak (inspiratory or expiratory) pressure
- airway pressure waveforms
  - ◊ pressure-volume
  - ◊ pressure-time
  - ◊ flow-volume
  - ◊ flow-time
  - ◊ airway occlusion pressure, maximum inspiratory pressure
  - ◊ estimation of the work of breathing

Measurement of lung water and anatomical relationships

- radiological examination

Monitoring gas exchange

Physical examination

Physical examination allows the examiner to identify the secondary effects of inadequate gas exchange

- tachypnoea
- pattern of breathing
  - ◊ fast and shallow breathing implies respiratory muscle fatigue
  - ◊ altered ventilatory pattern (Kussmaul breathing, Cheyne-Stokes breathing) implies an altered central ventilatory drive
- tachycardia
- use of secondary muscles of respiration
- central cyanosis
- clubbing (implies chronic disease)
- air hunger is a sign that requires urgent action by provision of supplemental oxygen

Pulse oximetry

Pulse oximetry is a method of estimating haemoglobin oxygen saturation. Light is transmitted through tissue containing blood. This light is absorbed by the tissue, as well as arterial, capillary and venous blood. Usually, only the arterial blood component is pulsatile, which then enables the absorption of pulsatile (arterial) blood at specific wavelengths to be measured. This can be used to derive a measure of the percentage of haemoglobin that is fully saturated with oxygen – the HbO_2 saturation (SpO_2).

Note: any waveform display is plethysmographic and represents the strength of electrical signal and NOT the degree of haemoglobin saturation nor perfusion pressure. The size of the display waveform can therefore be altered electrically by altering the gain, independently of SpO_2.

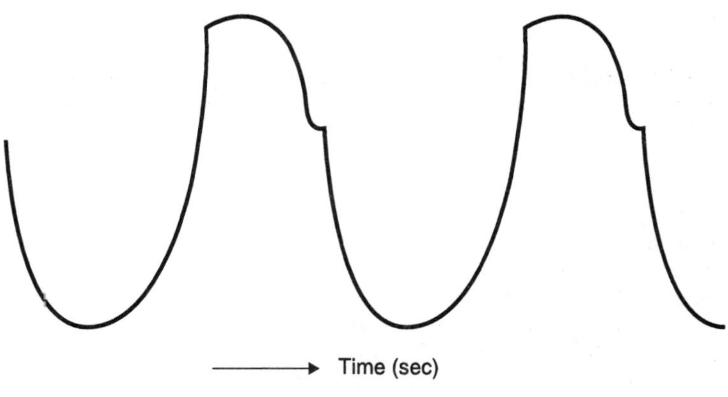

The plethysmographic waveform displayed on the pulse oximeter is* unrelated *to the blood oxygen saturation

In most clinical situations, the information provided by this technology is accurate but it cannot be relied upon in

- extreme hypoxia (S_PO2 < 70%)
- cardiac arrhythmias
- fluorescent lighting (falsely low)
- hypothermia (and peripheral vasoconstriction)
- motion
- surgical diathermy

Dyshaemoglobins

- carboxyhaemoglobin causes a false elevation of S_PO_2 and is of importance in chronic smokers and in long term ICU patients, where CO is a metabolic byproduct of haeme metabolism
- methaemoglobin levels >30–35%, S_PO_2 approaches 85% and becomes independent of the methaemoglobin level
- foetal haemoglobin does not affect the accuracy of the pulse oximeter
- severe anaemia (Hb < 5 g/dl) oxygen saturation does NOT reflect oxygen carrying capacity
- black, blue, green nail polish and jaundice give falsely low readings

Near infrared spectroscopy has been applied in a similar way to estimate the level of oxygenated and deoxygenated haemoglobin and cytochrome aa3 in the brain. Calculations are much more complex and require the use of expensive photomultiplier technology to sense the weak transmissions of light through the intact skull.

Arterial blood gases

Arterial blood gas measurements provide direct estimations of PaO_2, $PaCO_2$, pH and calculated values for bicarbonate, oxygen saturation and base excess. These values allow an inferred assessment of cardiac and respiratory status. Blood gas analysis is invasive, and usually intermittent, requiring repeated stabs or an arterial cannula.

Continuous, invasive arterial blood gas monitoring has recently become available and is useful in clinical situations where rapid changes in arterial blood gas parameters are encountered (Paratrend 7).

Interpretation

- Causes of $PaCO_2$ > 45 mmHg
  - increased production
    - increased physical activity (shivering)
    - increased metabolic rate and body temperature
    - hormones (catecholamines, thyroid hormone)
    - parenteral nutrition with high glucose content
    - malignant hyperpyrexia (malignant hyperthermia)
    - blood transfusion
  - decreased removal (hypoventilation)
    - inadequate alveolar ventilation (ventilatory failure)
    - inadequate tidal volume
    - inadequate respiratory rate
    - respiratory centre depression
    - increased dead space (the 'wasted' part of each tidal volume)
    - inside the lung (ventilation/perfusion inequality)
    - faulty equipment or poor circuit design

- Causes of $PaCO_2 < 35$ mmHg
  - ◊ decreased production
    - decreased physical activity (catatonia)
    - decreased metabolic rate and body temperature
    - hormones (decreased catecholamines, thyroid hormone)
  - ◊ increased removal (hyperventilation)
    - iatrogenic hyperventilation
    - altitude induced hyperventilation
    - hypoxaemia and carotid body stimulation
    - hypotension and/or acidosis
    - lung J-receptor stimulation
    - others – skeletal, muscle, joint proprioceptor stimuli

- Assessment of PaO_2
  - ◊ There are two major components to consider in evaluating the meaning of PaO_2
    - adequacy of arterial and venous oxygen content – important in considering adequacy of oxygen delivery to the tissues
    - assessment of lung function – ask, what is the expected PaO_2 for this patient, if lung function was normal?

The measurement of PaO_2 is of little value unless the inspired oxygen concentration (F_IO_2) and arterial (alveolar) PCO_2 are also known. An interpretation of lung function requires an application of the alveolar gas equation. In clinical practice, for patients breathing 30% oxygen or more at sea level, the alveolar gas equation can be simplified to:

$$P_AO_2 = [F_IO_2 \times 700] - PaCO_2$$

where P_AO_2 = alveolar partial pressure of oxygen
F_IO_2 = fraction of inspired gas that is oxygen (0.21 at room air)
$PaCO_2$ = arterial partial pressure of oxygen

The three main factors influencing P_AO_2 are:
- inspired oxygen concentration
- barometric pressure (decreased with altitude)
- arterial (alveolar) PCO_2

For every 10 mmHg change in $PaCO_2$, there is a change in the opposite direction of similar magnitude in the PaO_2

Alveolar-arterial oxygen gradient

Interpretation of PaO_2 and oxygen transfer requires assessment of P_AO_2 and is expressed as a gradient or a ratio:
- $D(A\text{-}a)O2 = P_AO2 - PaO2$
- normal A-a gradient varies from 5–10 mmHg at room air, to 100–150 mmHg on 100% oxygen
- $PaO2/P_AO2$
- normal a/A ratio is 0.75
  - ◊ lung oxygenation may be compared between two blood gas samples at different F_IO_2
  - ◊ change in lung oxygenation may be tracked over time
  - ◊ the effect of therapy manoeuvres can be assessed

'Rules of thumb' – acid-base analysis

- respiratory acidosis is secondary to ventilatory failure.
- metabolic acidosis is due to cell poisons or inadequate oxygen delivery.
- for every 10 mmHg change in $PaCO_2$, the pH should move 0.1 pH units in the opposite direction
  - ◊ For example, a pH of 7.3 can be completely explained by a $PaCO_2$ of 50 mmHg. If the pH were 50 mmHg and the pH were 7.2, there must be a metabolic component to the acidosis.
- the base excess and bicarbonate help to establish the magnitude and direction of any correction. The 'standardised' bicarbonate and base excess indicate the acid/base status that would pertain if there were no respiratory component to the acid/base change.

Transcutaneous blood gas measurements

- techniques have been developed for measurement of $PaCO_2$ and PaO_2 by heating skin and placing a sensor in close proximity to the warmed tissue. This technique is usually restricted to neonatal practice and is unreliable in adults.
- complications include the potential for skin burns, the need for calibration against arterial blood gas samples, and the need for re-positioning at frequent intervals.

Monitoring pulmonary ventilation

Physical examination

Many of the early signs of respiratory and ventilatory failure are seen first on physical examination.

- tachypnoea is often the first sign of respiratory failure.
- change in depth of respiration.
- fast and shallow ventilation is the most energy-efficient mode of breathing for exhausted respiratory muscles.
- nasal flaring
- accessory muscles of respiration with sternocleidomastoid and scalene muscle activity.
- 'respiratory arrest' (complete exhaustion lapsing into cessation of activity, unconsciousness and death) can be predicted before the event.
- pre-emptive management can be undertaken – elective tracheal intubation and mechanical ventilation commencing before a life-threatening episode.
- altered (central nervous system) ventilatory drive is manifested by altered patterns of breathing – Cheyne–Stokes and Kussmaul breathing.
- paradoxical respiration (abdominal protrusion and indrawing of the chest during inspiration) implies either a physical obstruction of the upper airway, or exhaustion of the respiratory muscles.
- stridor is produced by gas flow through a narrowed upper airway. If there is insufficient airflow it may not be heard even with severe upper airway obstruction.
  - ◊ if present during inspiration, it is more likely to be due to an extrathoracic lesion.
  - ◊ if present during expiration, it is more likely to be due to an intrathoracic lesion.
- Lung sounds should be monitored in conjunction with percussion, and each region of the lung attended to. A knowledge of the surface markings of the lung is important in differentiating pathology. Lung sounds are just as important when examining patients receiving mechanical support, although the sounds transmitted by the ventilatory apparatus need to be discounted when assessing lung pathology.
- Cyanosis
  - ◊ cyanosis is abnormal but this sign is neither sensitive nor specific enough to be reliable as a physical sign of hypoxia.
- carbon dioxide retention
  - ◊ venous dilatation, tachycardia, flushed skin.

CO_2 monitoring – capnography

The most commonly used monitor of ventilation was intermittent arterial carbon dioxide tension ($PaCO_2$), and although largely replaced by continuous end-tidal CO_2 monitoring, on-line, continuous blood gas sampling has now become clinically possible. An indirect measure of $PaCO_2$ is given by the end-tidal CO_2 concentration. The measurement of CO_2 concentration in the exhaled gas at the very end of exhalation provides a measure of alveolar CO_2 gas tension (P_ACO_2). When ventilation and perfusion are well matched $P_ACO_2 \approx PaCO_2 \approx P_{ET}CO_2$. The difference between $PaCO_2$ and $P_{ET}CO_2$ is usually less than 6 mmHg, but when lung perfusion is decreased, this gradient is increased. When there is maldistribution of ventilation, $P_{ET}CO_2$ no longer accurately reflects P_ACO_2.

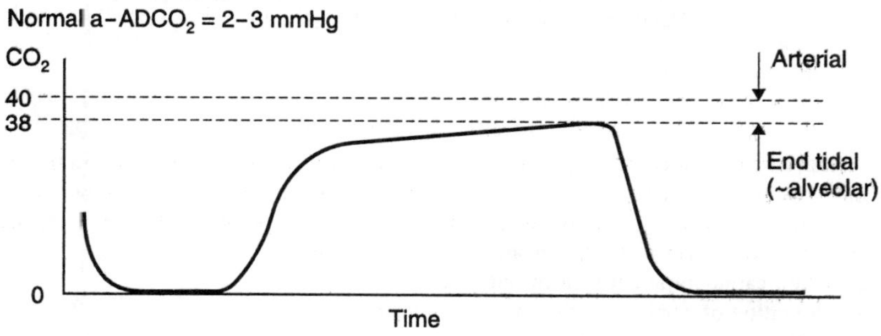

The effect of V/Q on ETCO₂

In mechanically ventilated patients, capnography is used as an indicator of the efficiency of ventilation. Changing the ventilation parameters affects $PaCO_2$, but rarely affects the PaO_2, because this depends more on the inspired oxygen concentration than lung ventilation.

The term 'capnogram' is used to define the waveform created by the carbon dioxide concentration over time and has four components:

- the ascending limb
  - ◊ represents the CO_2 concentration in gas from rapidly emptying alveoli
- the alveolar plateau
  - ◊ represents the CO_2 concentration in uniformly ventilated alveoli
- the descending limb
  - ◊ starts with the end-tidal point where the end-tidal PCO_2 is highest and represents the CO_2 concentration which most closely approximates true alveolar gas PCO_2
  - ◊ the rapidly descending limb corresponds to inspiration of fresh gas
- baseline
  - ◊ represents the CO_2 concentration of inspired gas.

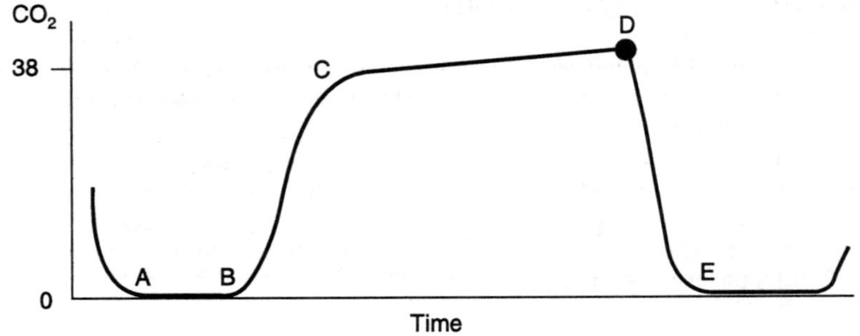

- Zero baseline (A–B)
- Rapid, sharp rise (B–C)
- Alveolar plateau (C–D)
- End-tidal value (D)
- Rapid, sharp downstroke (D–E)

The most commonly used method of gas analysis uses the principle of absorption spectrophotometry, where an infra-red light source is passed through a sample of gas. The amount of infra-red light absorbed is proportional to the CO_2 concentration in the sample. Mass spectroscopy and Raman gas analysis are used to measure volatile anaesthetic agents and other airway gases.

- Important capnographic waveform information:
  - ◊ confirmation of correct tracheal tube placement
  - ◊ adequacy of mechanical ventilation
  - ◊ shows respiratory obstruction
  - ◊ rebreathing of expired gases
- Limitations of capnography:
  - ◊ correlation between $PaCO_2$ and $P_{ET}CO_2$ is variable and may be poor in patients with a low cardiac output or altered ventilation/perfusion relationship
  - ◊ the correlation between $PaCO_2$ and $P_{ET}CO_2$ varies as the patient's condition changes over time
  - ◊ requires relatively expensive monitoring equipment

Monitoring pulmonary mechanics

These include:

- vital capacity (and forced vital capacity FVC)
- forced expiratory volume in 1 second (FEV_1) and FEV_1/FVC ratio
- peak airway pressure
- plateau airway pressure
- airway pressure waveforms
- lung/thorax compliance (static and dynamic)
- airway resistance

A useful 'rule of thumb': the FEV_1 should be greater than 1000 ml in an adult patient for safe general anaesthesia. It is possible to give anaesthetics to patients with poorer lung function but the combination of surgery and the residual effects of anaesthesia is extremely hazardous to the patient. Alternative analgesia to parenteral narcotics must be considered in patients with compromised respiratory reserve.

Ventilation/perfusion relationships

The development of 'Technigas' (an Australian initiative) has greatly simplified the conduct and improved the quality of ventilation-perfusion scans. Pulmonary angiography is much less used since the development of this relatively non-invasive nuclear medicine technique.

Respiratory centre drive

The following may be used:

- increased $PaCO_2$ should increase minute ventilation, and can be used to test respiratory centre integrity
- mean inspiratory flow (tidal volume/inspiratory time) – requires intact respiratory mechanics
- low ventilation rate
  - ◊ drug induced respiratory centre depression, hypothermia
- tidal volume
  - ◊ decreased with depression secondary to epidural narcotics while respiratory rate is preserved
- maximum negative inspiratory pressure obtained 100 milliseconds after temporary occlusion of the airway in a spontaneously breathing patient (P_{100} or $P_{0.1}$)
- apnoea monitoring
  - ◊ sleep apnoea, obesity hypoventilation, premature neonates

Lung water measurement

The following techniques may be used:

- chest radiography
  - ◊ approximately 35% increase in extravascular lung water may be required for a diagnosis of 'definite pulmonary oedema'
- CT scan – computerised tomography
  - ◊ useful for information regarding localised pathology
- MRI – magnetic resonance imaging
  - ◊ expensive, long data acquisition
- double indicator dilution
  - ◊ injection of ice-cold indocyanine green dye solution into the pulmonary artery and simultaneous thermal and green dye densitometry detection by constant withdrawal of blood from the femoral artery. Tends to overestimate extravascular lung water

Of these and other more esoteric techniques, the two most useful in clinical practice are:

- physical examination and chest auscultation at frequent intervals
- chest radiography

Chapter 10

Perioperative monitoring of cerebral function

Aim

To monitor the physiological conditions which determine brain integrity and to identify and quantify the effects of surgical and anaesthetic manoeuvres.

- the brain is 2% of body weight but receives 15% of cardiac output and uses 20% of the body's oxygen stores at rest
- electrical activity disappears before irreversible brain damage, as most energy is used to maintain ionic electrical gradients
- the brain is totally oxygen dependent with virtually no capacity to store oxygen or convert to anaerobic metabolism
- the cerebral cortex and basal ganglia are most sensitive to hypoxia and patient recovery after an hypoxic incident is often associated with a severe intellectual deficit or Parkinsonism

Clinical monitoring (optimising the milieu)

Adequate cerebral oxygen flux i.e.

- adequate oxygen delivery
- adequate blood delivery
    - ◊ blood pressure within the auto-regulatory range for the particular patient (normal MAP 50–150 mmHg)
    - ◊ no obstruction to venous drainage

Biochemistry

- normal blood sugar; serum sodium; serum osmolarity; blood gases
- appropriate drug levels of anticonvulsants or antibiotics
- $PaCO_2$ less than that which will cause a rise in intracranial blood volume and therefore intracranial pressure (ICP), and greater than that which will result in ischaemic vasoconstriction but appropriate for the particular patient's condition (35-45 mmHg)

Pre-existing conditions which compromise CNS integrity

- carotid artery disease
- raised ICP
    - ◊ space occupying lesions
        - bleeding
        - tumour
        - hydrocephalus
        - cerebral oedema
    - ◊ diffuse brain injury (traumatic or ischaemic insults)
    - ◊ the effects of secondary insults are more than additive

Clinical monitoring

- clinical neurological responses are obtunded or unpredictably altered by anaesthesia and therefore a high index of suspicion must be exercised, particularly in the high risk anaesthetised patient.
- changes of pulse rate, blood pressure, respiratory rate and rhythm, spinal reflexes and symmetrical change in pupil size or response to bright light, may be due to anaesthetic technique, depth of anaesthesia or response to surgical stimulus.
- asymmetrical changes in pupil size, particularly in an '*at risk*' patient, warrants a brain scan (computerised axial tomography – CAT scan), provided that trauma and the effects of pharmacological agents directly on the eye are first excluded, and it is not feasible to waken the patient for clinical assessment of conscious state.
- cardiovascular changes (BP, HR) are relatively late and unreliable when associated with raised intracranial pressure. The classic 'Cushing Reflex' of bradycardia and hypertension is probably due to brain stem ischaemia, associated with a rise in ICP, and while highly suggestive of intracranial pathology, is not infallibly so.
- hypotension is rarely a sign of intracranial pathology (except haemorrhage in small infants and in brain stem death). Look for another cause of the hypotension!!!
- erect and supine blood pressure and response to Valsalva may be used to assess the integrity of autonomic nervous system function.
- The Glasgow Coma Score (GCS) is now used to monitor coma and a score less than 9 requires careful attention to airway patency and protection; ventilation and oxygenation.
- spontaneous ventilation may be used to monitor brain stem function with some surgical procedures in this region.
- hyperthermia is a major determinant of cerebral metabolic rate and may occur in response to intrinsic hypothalamic/brain stem injury or external disease such as infection. Mild hypothermia may lessen cerebral oxygen demands but may also increase susceptibility to infection.
- general anaesthesia and sedation may increase ICP due to hypercarbia associated with respiratory depression or hypoxia from pulmonary atelectasis and infection.

ALWAYS SUSPECT CONCOMITANT CERVICAL SPINE INJURY IN:

◊ trauma
◊ rheumatoid arthritis
◊ achondroplastic dwarfs
◊ Down's syndrome

Device monitoring

Many attempts have been made to monitor different aspects of the nervous system in anaesthetised patients because of the limitations of clinical monitoring described above. These techniques are not readily available, require expensive equipment and are difficult to interpret even for experienced operators because of false negatives, false positives and failure reliably to reproduce data. Comparisons between patients are subject to inaccuracy because of varying anaesthetic techniques, depth of anaesthesia, surgical conditions, theatre electrical environment, not to mention interpatient variability.

Electrophysiological

The electroencephalogram (EEG)

- is a recording of the simultaneous scrambled electrical activity of many organised rhythmic activities arising from lots of post synaptic action potentials from little tissue masses.
  - ◊ the signal size is in the 10–100 mV range and the frequencies are banded and filtered by convention into 4 groups (δ < 4 Hz; θ 4–7 Hz; α 7–13 Hz; β > 13 Hz).
  - ◊ recordings are made from a series of electrode pairs over the skull usually positioned in accordance with international convention (the 10:20 montage).

◊ spikes of high voltage may be associated with seizure activity over specific areas, but the EEG may show ischaemic, metabolic, infective, degenerative and drug changes.
◊ general anaesthesia usually is associated with a general slowing.

Many attempts have been made to make the EEG more intelligible and user friendly with varying degrees of lack of success.

The processed EEG (pEEG)

◊ loses raw data and fine detail for ease of interpretation.
◊ these are generally based on making power graphs of the different frequencies and displaying them as brief temporal epochs of graphs or '*mountain ranges*'.
◊ the power spectra are analysed for changes in spectral edge (associated with cerebral perfusion) or in median frequency (associated with anaesthetic depth).

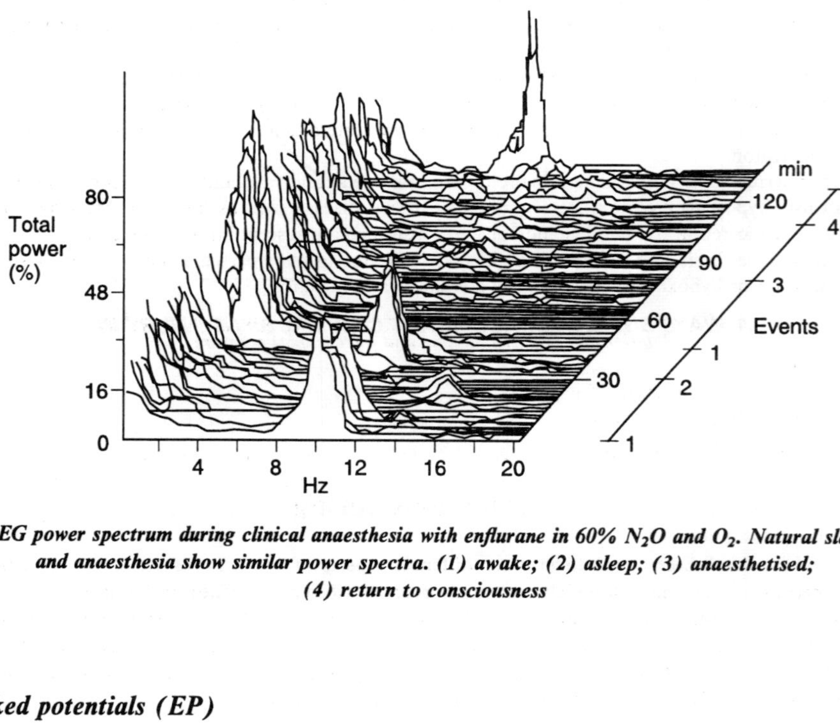

EEG power spectrum during clinical anaesthesia with enflurane in 60% N_2O and O_2. Natural sleep and anaesthesia show similar power spectra. (1) awake; (2) asleep; (3) anaesthetised; (4) return to consciousness

Evoked potentials (EP)

- investigate the integrity and functional status of specific tracts by filtering and amplifying minute central signals in the EEG related temporally to repetitive peripheral stimuli and looking for changes in amplitude and latency of specific waveforms correlated with synapses along the tract.
  ◊ different types of evoked potentials are used to assess different pathways – somatosensory (SSEP), motor (MEP), visual (VEP), brain stem auditory (BAER).

Cerebrovascular mechanics

- the adult skull is a rigid box containing non-compressible brain tissue (85%) and the displaceable fluids blood (5%) and CSF (10%).
- intracranial pressure rises rapidly when brain swelling or a space occupying lesion displaces the intracranial fluids, thereby inhibiting cerebral perfusion (see cerebral compliance diagram below).

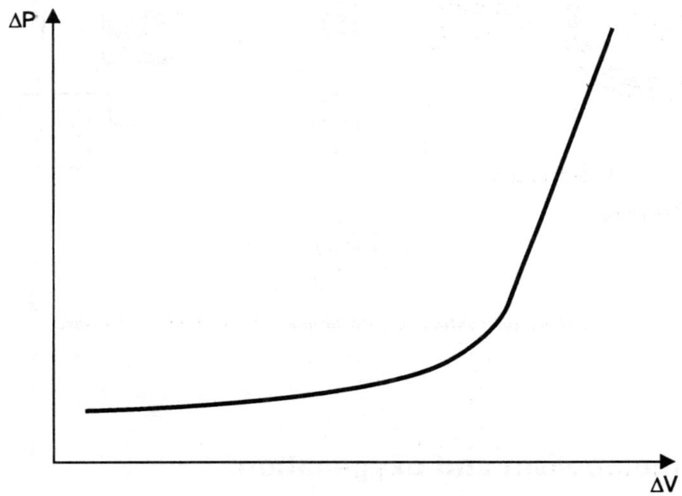

Relationship between volume and intracranial pressure

- cerebral blood flow is traditionally measured by indicator dilution by applying the Fick technique.
- Transcranial Doppler (TCD) pulsed low frequency ultrasound can be used non invasively and continuously to estimate flow velocity in intracranial vessels which under many conditions is proportional to blood flow.
  - ◊ TCD can also show vessel spasm or obstruction.
- intracranial pressure monitoring is necessary to determine cerebral perfusion pressure (CPP = MAP – ICP), which should be kept above 70 mmHg.

Waveforms

- ◊ A waves or plateau waves rise suddenly and persist for at least 5 minutes above 50 mmHg before falling precipitously, even to below the original level. These waves emerge at variable intervals from a background of elevated pressure and may be precipitated by seizure activity, elevation of $PaCO_2$ or stimulation. Neurological deterioration may be associated but plateau waves can usually be rapidly aborted by CSF withdrawal, barbiturate bolus and acute hyperventilation
- ◊ B waves are rhythmic oscillations at 0.5 to 2 / minute with an amplitude range of 10–50 mmHg. They are related to Cheyne–Stokes breathing but their precise origin is still debated.
- ◊ C waves have a frequency of 4 to 8 per minute and are of small amplitude, corresponding to blood pressure variations of the Traube–Herring–Meyer type.

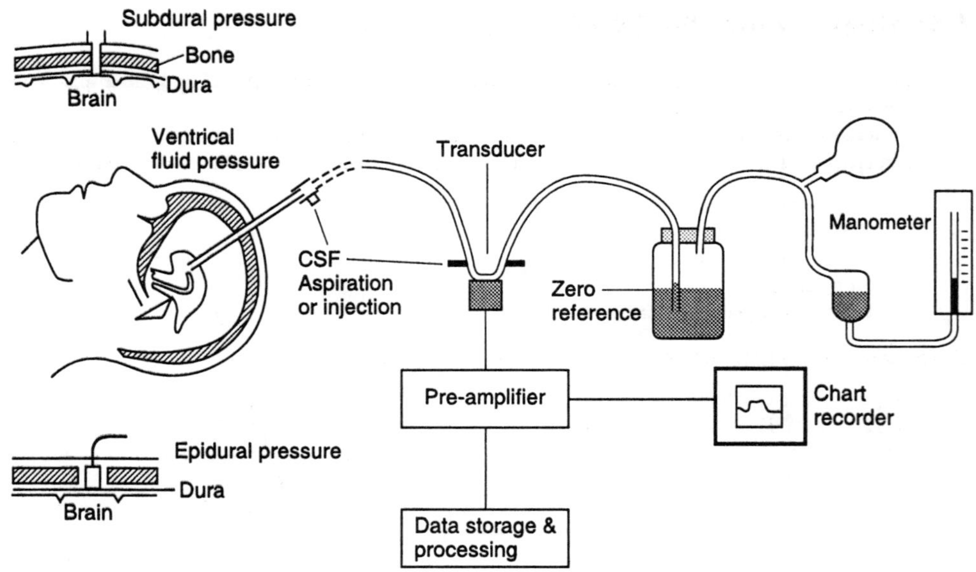

Techniques for continuous measurement of intracranial pressure

Cerebral metabolism and oxygenation

- global ***cerebral oxygen extraction*** is used to estimate cerebral metabolism.
  - ◊ an oximetry catheter is placed in the jugular venous bulb via the jugular vein and arteriovenous oxygen difference (A-Jv ΔO_2) and lactate production may be measured continuously to provide an early warning of cerebral metabolic compromise
- ***transcranial reflectance oximetry*** remains to be proven reliable as a monitor of cerebral oxygenation, as does the use of ***continuous intravascular blood gas analysis***.
- CSF biochemistry is intermittent, invasive, slow and often difficult to interpret.

Electromyography

- EMG monitoring is useful for identification of the facial nerve in parotid and acoustic tumour surgery but will be of no use if the patient has received muscle relaxant drugs.

End tidal carbon dioxide tension ($P_{ET}CO_2$):

- venous air embolism or paradoxical air embolism may be serious problems in surgery of the:
  - ◊ head and neck
  - ◊ posterior fossa
  - ◊ spine
- monitored with varying degrees of sensitivity by:
  - ◊ $F_{ET}CO_2$
  - ◊ praecordial stethoscope
  - ◊ Doppler
  - ◊ transoesophageal echocardiography

There are more elaborate forms of cerebral monitoring such as:

- computerised axial tomography (CAT), magnetic resonance imaging (MRI), positron emission tomography (PET) and single-photon emission computed tomography (SPECT) scans, and angiography, but they are not available in the operating suite, are time consuming and provide peculiarly difficult environments for anaesthesia.
- selective anaesthesia through cerebral angiography catheters or temporary balloon occlusion of vessels may be used to predict the effects of future surgery.

Seizures

- most anaesthetic drugs are anticonvulsant but, under some circumstances, several have been reported to cause fitting in some patients.
- seizures increase ***focal ischaemia*** and cause ***regional oedema***. Clinical signs of fitting may be masked by muscle relaxant administration, however the cerebral metabolic consequences remain.
- airway control and oxygenation should be established before looking to medication.
- fitting may be one of several causes of prolonged unconsciousness after anaesthesia.
- focal twitching, eye movements or pupillary dilatation may be suggestive, an EEG may be necessary to confirm the diagnosis.

Seizures are frequently associated with one or more of the following:

- ◊ hypoxia
- ◊ hypocarbia and alkalosis
- ◊ hypoglycaemia
- ◊ hyponatraemia
- ◊ inadequate anticonvulsant levels
- ◊ surgical trauma
- ◊ intracranial tumour, trauma or bleeding
- ◊ history of epilepsy
- ◊ drugs – pethidine, penicillins

If oxygenation is adequate, blood pressure, carbon dioxide and temperature are maintained within normal limits and due consideration is given to cervical spine injury, then anaesthesia per se will not compromise the central nervous system. However failure to observe these basic tenets of care augurs badly for the neurosurgical patient.

Chapter 11

Recovery from anaesthesia

The recovery room

One of the most significant advances in anaesthesia has been the incorporation into all modern operating suites of a Recovery Room, in which patients are detained during the transition from anaesthesia to full consciousness, return of muscle power and circulatory stability. The effectiveness of this environment in detecting and successfully managing problems which can arise during the early post-anaesthetic period depends on the presence of 1:1 nursing staff specifically trained in the care of the unconscious and the availability nearby of anaesthetists with the necessary resuscitative skills and specialised equipment – oxygen, a means of inflating the lungs, a defibrillator and suction.

The commonest cause of death in the recovery room is hypoxia, due to unrecognised respiratory depression or obstruction. Monitoring of haemoglobin oxygen saturation, end tidal carbon dioxide concentration and automatic non-invasive blood pressure should be continued into the recovery period. A period in the Recovery Room should follow both regional and general anaesthesia, especially if the former has involved significant autonomic blockade.

When

- the patient can maintain an airway without support
- the upper airway protective reflexes have returned
- respiratory and cardiovascular systems are stable
- the patient demonstrates a satisfactory elevation of conscious state
- there are no untoward losses from any body cavity

only then can the patient be returned to the ward.

The most important aspects of care in the recovery room such as management of the unconscious patient, acute pain, monitoring and fluids are covered in other chapters of this book.

Delayed recovery of consciousness

This results from drug administration, physiological disturbances (hypoxia) or incidental disease:

- relative premedicant overdose in recovery due to
  - ◊ dose or timing of administration, delayed drug absorption
- delayed drug clearance
  - ◊ volatile agent
    - respiratory depression or disease
    - depressed cardiac output
  - ◊ intravenous agents
    - depressed cardiac, renal or hepatic function
    - abnormal enzyme activity
  - ◊ age, obesity, poor physical status
- carotid endarterectomy and cardiopulmonary bypass have an increased risk of postoperative neurological dysfunction associated with cerebral emboli or hypoperfusion

- postoperative delirium
  - ◊ cerebral hypoxia
  - ◊ anaesthetic drugs – ketamine, scopolamine, propofol
  - ◊ pain
  - ◊ drug abuse
  - ◊ extremes of age
  - ◊ organic brain disease
  - ◊ psychiatric disorder

THERE IS NO SUCH THING AS A 'TRIVIAL' ANAESTHETIC,

NO MATTER HOW BRIEF OR STRAIGHTFORWARD THE SURGICAL PROCEDURE.

Chapter 12

Oxygen therapy

Oxygen is a drug. It has:

- physiological actions
- pharmacological actions
- a dose–response relationship
- adverse effects

Supplemental oxygen should be administered when tissue oxygenation is inadequate or threatened.

Physiology

Oxygen is utilized in aerobic metabolic pathways to produce biological energy from food fuels. Anaerobic metabolism produces fewer high-energy molecules for an equivalent amount of substrate. Conversely, greater glucose consumption is required to produce an equivalent amount of energy, because the cellular uptake of glucose is enzyme limited. A decrease in biological energy results from anaerobic metabolism and those tissues that have a high utilization of energy and limited cellular stores (cerebral, adrenal, hepatic and renal) will be damaged by hypoxia. The accumulation of biological acids as a consequence of anaerobic metabolism has further deleterious effects on cellular performance.

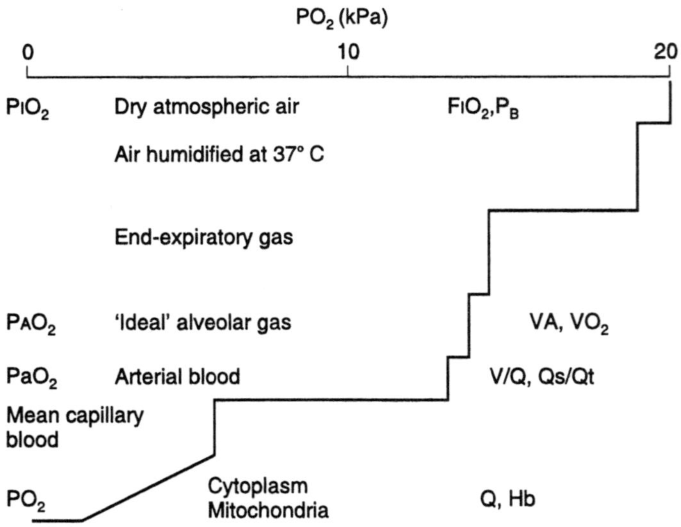

Oxygen cascade with PO_2 falling from ambient air to mitochondria. On the right are shown the factors influencing oxygenation at different levels in the cascade : FiO_2 – inspired oxygen concentration, PB – barometric pressure, VA – alveolar ventilation, VO_2 – oxygen consumption, V/Q – scatter of perfusion and ventilation matching, Qs/Qt – venous admixture, Q – blood flow, Hb – haemoglobin

The '**oxygen cascade**' (oxygen-tension gradient from the inspired gases to the mitochondria) acts as a pressure head of oxygen which determines the oxygen supply to the mitochondria where major oxidative enzymatic processes occur at a partial pressure of around 1–5 kPa. Anaerobic metabolism occurs when the oxygen tension falls below the Pasteur point which is about 0.27 kPa.

Oxygen is delivered by ventilation and pulmonary gas exchange to arterial blood and then is carried to the tissues via the vascular system. Oxygen passes from capillaries by diffusion to the mitochondria. This diffusion requires a pressure head of at least 2.7 kPa and an arterial oxygen tension of less than 4.0 kPa will jeopardize mitochondrial function, particularly if regional blood flow is also compromised.

Arterial oxygen content (CaO_2)

The normal value of 18 to 20 volumes % is a measure of the number of ml of oxygen contained in 100ml of blood. Since oxygen is both dissolved in plasma and bound to haemoglobin, the calculation of oxygen content has two components.

$$CaO_2 = 1.37 \times Hb \times SaO_2 + 0.003 \times PaO_2$$

$$19.7 + 0.3$$

Hb = haemoglobin in gram per 100ml blood
SaO_2 = % haemoglobin saturation

1.37 = number of ml of oxygen bound to one gram of fully saturated haemoglobin

PaO_2 = arterial oxygen partial pressure in mmHg

0.003 = solubility of O_2 in plasma, vol%/mmHg

From the above equation it can be seen that the haemoglobin term is much larger than the dissolved term and therefore CaO_2 should not be very sensitive to PaO_2. This would be true except for the dependence of SaO_2 on PaO_2 expressed in the oxyhaemoglobin dissociation curve.

The points to remember are:

- 90% saturation with PaO_2 60mmHg (7.9kPa) (shoulder of curve)
- 75% saturation with PaO_2 40mmHg (5.3kPa) (venous point)
- 50% saturation with PaO_2 26mmHg (3.4kPa) (P_{50})

The curve is displaced to the right by four factors:

- increasing $PaCO_2$ (Bohr effect)
- increasing hydrogen ion concentration (decreasing pH)
- increasing temperature
- increasing 2, 3 DPG concentration

The position of the curve is defined by the 50% saturation point known as the P_{50}.

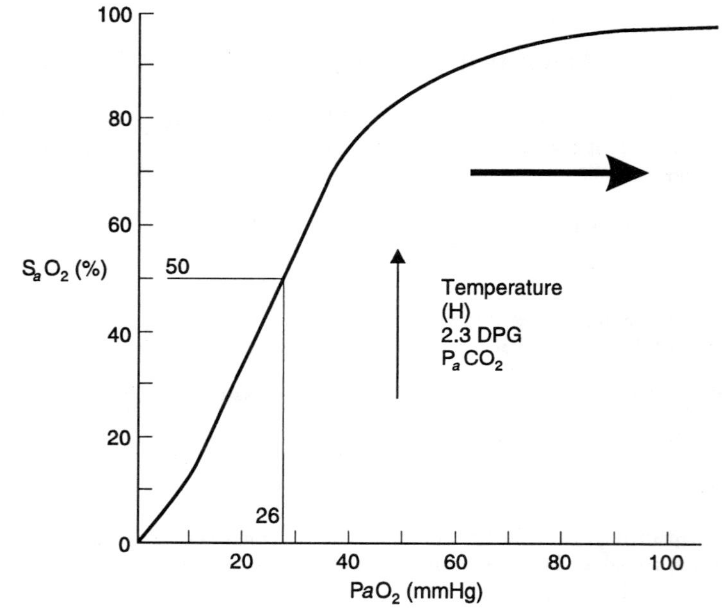

Oxygen flux

Oxygen flux is the amount of oxygen delivered to the tissues per minute. Oxygen flux equation describes the global oxygen availability and illustrates the reservoir above the average resting oxygen consumption of 115-165 ml/min m^2. As the amount of oxygen in the arterial blood is known (CaO_2) and the rate at which this oxygen is delivered to the tissues is determined by the cardiac output, and the body surface area is used to index the cardiac output for patients of different size, then the oxygen delivery index can be calculated.

Oxygen Flux = Cardiac Index (CI) x CaO_2 x 10 = 550–650 ml O_2/min m^2

Sufficient oxygen must be available to provide for the capillary cell diffusion gradient and tissue differences in oxygen extraction may be important. The normal range given above is for a patient at rest and is not necessarily adequate to meet the oxygen delivery demands of the tissues during periods of stress.

Oxygen consumption (VO_2)

This is a relatively stable parameter for a patient at rest and is calculated from the oxygen balance:

oxygen in – oxygen out	$= VO_2 = CI \times CaO_2 - CI \times CvO_2$
therefore, VO_2	$= CI\ (CaO_2 - CvO_2)$
where CvO_2	= mixed venous blood oxygen content (sampled from the pulmonary artery)

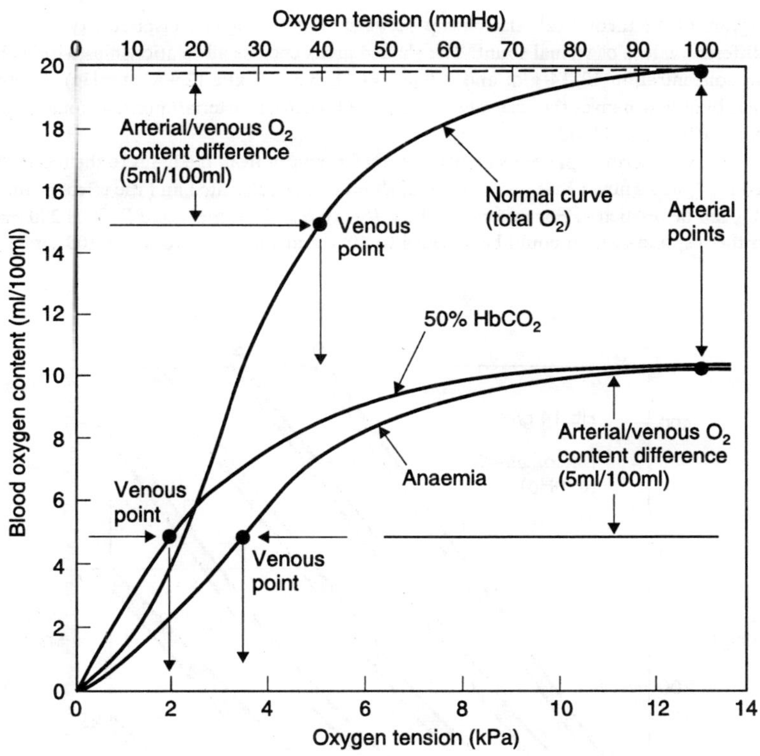

The tissues usually consume an average of 5ml of O_2 per 100ml of circulating blood. The mixed venous O_2 is a global measure of the adequacy of oxygen supply relative to oxygen demand. If the oxygen delivery decreases, more O_2 will be extracted from the arterial blood, therefore lowering the CvO_2. An increase in oxygen consumption will produce the same result if there is no compensating increase in oxygen delivery.

Mixed venous oxygen (physiological values)

Oxygen content CvO_2	= 12 to 15 vol%
Hb Saturation SvO_2	= 72 to 78%
Partial Pressure of Oxygen PvO_2	= 5.5 to 6.5 kPa

The iso-shunt chart

This is a diagram of the theoretical relationship between arterial PO_2 and inspired oxygen concentration (F_IO_2) for different values of virtual shunt. The shaded areas enclose all relationships within the limits of haemoglobin concentration 10–14 g/dl and arterial PCO_2 3.3–5.3 kPa (25–40 mmHg). Virtual shunt is defined as the shunt which gives the relationships depicted when the arterial/mixed venous oxygen content difference is 5 ml/100ml of blood.
This graph is used to describe a patient's ability to transfer oxygen from the lungs to the blood. By plotting the measured PaO_2 at a known F_IO_2, the degree of shunt can be estimated and the effect of increasing the F_IO_2 on PaO_2 can be predicted. For instance if the F_IO_2 is 0.6 and the measured PaO_2 is 200 mmHg (12% shunt), then the inspired oxygen could be reduced to 40% and the PaO_2 would be 100 mmHg.

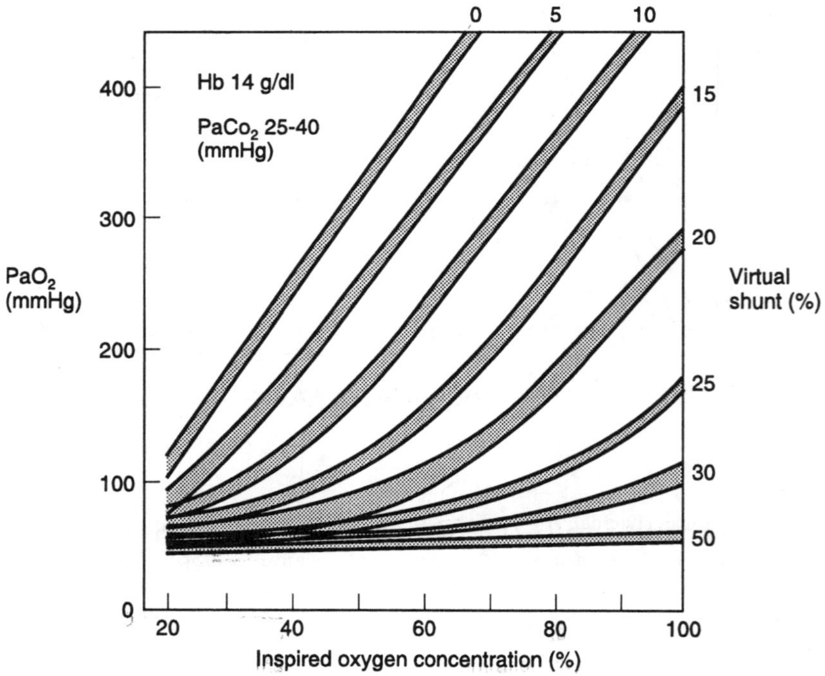

Hypoxia

Hypoxia is defined as inadequate tissue oxygenation. The types of hypoxia are:

- **Ischaemic hypoxia** — decreased blood flow, normal CaO_2
- **Hypoxaemic hypoxia** — decreased CaO_2
  - ◊ Hypoxic hypoxia — decreased PaO_2, decreased SaO_2, normal Hb
  - ◊ Anaemic hypoxia — decreased Hb, normal PaO_2, normal SaO_2
  - ◊ Toxic hypoxia — decreased SaO_2, normal PaO_2, (increased metHb, COHb)

Hypoxic hypoxia is caused by:

- ◊ hypoventilation
- ◊ impaired diffusion
- ◊ shunts (Qs/Qt)
- ◊ ventilation/perfusion mismatch V/Q

When a pulmonary shunt is present, poorly oxygenated venous blood mixes with well oxygenated end pulmonary capillary blood to produce a lower PaO_2 (i.e. venous admixture). The larger the shunt the greater the effect of PvO_2 on PaO_2. Consequently, in the presence of a shunt, any further decrease in PvO_2 will also lower PaO_2.

Clinically, venous admixture is due to:

- anatomical shunts (bronchial and thebesian veins)
- pulmonary atelectasis, oedema and infection
- pulmonary arteriovenous shunts
- congenital right-to-left heart disease
- ventilation/perfusion mismatch

Equipment to administer oxygen

Oxygen may be delivered to spontaneously breathing patients by:

- facial mask
- nasal cannulae
- anaesthetic circuits (via a mask or tracheal tube)
- resuscitation devices (Laerdal, Air-Viva and Ambu)
- headboxes
- cots
- tents
- incubators

Favourable specifications

- patient comfort
- low resistance to breathing
- no accumulation of carbon dioxide
- accurate control of FiO_2

A patient's alveoli can only receive 100% oxygen if

- $F_{IO_2} = 1.0$
- Oxygen delivery flow > patient's peak inspiratory flow rate (PIFR)
  (Adult, at rest = 25–35 l/min)
- Circuit has a reservoir bag and is 'closed' (i.e. airtight seal)

Therefore patients CANNOT inspire 100% oxygen with a standard bedside mask because the maximum flow of a conventional flowmeter is only 14 l/min.

There are two categories of oxygen delivery devices:

- Fixed performance systems : the F_{IO_2} will remain constant and independent of patient factors
- Variable performance system : the F_{IO_2} varies with the patient's ventilation

Fixed performance systems

The inspired oxygen concentration is determined by the oxygen flow rate and is independent of the patient's ventilation. To accomplish this, the system must deliver the prescribed gas mixture at a flow greater than the patient's peak inspiratory flow rate (PIFR), e.g. anaesthetic machines, continuous positive airway pressure (CPAP) masks, venturi-type masks.

Venturi-type masks

The oxygen flow to a venturi-type mask entrains room air by the venturi principle, resulting in a high total flow of gas which provides an accurate fractional inspired oxygen concentration. There are many brands of mask which utilise this principle. Some have colour-coded interchangeable components with varying bore; others use a rotating ferrule which alters the size of the entrainment aperture. Oxygen flow rate is usually set at 6–8 l/min and will produce gas flows of approximately 40–60 l/min, depending on the oxygen concentration which is prescribed. High flows maintain a constant F_{IO_2} without rebreathing and a tight fitting face mask is unnecessary. In severe dyspnoea with high PIFRs, the oxygen flow rate should be increased to 14 l/min to maintain the intended F_{IO_2}.

CPAP mask

A continuous positive pressure delivered throughout the respiratory cycle can improve oxygenation by increasing functional residual capacity, reducing shunt and thereby reducing venous admixture in patients who have a diminished FRC and are hypoxic. The supply of air/O_2 mixture must be greater than the patient's minute ventilation. A CPAP circuit and reservoir bag will allow the F_{IO_2} to be set by the fresh gas mixture.

Variable performance systems

The F_{IO_2} depends on the oxygen flow rate, patient ventilation and device factors.

Nasal cannulae

Oxygen flow rate of 0.5–4 l/min delivers a F_{IO_2} 0.22–0.4, however an accurate prediction of the F_{IO_2} is not possible. The F_{IO_2} will vary from breath to breath depending on the rate and depth of breathing, nose or mouth breathing and the length of the expiratory pause. High oxygen flow rates are very uncomfortable and dry the mucosa. In infants, a high F_{IO_2} can be achieved by a catheter tip placed at the uvula and taped to the side of the face. The nasopharynx acts as a reservoir and is loaded with oxygen for the next breath during the expiratory pause.

Standard face masks

These are simple, semi-rigid, plastic and disposable. Oxygen is fed to the mask and the patient expires via lateral perforations and between the mask and the face. On inspiration the patient entrains a variable amount of air and so the F_{IO_2} varies, but is always less than 100%. Provided the oxygen flow rate is greater than 4 l/min rebreathing is not a problem and flow rates between 4 and 14 l/min provide $F_{I}O_2$ 0.35–0.6. In severely dyspnoeic patients, the actual oxygen concentration that is inspired may be considerably less than intended. Dual flowmeters can give a maximum flow of 28 l/min in an attempt to match the patient's PIFR. In children, by virtue of their small size, PIFR approximates more closely with a flowmeter flow rate and $F_{I}O_2$ 0.8 can be achieved with a flow rate of 8 l/min.

High concentration masks

Masks with unidirectional expiratory valves and a reservoir bag can deliver $F_{I}O_2$ 0.9. These masks have to be used with great care as the rebreathing of carbon dioxide and asphyxia are potentially lethal complications if the rather primitive valves malfunction.

Face tents, tracheostomy mask and T-pieces

Artificial humidification should be supplied if the normal humidifying mechanisms are bypassed, laryngeal oedema or thick tracheobronchial secretions are present. The humidified oxygen mixture is delivered from the apex of the face tent and gases are expired through the open upper part. A T-piece is a non-rebreathing, large bore circuit that is attached directly onto the tracheal tube. The oxygen mixture is delivered by way of one limb of the T-piece and the expired gas leaves by way of the other limb, which also acts as a reservoir. Rebreathing is prevented by having sufficient flow rate (approximately 3 x minute volume) to wash expired gases out of the expiratory limb. A tracheostomy mask is a small, plastic mask placed over the tracheostomy stoma. The patient will inspire less humidified oxygen than that delivered, because dilution from room air occurs.

Oxygen headbox

The $F_{I}O_2$ depends on the oxygen flow rate, size of the headbox, size of the leak around the neck, the position of the head, the frequency of lid-opening and the neonate's respiratory pathology. An $F_{I}O_2$ of 1.0 can be achieved but falls rapidly on box opening, and the recovery half-life is long. Rebreathing of carbon dioxide can occur at low flow rates and with a seal around the neck.

Incubators

These are a means to deliver oxygen and provide a neutral thermal environment. It is possible to deliver $F_{I}O_2$ 0.85, however the need for high oxygen flow rates, patient access and the long recovery after each opening are major problems.

Oxygen tents and cots

Larger children can be nursed in these devices, however oxygen concentrations above $F_{I}O_2$ 0.4 are difficult to achieve. Recovery after opening the tent is very slow and access and observation of a sick child is severely restricted.

Clinical aspects of oxygen administration

- Oxygen should be administered when oxygen flux is decreased and the PaO_2 falls below 8.0 kPa. Haemoglobin saturation falls steeply with oxygen tensions below this because of the shape of the oxy-haemoglobin dissociation curve. Profound hypoxaemia is present and death is imminent when the PaO_2 is less than 4.0 kPa.
- Patients who are seriously ill from non-respiratory causes **require** oxygen therapy:
  - ◊ shock
  - ◊ sepsis
  - ◊ cardiac failure
  - ◊ acute myocardial infarction
  - ◊ burns
  - ◊ trauma
  - ◊ unconscious patient

◊ neuromuscular disease
◊ immediately post-anaesthesia

- Physiological humidification of gases requires a heated humidifier. Cold water bubble-humidifiers are inefficient and potential sources of infection. Humidification is not necessary for venturi masks where large volumes of room air are entrained, nor for other masks which effectively trap expired moisture.

Arterial partial pressure of oxygen (kPa)	**(mmHg)**	**Saturation (%)**	**Clinical significance**
20.0	150.00	99.00	inspired air at sea-level
12.9	97.00	97.00	young normal adult
10.6	80.00	95.00	young normal adult asleep, old normal adult awake; inspired air at 5,800 m
9.3	70.00	93.00	lower limit of normal
8.0	60.00	90.00	respiratory failure
6.7	50.00	85.00	moderate-to-severe respiratory failure requiring hospital admission
5.3	40.00	75.00	normal venous blood values; severe respiratory failure; acclimatized adult at rest at 5,800 m
4.0	30.00	60.00	usually unconscious if not acclimatized
3.5	26.00	50.00	P_{50} (50% saturation) value
2.7	20.00	36.00	acclimatized adult exercising at 5,800 m; hypoxic death

- Patients with severe chronic obstructive airways disease (COAD) may rely on a hypoxic stimulus to the medullary respiratory centre, whose normal hypercarbic drive is depressed by chronic carbon dioxide elevation. The uncontrolled administration of oxygen **may** lead to respiratory depression and death. These patients require accurately metered concentrations of oxygen which are titrated against PaO_2 and close patient observation.

COAD patients should receive controlled oxygen therapy commencing with FIO_2 0.24 via a venturi mask and blood gas analysis after 30 minutes. If the $PaCO_2$ remains below 10kPa and the rise in $PaCO_2$ is less than 1.3kPa, the FIO_2 should be increased to 0.28 and later to 0.35 if required. It is unnecessary and hazardous to aim for large improvements in PaO_2, remembering that a small increase in PaO_2 will provide a large increase in tissue oxygen availability because of the shape of the oxy-haemoglobin dissociation curve. Many patients with COAD are **NOT** sensitive to oxygen and their $PaCO_2$ does not rise with increases in FIO_2.

Rationing of oxygen to every hypoxic patient who has a raised $PaCO_2$ is illogical, as the central depression may be associated with another cause. Profound hypoxaemia is commonly associated with acute asthma which may be aggravated by beta-adrenergic bronchodilators and methylxanthine substances. Adequate oxygen, with simple masks (not low concentration venturi masks) should be administered to patients in acute asthma, many of whom have low $PaCO_2$ anyway.

- Inspired oxygen displaces air in alveoli, and being more soluble than nitrogen, will lead to increased pulmonary microatelectasis. Acute cessation of supplementary oxygen may cause substantial hypoxaemia and is hazardous.
- Facemasks should be replaced by nasal cannulae with restless patients, during meals and physiotherapy sessions to maintain a continuous oxygen supply.

Complications of oxygen therapy

Barotrauma

This is uncommon provided the equipment is used correctly. It is important to realise that oxygen from wall or cylinder supply is delivered at a **high pressure** (450 kPa) even if the flow rate is low. Hence it is lethal to connect an oxygen supply to a closed cavity, such as an intubated patient, without providing a vent to atmosphere. High flows suddenly applied to the lung may generate dangerous pressures unless the apparatus contains a distensible component, such as a rebreathing bag, as well as an expiratory valve. Occasionally tragedies occur when a nasal catheter is inserted too far and enters the oesophagus.

Retrolental fibroplasia

May occur when the PaO_2 in premature infants exceeds 90 mm Hg or 12.5 kPa. Hence it is important to monitor the PaO_2 of these infants when they are receiving oxygen therapy. This may be done by the use of percutaneous blood gas analysers, but oximeters may also be used, and if the SaO_2 is kept within the range 90-95%, the retina is not in danger.

Pulmonary oxygen toxicity

Does not occur in patients who are breathing spontaneously from standard oxygen therapy appliances, since it requires an FIO_2 of 1.0 for more than 24 hours, and in practice this is impossible under normal clinical circumstances. However, increasing alveolar-arterial oxygen differences occur when patients are **ventilated** with 100% oxygen for more than a short time.

Cerebral oxygen toxicity

Cannot occur unless oxygen is administered at hyperbaric pressure.

Carbon dioxide narcosis

Can occur in some COAD patients but not if oxygen therapy is controlled according to the principles outlined above.

Oxygen measurement and monitoring

Oxygen measuring devices can be divided into two groups, those which measure partial pressure and those which measure haemoglobin saturation. Oxygen therapy is titrated against frequent arterial blood-gas estimations, continuous transcutaneous PaO_2 measurement or pulse oximetry. The oxygen flow rate, FIO_2, device used, ventilation mode should be quoted with each arterial oxygen tension measured. A solitary PaO_2 represents oxygenation at one specific point in time and is meaningless without the concomitant information.

Chapter 13

Regional anaesthesia and analgesia

Definitions

Regional anaesthesia is the reversible abolition of sensation in a part of the body, without loss of consciousness.

Regional analgesia is the reversible reduction or abolition of pain in a part of the body, without loss of consciousness.

To obtain the above conditions, drugs are used which, when placed in the proximity of nerve fibres, interrupt impulses passing along those fibres by blocking the sodium channels of the axonal membrane.

Physico-chemical structure of local anaesthetic agents

Clinically useful compounds that demonstrate local anaesthetic (LA) activity usually possess the chemical arrangement:

Aromatic portion – Intermediate chain – Amine portion

There are two distinct chemical groups:

- AMINO-**ESTERS** - ester linkage between the aromatic portion and the intermediate chain. (e.g. procaine, 2-chloroprocaine, amethocaine, cocaine and benzocaine)
- AMINO-**AMIDES** - amide link between the aromatic end and the intermediate chain. (e.g. lignocaine, mepivacaine, prilocaine, bupivacaine and etidocaine)

The differences between these two groups of compounds are:

- their metabolism
  - ◊ esters are hydrolysed in the plasma by pseudocholinesterase
  - ◊ amides undergo enzymatic degradation in the liver
- their allergic potential:
  - ◊ ester hydrolysis forms para-aminobenzoic acid which will induce allergic phenomena in a small number of patients
  - ◊ the amides do not form para-aminobenzoic acid and allergic reactions to these agents are extremely rare

Except for cocaine, all local anaesthetic agents are **vasodilators**. Following injection of a local anaesthetic agent, some of the drug is taken up by the nerve and some is absorbed by the vascular system. The degree of vascular absorption is related to blood flow through the area into which the drug is deposited.

Duration of action is affected by the ***site*** in the body into which the drug is deposited (greater vascularity produces a briefer block) and by the addition of ***vasoconstrictors*** (such as adrenaline), which by delaying absorption, prolong the duration of action.

Anaesthetic characteristics of local anaesthetics

The anaesthetic profile of a chemical compound is dependent on:

Lipid solubility

- primary determinant of intrinsic anaesthetic **potency**.
- lipid solubility is proportional to the drug's partition coefficient and therefore procaine with a partition coefficient less than one is the least lipid soluble of the local anaesthetics and is therefore the least potent.
- partition coefficients of bupivacaine, tetracaine and etidocaine vary from 30–140, indicating a high lipid solubility and an intrinsic anaesthetic potency approximately 15 times greater than procaine.
- the relationship between lipid solubility and anaesthetic potency is consistent with the lipoprotein composition of the nerve membrane.

Protein binding

- primary determinant of **duration** of action.
- the less protein binding, the shorter the duration of action. Procaine is poorly bound to protein and therefore short acting (less than one hour) whereas bupivacaine and tetracaine are highly protein bound and therefore long acting (>2 hours).
- the relationship between protein-binding of local anaesthetic agents and their duration of action is again consistent with the basic structure of the nerve membrane.

pK_a

- pK_a of a chemical compound is the pH at which its ionized and non-ionized forms are in equilibrium, i.e. 50% in ionized form and 50% in non-ionized form.
- the unchanged base form of a local anaesthetic is primarily responsible for diffusion across the nerve sheath.
- **onset** of anaesthesia is directly related to the rate of epineural diffusion which depends upon the amount of free (un-ionised) base present at a pH of 7.4.
- lignocaine has a pKa of 7.74, is 65% ionized and 35% non-ionized at pH 7.4 and therefore, as the pKa is relatively close to the pH, the onset time is rapid.

Toxicity of local anaesthetic agents

All excitable membranes will be affected by local anaesthetic agents if they achieve a sufficient tissue concentration.

- Toxicity may be due to:
  - ◊ inadvertent intravascular administration of the correct dose of local anaesthetic(s)
  - ◊ administration of an excessive dose of local anaesthetic(s)
  - ◊ direct tissue toxicity due to the agent or its associated preservatives
  - ◊ rarely, an anaphylactoid or anaphylactic reaction
- The signs and symptoms of toxicity will depend upon:
  - ◊ the dosage of the drug administered and
  - ◊ the rate at which the agent enters the intravascular compartment

Effects on the central nervous system

- Initially – circumoral numbness, dizziness, difficulty in focusing and tinnitus
- Excitation phase – shivering, muscle twitching and tremors, generalised tonic-clonic convulsions
- Depression phase – unconsciousness, respiratory arrest

The excitatory phase is due to selective blockade of inhibitory pathways, however with large doses of local anaesthetic(s) there is inhibition of both excitatory and inhibitory pathways producing generalised CNS depression.

◊ the relative CNS toxicity of bupivacaine, etidocaine and lignocaine is approximately 4:2:1, which is similar to the relative intrinsic anaesthetic potency of these agents for the production of epidural anaesthesia in man.

Effects on the cardiovascular system

- The doses and blood levels of local anaesthetic(s) which cause significant CVS depression are approximately 2 to 7 times higher than those which will produce convulsions.
  - ◊ Initially – hypertension and tachycardia during CNS excitation.
  - ◊ Intermediate phase –
    - prolongation of conduction time
    - negative inotropic effect decreases cardiac output and results in moderate hypotension
  - ◊ Terminal phase – peripheral vasodilatation, profound hypotension, sinus bradycardia, conduction defects, ventricular arrhythmias and circulatory collapse.
- all local anaesthetic(s) exert a dose dependent negative inotropic action which correlates with their local anaesthetic activity.
- the more potent, highly lipid soluble, highly protein bound local anaesthetic(s) are more cardiotoxic (e.g. inadvertent IV bupivacaine).
- bupivacaine markedly inhibits sodium conductance in cardiac muscle, and whereas lignocaine's action is short, the bupivacaine action persists for a prolonged period (so called 'fast-in, slow out' drug).
- ultimately, the combined peripheral vasodilatation, decreased myocardial contractility and depressant effects on rate and conductivity lead to cardiac arrest.

Local tissue toxicity

The potential for local anaesthetic agents to cause localised nerve damage is very low; however the local neural toxicity reported with 2-chloroprocaine solutions is believed to be related to the antioxidant, sodium bisulphite, and the low pH of the anaesthetic solution. Local anaesthetics are relatively safe if administered properly. However, comparison of the dose required to produce a clinically useful blockade and that which will produce toxic symptoms reveals a poor therapeutic ratio.

Adding a vasoconstrictor

- the vasoconstrictor of choice is adrenaline.
- it should **never** be used in concentrations greater than 1:200,000, and
- the total dose should not exceed 0.5 mg at a single session.
- never use a vasoconstrictor in an end-artery situation.
- it is neither necessary, nor desirable to use adrenaline in the subarachnoid space.

Prevention of toxicity

Guidelines

- **never** use a more concentrated solution than is necessary. For infiltration anaesthesia in peripheral lesions, 0.5% lignocaine is sufficient.
- for vascular areas, stronger concentrations and large volumes, **always** use a vasoconstrictor.
- **always** aspirate before injecting. Do not inject if blood is aspirated.
- **always** have another person check the identity and concentration of the drug intended for use.
- **always** calculate the maximum dose (on a per kg basis) and verify that the dose to be administered is within the safe range.
- IV line **must** be in place for all regional blocks except for limited topical and infiltration anaesthetics.
- a sucker and a means of ventilating the patient with oxygen **must** be close at hand.

Local anaesthetic agents

A wide variety of local anaesthetic agents is available.

Agent	Duration	Onset	Toxicity	Applications
Lignocaine	medium	rapid	medium	topical nerve block spinal
Bupivacaine	long	slow	high	infiltration nerve block plexus block epidural, spinal
Cinchocaine	long	rapid	high	epidural, spinal
Prilocaine	short	rapid	medium	Bier's block
Cocaine	medium	rapid	very high	topical only

Dosage of local anaesthetic agents

It is inadvisable to exceed:

- Lignocaine plain 3mg/kg — Lignocaine with adrenaline 5mg/kg
- Prilocaine with adrenaline 7mg/kg
- Bupivacaine plain or with adrenaline 2 mg/kg
- Mepivacaine plain 3mg/kg — Mepivacaine with adrenaline 5mg/kg

Factors influencing the choice of regional anaesthesia

Controversy has long existed as to the optimal and appropriate use of regional as opposed to general anaesthesia for a variety of surgical operations.

- Patient suitability.
- Skilled anaesthesiologist.
- Other personnel – surgeons, nursing staff.
- Operative site – the periphery is easier.
- Special risks associated with unconsciousness, e.g. in obstetrics.

But in the long run the choice must be made principally on the basis of what is safer for the patient, whilst at the same time providing effective anaesthesia.

Techniques

Local anaesthetic agents may be:

- Applied to a surface; this is TOPICAL anaesthesia
- Injected into the vicinity of a lesion; this is INFILTRATION.
- Injected around the trunk of a major nerve; this is a NERVE BLOCK.
- Injected around a plexus of nerves; this is a PLEXUS BLOCK.
- Injected into the extradural space; this is an EPIDURAL BLOCK.
- Injected into the subarachnoid space; this is a SPINAL BLOCK.
- Injected into the exsanguinated veins of a limb distal to an arterial tourniquet; this is INTRAVENOUS REGIONAL ANAESTHESIA (Bier's block).
- Refrigeration.

Topical anaesthesia

Cocaine, a very powerful surface anaesthetic, is used by ENT surgeons in the nose because of its additional vasoconstrictor activity. It is, however, a very difficult drug to use without producing toxicity. Many junior medical officers will use amethocaine 0.5% on the cornea to allow the painless removal of embedded foreign bodies, or the examination of a painful eye. Remember that the continuing anaesthesia renders the eye vulnerable to damage, and that it must be covered until sensation returns.

When mucous surfaces, as in the nose or throat, are anaesthetised topically, absorption may be very rapid, especially in the presence of inflammation. Very careful attention must therefore be paid to dosage, particularly using Xylocaine aerosol in children, as it contains lignocaine 10% delivered as a metered dose of 10 mg per puff.

EMLA emulsion cream – eutectic mixture of lignocaine 25 mg/g and prilocaine 25mg/g – when applied to the skin (30g/100cm^2) produces anaesthesia in 30 minutes. Some uses are: intravenous cannula insertion in children, split-skin harvesting, reduction of nasal fracture, wart curettage, tattoo removal, lumbar puncture and bone marrow aspiration.

Infiltration

Infiltration with a local anaesthetic solution via a syringe and hypodermic needle is the commonest anaesthetic procedure in the world, and one of the few techniques which non-anaesthetists can carry out safely and effectively provided they observe a few simple rules.

Because of the limitations of dosage, only a relatively small area of the body can be anaesthetised in this way at one time. Peripheral lesion excisions, cannulations, dental procedures and blood donations are painlessly performed every day using this technique.

Nerve block

By placing a relatively small quantity of local anaesthetic agent in close proximity to the nerve trunk, a block of all the sensation in the distribution of that nerve can be achieved (e.g. femoral nerve block – adult dose: 10ml of 0.5% bupivacaine with adrenaline). The advantages of this technique are:

- the small amount of drug used and the reduced likelihood of toxicity.
- the nerve block is remote from the area on which the operation is to be performed. This is particularly useful if the operation site is infected.

Nerve block techniques vary with respect to the precision of anatomical knowledge they require for success. Some, such as maxillary nerve block, are technically very challenging; others, such as digital nerve block, can be easily performed.

Higher concentrations of local anaesthetic agent are required for a successful nerve block compared to infiltration. Vasoconstrictors are useful, but must **never** be used in the 'end-artery' situations of the digits or penis.

Plexus block

Even larger body areas can be anaesthetised by blocking the plexus of nerves which supply them. This is particularly the case with the upper limb, where the accessibility and anatomical constancy of the brachial plexus in the root of the neck make it feasible. Interscalene, supraclavicular and axillary approaches have been described; the most popular is the axillary approach which is virtually free of anatomical complications.

Relatively large volumes of local anaesthetic solution are necessary for successful plexus blocks, and careful attention must be paid to dosage (e.g. axillary plexus block – adult 30–40ml lignocaine 1% with adrenaline 1:200,000). Once again, vasoconstrictors are a big help in controlling absorption and prolonging block.

IMPORTANT
In both plexus and major nerve blocks, time must be allowed for penetration of the nerve trunks by the local agent, and up to 20 minutes must elapse before the larger nerves will be completely blocked. Surgery must therefore not be commenced prematurely.

Epidural anaesthesia/analgesia

Amongst the most useful of all regional techniques is that of epidural anaesthesia and analgesia. The former is suitable for a wide range of surgery below the umbilicus, whilst the latter can be used for the abolition of pain in labour or for postoperative pain relief.

Before epidural block is attempted, an intravenous cannula must be placed, and a fluid load of 500ml of crystalloid solution is administered before the onset of sympathetic blockade. If extensive block is intended, a systemic vasoconstrictor such as ephedrine IV may be required. The procedure is technically difficult until practice has been acquired. Placement of the needle in the epidural space is via the interspinous route from the back, and several tests for entry of the needle tip to the extradural space have been described. The most common in use is the loss of resistance test, in which an air or fluid-filled syringe is attached to the needle as it is advanced through the ligaments, whilst firm pressure is maintained on the plunger. As the space is entered, resistance falls and a quantity of air or solution (usually saline) is injected. Local anaesthetic solution may now be injected, or a catheter may be introduced to allow more than one dose to be given. This is especially useful in obstetrics, since longer periods of analgesia may be required than a single dose of bupivacaine is capable of producing. Successful epidural blockade of a number of segments requires volumes and concentrations verging on the toxic threshold; many anaesthetists therefore believe that addition of vasoconstrictor to the solution is essential.

The bilateral block which results includes the sympathetic outflow. The denervation eventually produces sufficient vasodilatation for blood pressure to fall. In fit patients, even extensive sympathetic block is of little consequence, although if the hypotension is sudden, nausea may result. In old, sick and compromised patients, sudden, extensive sympathetic blockade may be lethal. Very careful consideration must therefore be given to the choice of agent and extent of epidural anaesthesia in poor risk patients. The difference between anaesthesia and analgesia is largely a matter of the strength of solution employed. For caesarean section (anaesthesia) 0.5% bupivacaine is necessary, whereas for pain relief during labour, the concentration is reduced to 0.25%. Very careful attention must be paid to charting the total dose of drug given if repeated injections are necessary, as well as BP, pulse, respiratory rate and sensory level of blockade at frequent intervals. There is a limit to the amount of agent which the patient can metabolise, and the manufacturers' literature should be consulted for the amount which is safe to administer within a 24 hour period.

Spinal block

Essentially similar results to that of epidural block can be obtained from introducing a much smaller volume (e.g. 2–3ml of isobaric bupivacaine 0.5%) of local anaesthetic solution into the subarachnoid space, and bringing it into contact with the spinal cord. All sensation below that level will be lost, as well as vasomotor tone, as in epidural block. The concentrations of solution required are high, but the total dose of drug is less. Spinal block is technically simpler, and more likely to succeed in less experienced hands. Its principal drawbacks are that it cannot easily be prolonged via a catheter and the dural integrity is breached. All of the problems of sympathetic blockade are the same as in epidural anaesthesia, and similar precautions apply. Very fine needles (25G) are used to minimise post spinal puncture leakage of CSF and consequent low pressure headache.

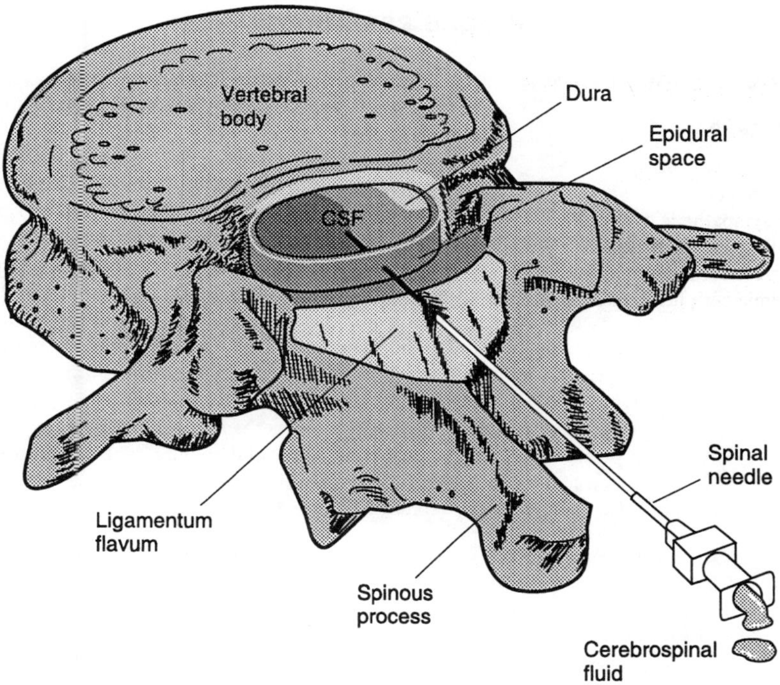

Insertion of a spinal needle through both the epidural space and the dura mater into the cerebrospinal fluid

Intravenous regional perfusion (Bier's) block

If a limb is exsanguinated and an arterial tourniquet applied, dilute local anaesthetic solution (e.g. 30ml prilocaine 1.0%) introduced into the veins below the tourniquet produces anaesthesia for as long as the tourniquet is left on. Removal of the tourniquet terminates anaesthesia within a few minutes. This simple technique is especially applicable to the upper limb, and can be carried out as an outpatient procedure. It is essential that a second intravenous cannula is sited in a limb, other than the operative limb, prior to commencement of the procedure. Risks are present from local anaesthetic toxicity, especially if any defect develops in the tourniquet within 15 minutes of the drug having been administered. Bupivacaine is especially dangerous and should never be used for this block. Prilocaine is recommended.

Painful conditions

Relief by regional block

some examples:

- fractured shaft of femur – femoral nerve block
- herpes zoster – thoracic epidural
- reflex sympathetic dystrophy – cervico-thoracic sympathetic block
- carcinoma of the pancreas – coeliac plexus block
- skin graft donor site – topical bupivacaine 0.25% with adrenaline 1:200,000
- ischaemic peripheral vascular disease – lumbar sympathetic blockade

Chapter 14

The management of acute pain

The treatment of chronic pain has improved considerably over the past 10 years. Too little time, staff resources and funding have been devoted to acute pain, which in practical terms is still a largely unresolved problem. Many forms of acute pain are equally in need of attention. e.g.

- post traumatic pain
- acute 'medical' pain (e.g. AMI, acute pancreatitis)
- obstetric pain
- paediatric pain

Harmful effects of unrelieved pain

Adverse psychological effects

- unrelieved acute pain progressively results in increasing anxiety and interferes with sleep. This rapidly demoralises patients and depletes their psychological reserves.
- children tend to become withdrawn and appear not to be in any discomfort. However, in reality they are in a state of catatonia and severe depression caused by unrelieved pain.

Adverse physiological effects

- atelectasis, hypoxia and hypercarbia
- inability to cough, sputum retention, lobar collapse and pneumonia
- increased sympathetic activity, increased myocardial work, increased myocardial oxygen consumption can produce myocardial ischaemia
- compromised regional blood flow to the brain, kidney & uterus
- gastric stasis, activation of neuro-humoural stress response resulting in vasoconstriction, decreased urine flow, decreased insulin, increased cortisol
- increased platelet aggregation, decreased venous blood flow and skeletal muscle spasm producing splinting and giving rise to deep vein thrombosis and pulmonary embolism

Physiology of pain

It is important to emphasise **individual variability** in the pain response, which may be substantially due to psychological factors, and also possibly due to individual differences in levels of endogenous opioids and in receptor responses. Therefore each patient requires an **individual pain treatment regimen**.

Central mechanisms

Melzack and Wall demonstrated that pain can be modulated in the spinal cord and brain to produce powerful influences on pain perception. This 'descending modulation' may help to explain the influence of psychological factors and is certainly important with the centrally acting analgesics. Modulation also occurs as a result of ascending input due to collaterals at several levels.

Interest in acute pain management has focused on spinal modulation at the level of the substantia gelatinosa (SG), in the dorsal horn of the grey matter.

Recent work has indicated the following possibilities for postoperative pain control:

- at least two different populations of opioid receptors.
- a noradrenergic system (e.g. relief of postoperative pain by the agonist epidural clonidine).
- a serotonergic system.
- possibly a GABA-ergic system.
- the eleven amino acid peptide, substance P, may be depleted or blocked, to interfere with primary afferent transmission.

Since the discovery of opiate receptors, it has been possible to identify endogenous opiate substances (e.g. endorphins, enkephalins) and to increase the understanding of the analgesic actions of endogenously administered opioids. A high density of opiate receptors is found in the limbic system, medial thalamic nuclei, periaqueductal and periventricular grey matter, midbrain reticular formation and the substantia gelatinosa of the spinal cord. The density of opiate receptors increases 20 times between birth and adulthood. Differences in the pharmacological effects of opiates have been ascribed to interactions with different receptor sites, e.g. mu (responsible for analgesia and sedation) and sigma (responsible for tachycardia, hypertonia and tachypnoea). Compounds that preferentially interact with the kappa receptor are of potential interest because they would be capable of inducing analgesia and sedation without respiratory depression. The relative efficiency and safety of these options remains to be evaluated in comparison to older techniques.

Peripheral mechanisms

There are various factors which decrease or increase the sensitivity of peripheral nociceptors. One example of modifying pain at this level is the inhibition of prostaglandin synthetase by aspirin-like drugs. Local anaesthetics can be applied directly at the receptor level using subcutaneously implanted catheters for wound pain, or at the level of afferent fibres.

Reflex activity

Since afferent fibres ascend or descend at least three segments before synapsing in the substantia gelatinosa, reflex activity may extend well beyond the level of noxious stimuli. Such reflexes may include viscero-somatic, viscero-sympathetic and viscero-visceral reflexes.

Visceral sympathetic afferents converge on the same dorsal horn neurone as somatic nociceptive afferents. Visceral noxious stimuli are then conveyed, together with somatic noxious stimuli via the spinothalamic pathway to the brain. Note the following:

- 'referred' pain is felt in the cutaneous area corresponding to the dorsal horn neurones upon which visceral afferents converge. It is accompanied by hyperalgesia in this skin area.
- reflex somatic motor activity results in muscle spasm which may stimulate parietal peritoneum and initiate somatic noxious input to the dorsal horn.
- reflex sympathetic efferent activity may result in spasm of sphincters over a wide area.
- reflex sympathetic efferent activity may result in visceral ischaemia, and further noxious stimulation. Also, visceral nociceptors may be sensitized by norepinephrine release and microcirculatory changes.
- increased sympathetic activity may influence cutaneous nociceptors and this may be at least partly responsible for 'referred pain'.

Narcotic pharmacokinetics

The absorption, distribution and elimination of opioid compounds determines their onset, intensity and duration of action. Pharmacokinetic data are most useful clinically when there is a close relationship between the plasma drug concentration and its effect on the CNS. Analgesics that rapidly equilibrate between the plasma and neuronal tissue will enable effects in the CNS to parallel changes in the plasma levels.

- CNS opioid penetration is dependent upon
  - ◊ free, non-ionized fraction (non protein-bound)
  - ◊ oil/water partition coefficient at pH 7.4 (lipophilicity)
    - ➲ fentanyl therefore enters the CNS approximately 150 times faster than morphine.
- pharmacokinetic data provide the anaesthetist with an understanding of how the body handles a given drug.

The $t_{1/2}\alpha$ = distribution phase (rapidity of drug uptake)
- $t_{1/2}\beta$ = elimination phase (persistence of the drug in the body)
- Vd_c = central volume of distribution
- Vd_{ss} = steady state volume of distribution
- CL = clearance (high hepatic clearance of opioids is dependent on liver blood flow)
- $t_{1/2} = \frac{0.69\ Vd}{CL}$

Opioid pharmacokinetics and related data

- fentanyl undergoes extensive redistribution in the body. This results in a short duration of action after small or infrequent doses. However, after large or frequent doses, the slow half-life may be > 13 hours.
- buprenorphine blood concentration and slow half-life do not determine analgesic response. This is determined by rate of dissociation from receptors.
- methadone can provide up to 24 hours of pain relief after a single IV dose, due to its long elimination half-life which reflects the drug's large volume of distribution and low clearance rate.

A summary of mean pharmacokinetic properties of various opioids following intravenous administration

Opioid property	Fentanyl	Alfentanil	Sufentanil	Pethidine	Morphine	Methadone	Buprenorphine
IV potency ratio	292	73	4521	0.53	1.0	1.0	33
Ionized at pH 7.4 (%)	91	11	80	95	76	99	91
Plasma protein binding at pH 7.4	83	91	92	65	35	85	96
Typical fast half-life $T_{1/2}\ \alpha$ (min)	2.3	3	1	4.2–11	25	10	3
Slow half-life $T_{1/2}\ \beta$ (hr)	2.5	1.3-3.3	2.5	3–7	1.4–4.0	25–45	2–4.5
CL (l/min)	1	0.92	0.73	0.5–1.8	0.9–1.5	0.1–0.2	1.1–1.5
Vd_{ss} (l)	375	36	98	250	200	420	180
Vd_c (l)	40–80	9–15	7–10	40–80	15–30	50–100	12–18
MEC (ng/ml)	1–3	100–300		300–650	12–24	30–70	

Vdss = total volume of distribution at steady-state equilibrium
CL = mean total body clearance
V = initial dilution volume
MEC = minimum effective analgesic blood concentration

The durations of analgesia produced by various opioids are related to redistribution (fentanyl) and elimination (methadone) processes. For the short acting alfentanil, both processes are important. Although fentanyl is generally considered to be short-acting as a result of its rapid redistribution, if given in high-dose, repeated or continuous administration, fentanyl can become long acting because of its long elimination half-life ($t_{1/2}\beta$).

The therapeutic plasma concentration (Cp) or MEC (minimum effective analgesic blood concentration) has a wide range depending on the surgical stimulus and anaesthetic conditions. The required Cp depends upon an individual's:

- CNS sensitivity
- type of operation
- presence of adjunctive drugs (sedatives, muscle relaxants, N_2O)

Pharmacokinetic knowledge has now provided the rational basis for **increased efficiency** and **safety** of opioids delivered as:

- controlled rate of IV infusion
- on demand patient activated infusion
- orally
- regular, prescribed intramuscular injection (NOT p.r.n.)
- transdermally.

By using a continuous infusion technique, a drug can be titrated to the patient's needs and thereby:

- minimise the amount of drug administered
- improve pain relief
- decrease recovery time.

The loading dose (LD) and initial maintenance infusion rate (MIR) are calculated as follows:

$$\text{LD } (\mu g/kg) = \text{CP } (\mu g/ml) \times \text{Vd } (ml/kg)$$

$$\text{MIR } (\mu g/kg/min) = \text{CP } (\mu g/ml) \times \text{CL } (ml/kg/min)$$

Because achievement of a steady state drug concentration is slow with a constant infusion, a loading dose is required to boost plasma levels of the drug initially. This can be administered as a bolus or short priming infusion. If a smaller LD is given then a higher initial MIR will be required because the amount of drug infused must equal that which is effectively removed from the brain by both redistribution and elimination.

In time, redistribution becomes less important and the infusion rate is dependent on the drug's clearance from plasma. Thus the MIR decreases during the infusion. Clearance is often lower than predicted in steady state infusions, particularly in the critically ill, morbidly obese and with cardiopulmonary bypass.

Further reading

- Prys-Roberts C, Hug CC Jr (eds). *Pharmacokinetics* of *Anaesthesia*, Blackwell Scientific, London, 1984.

Narcotic pharmacodynamics

The pharmacological effects of opioid compounds on the various organ systems include:

- CNS – opioid compounds produce a similar spectrum of action on the CNS, with dose-dependent depression resulting in analgesia, sedation, and ultimately, loss of consciousness.
- Cardiovascular – haemodynamic stability is usually associated with the opiates. However, bradycardia (due to stimulation of the medullary vagal nucleus) and hypotension (due to arterial and particularly venous dilatation) can occur during high dose narcotic techniques.
- Respiratory – a dose-dependent decrease in the responsiveness of the respiratory centre to carbon dioxide is seen with all opioid agonist compounds.
- Gastrointestinal – narcotic analgesics directly stimulate the emetic chemoreceptor trigger zone and increase smooth muscle tone (e.g. pylorus, sphincter of Oddi, ileocaecal valves).
- Renal – opiates increase bladder detrusor and urethral sphincter tone, which can result in urinary retention.
- Neuromuscular – truncal muscle rigidity may occur when opiates are rapidly administered in high doses and may be further enhanced by N_2O.
- Metabolic – high-dose narcotic anaesthesia (e.g. fentanyl) is alleged to be more effective than inhalation anaesthesia in blunting the release of 'stress' hormones (e.g. catecholamines, glucocorticoids, aldosterone) in response to surgical stimulation.

All the opioids are readily absorbed from the gastrointestinal tract, nasal mucosa, lungs and of course parenterally. The oral dose of morphine is considerably less effective than the equivalent IV dose because the drug undergoes 'first pass' hepatic metabolism. Less of the drug reaches the systemic circulation, and that which does is mostly as the pharmacologically inactive glucuronide. It must also be remembered that the majority of strong analgesics are excreted by the kidneys to a clinically significant extent as the unchanged drug.

Spectrum of activity of opioids

Alfentanil is a rapid, short-acting analgesic useful in outpatient anaesthesia and to block the stress response of intubation. Sufentanil is a potent, rapid, but longer acting analgesic. The agonist-antagonist compounds have a 'ceiling' effect on respiratory depression and a lower incidence of side effects, however their analgesic potency is limited.

Agonist <--------------------------- (strong narcotic analgesic)				------------------------------> **Antagonist** (narcotic antagonist)
Fentanyl	Morphine	Pethidine	Pentazocine	Naloxone
Sufentanil	Methadone		Butorphanol	
Alfentanil			Nalbuphine	

Classification of analgesics according to time to peak effect

Ultrashort	Short	Intermediate
Alfentanil	Fentanyl Sufentanil Pethidine Methadone	Morphine

Classification according to duration of action

Ultrashort	Short	Long
Alfentanil	Fentanyl Sufentanil Pethidine Butorphanol Nalbuphine	Morphine Methadone Buprenorphine

In spite of all the physiological, pharmacokinetic and dynamic data, if the drug is not administered, the patient's pain remains unalleviated.

Administrative and logistical problems in opioid use:

Dose too small, interval too long	Inadequate pharmacokinetic knowledge and failure to observe analgesic effect
Range of doses ordered Opioid order prn Alternative non-opioid analgesics ordered	Unwillingness or inability to assess Opioid needs of individual patients

Inadequate implementation of orders by nurses

Use of lower range of opioid dose, encourage long intervals between doses. Interpretation of prn as 'as little and infrequently as possible'	Fear of addiction and respiratory depression
Delay in administering opioid when patients report pain	Delays due to: Deciding if nurse thinks patient has pain Convincing senior nurse Staff attitude to that patient Availability of senior nurse Finding key to drug cupboard Demands of other patients

Difficulties in patient communicating analgesic needs

- Problems due to language, intelligence, or age (e.g. very young and old).
- Ethnic, cultural, and psychological background leading to over, or under reporting of pain.

Misconceptions in the use of opioid drugs in acute pain

Most of the non-compliance of medical practitioners in administering narcotics is due to ignorance.

- Doses should be as small and infrequent as possible to avoid development of addiction.
- Doses larger than the standard do not increase pain relief and cause heavy sedation and respiratory depression.
- Nursing and/or medical staff know when and how much pain relief each patient needs.
- Patients requesting more pain relief than the standard are psychologically abnormal or are becoming addicted.
- If non-opioid drugs are also ordered, these should be tried in preference to opioids.
- What is needed is a powerful non-addictive pain reliever.

THE ABOVE ATTITUDES ARE WRONG AND INAPPROPRIATE

TO THE PATIENT'S REQUIREMENTS!!

Clinical uses of narcotics

Preoperative administration

The major problem with the routine use of analgesics preoperatively is the high incidence of side effects (nausea, retching, dizziness, flushing, chest tightness, dysphoria). Sedative-anxiolytic drugs can potentiate opioids and therefore in combination can allow a reduced dose to be administered. The side effects which are dose dependent may be reduced, but excessive sedation can occur. An opiate (e.g. alfentanil 0.3mg/kg IV) can be administered 90 seconds prior to induction to blunt the haemodynamic response to intubation and if continued as an alfentanil infusion will decrease subsequent anaesthetic requirements.

Intraoperative analgesics

Advantages claimed for the use of narcotic anaesthesia:

- minimal cardiac depression.
- no sensitization of the heart to catecholamines.
- preservation of blood flow autoregulation (CNS, heart, kidney).
- no interference with autonomic or cardiovascular drug actions.
- tolerance of a tracheal tube and airway manipulation.
- facilitation of mechanical ventilation.
- postoperative analgesia.
- arousable patient.
- antagonist available.
- no primary hepatic or renal toxicity.
- not a trigger of malignant hyperpyrexia.
- not teratogenic – but newborn depression after maternal dose.
- no environmental pollution – but potential for abuse and dependence.

To exert their 'sole anaesthetic' properties, analgesics must be administered in doses 10-30 times more than those used for conventional analgesia. Of the available analgesics, fentanyl has been the most successful for the induction and maintenance of anaesthesia. When a high dose fentanyl technique is used, plasma concentrations in excess of 18ng/ml are required to maintain haemodynamic stability during cardiovascular surgery. A loading dose equal to 50–70 μg/kg followed by a MIR of 0.3–0.6 μg/kg/min would be expected to achieve a steady state fentanyl level of >20 ng/ml.

One of the most serious problems associated with opiate 'anaesthesia' is the high incidence of inadequate anaesthesia (awareness, movement, sympathetic autonomic hyperactivity). Supplementary drugs are added to provide greater depth of anaesthesia without increasing the incidence of intraoperative hypotension or producing prolonged postoperative depression.

Supplementation of narcotic anaesthesia

To prevent or control	Supplemental drugs
Awareness intraoperatively	Hypnotic, nitrous oxide, or volatile anaesthetic
Recall of perioperative events	Nitrous oxide, benzodiazepine, or hyoscine
Hypertension	Vasodilator or volatile anaesthetic
Tachycardia	β-sympatholytic or volatile anaesthetic
Muscular rigidity	Muscle relaxant or volatile anaesthetic

Opioid infusions are now frequently used in 'balanced' anaesthesia with N_2O and muscle relaxants. In fact, pharmacokinetic/dynamic studies with fentanyl and alfentanil have defined therapeutic plasma concentrations for a variety of surgical procedures.

Postoperative analgesic therapy

Intermittent intramuscular injection

- this often results in inadequate control of postoperative pain because of widely fluctuating blood levels, especially if administered p.r.n. The minimum effective blood concentration has been shown to be exceeded for only 35% of a 4 hour period, when the patient actually required analgesia.

Opioid infusions

- the use of an infusion of a medium to high clearance opioid with a short terminal half-life has become a routine in some surgical wards and intensive care units. The infusion is adjusted until the MEC for analgesia has been exceeded and this blood level is maintained. In this way continuous analgesia is given with minimum side effects. Repeated injections, discomfort and fluctuating blood levels are avoided.
- the risk of overdosage must be carefully monitored by
  - ◊ analgesic response
  - ◊ respiratory rate
- therefore the infusion equipment must be simple, safe, reliable and the opioid infusion should follow a prescribed protocol. Trained personnel should recognise and treat appropriately both inadequate and excessive blood narcotic levels.

Patient controlled analgesia (PCA)

- PCA may be by bolus only, bolus + fixed background infusion or bolus + variable background infusion rate
  - ◊ provides for variability in interpatient requirements and 'incident' pain (e.g. physiotherapy) can be treated
- PCA allows patients to increase the dose rate when the pain increases and reduce it when they have less pain. Hourly usage rates are similar to those for 'maintenance infusions'.

Single dose analgesia

- methadone has a long elimination half-life. Stable 'analgesia' blood concentration lasting 20-30 hours after a 20 mg bolus dose is possible. There is however considerable patient variability and initial doses must be carefully titrated.
- supplementary doses must be given by:
  - ◊ trained personnel
  - ◊ only if pain is reported spontaneously
  - ◊ only if the unstimulated respiratory rate is greater than 12/min
- a further feature of methadone is its high bioavailability when given orally.

Intrathecal opioids

- morphine 0.25–0.5 mg gives good analgesia after an onset time of 15–45 minutes, with a duration of about 12 hours. Delayed respiratory depression occurs in 0.36% of patients. The slow onset (3-6 hours) relates to the slow cephalad spread of the drug to the brain stem. This is predisposed to by high dose, sensitivity to opioids, administration of other opioids, serious illness and advanced age. The incidence of respiratory depression with the more lipid soluble drugs (fentanyl) appears much lower. Other problems such as urinary retention, itching, nausea and vomiting do, however, occur.

Epidural opioids

- low dose epidural opioid infusion as a mixture with dilute bupivacaine is very effective and has a low incidence of side effects. Epidural morphine seems most appropriate for acute pain of widespread origin (post thoracotory, upper abdominal surgery) and a lumbar catheter is just as effective as a thoracic one because of morphine's CSF migration. Lipid soluble opioids such as fentanyl or pethidine may be more appropriate with pain from a more limited segmental area.

Transdermal fentanyl

- effective blood concentrations can be achieved and sustained, with an efficacy similar to IV infusion, however there is a 6-8 hour 'lag time' in achieving analgesia and a slow washout time from the skin after removal of the patches.

Sublingual, oral 'lollipop', subcutaneous infusion of buprenorphine

Local anaesthetic neural blockade

- local anaesthetic drugs provide the best quality analgesia as pain can be abolished rather than diminished. However there is always some degree of motor and sympathetic block accompanying the sensory block. Some examples are:
  - ◊ intercostal nerve blocks, paravertebral block
  - ◊ femoral nerve block, continuous branchial plexus block

Transcutaneous electrical nerve stimulation (TENS)

- there is a 50% reduction in opioid requirements, though TENS is not effective by itself.

Cryoanalgesia

- post thoracotomy and inguinal herniorraphy but some incidence of chronic neuralgia.

Non-steroidal anti-inflammatory drugs (NSAIDS)

- these are particularly useful when mild to moderate pain is anticipated, such as following minor orthopaedic and gynaecological surgery
- are contra-indicated with
  - ◊ concurrent dehydration or hypovolaemia
  - ◊ renal impairment
  - ◊ risk of haemorrhage or incomplete haemostasis
  - ◊ hypersensitivity to any NSAID and asthma in conjunction with nasal polyps
  - ◊ history of gastrointestinal bleeding
  - ◊ pregnancy, children

Guidelines for management of severe postoperative pain

Principles

- multimodal – local anaesthetic + opiate + NSAID
- pre-emptive
- continuous delivery

First 24 hours

- epidural local anaesthetic by infusion (± epidural opioid) in a high dependency care area

From 24 hours onwards

- lower abdominal and lower limb surgery. Lumbar epidural catheter and fentanyl or pethidine infusion or top-ups by trained staff in medium care area. Naloxone available.
- upper abdominal-thoracic surgery (extensive pain stimulus). Epidural morphine tops-ups by trained staff in critical care area. (Lumbar catheter as effective as thoracic.) Naloxone available.

for marked increase in pain stimulus (e.g. vigorous physiotherapy to chest, hip or knee). Epidural local anaesthetic, 0.25% bupivacaine (avoids problems of additive respiratory depression of epidural and parenteral opioids).

Comparison of side effects

	Spinal Opioids v	**Local Anaesthetics**
CVS	No change in HR, CO or BP unless toxic dose	HR, CO and BP may be decreased with high dose
	Vasoconstrictor response intact	Postural hypotension
RESP	Early decrease (1–2h) – due to drug in *plasma* Late decrease (6–24h) – due to drug in CSF	Usually unimpaired

In summary, there are now many drugs, techniques and a considerable amount of pharmacokinetic data available for pain control. To utilise these techniques properly there must be:

- commitment to provide staff and equipment to supervise and deliver acute pain relief.
- training of medical and nursing staff in the basic principles of pain control.

Chapter 15

The management of chronic pain

Non-cancer pain

- avoid the use of opioids
- avoid the use of destructive procedures to interrupt the pain pathways

There are four basic types of pain:

- inflammatory
  - ◊ classical and responds to simple analgesics and opioids
- neural damage
  - ◊ pain is a shooting neuralgic type
    - post-herpetic, trigeminal or nerve compression
  - ◊ or a constant burning type
    - lesion in a sensory ganglion or spinal cord
    - treated with flecainide or mexiletine – neuronal stabilising properties
- sympathetically maintained pain
  - ◊ abnormal sympathetic efferent activity stimulates the peripheral sensory C fibres producing pain
  - ◊ non-dermatomal, burning, cold and blue limb
  - ◊ treatment is sympathetic nerve block and physiotherapy
- psychogenic
  - ◊ pain without an organic basis is rare
  - ◊ minor pain may result in hypersensitivity of the dorsal horn neurones and magnification of the pain severity out of proportion to the pain stimulus

Cancer pain

Incidence

- 50% of patients with cancer have no pain
- 15% of patients with non-metastatic cancer pain require opioids
- 33% of patients with metastases require opioids
- nociception (pain from tissue damage) and suffering (emotional response) require a comprehensive treatment plan

Nociceptive component

- onset, location, duration, severity, factors affecting intensity
- 75% pain due to cancer, 20% pain due to treatment

Suffering component

- fear, anxiety, depression, physical, social, emotional, spiritual needs

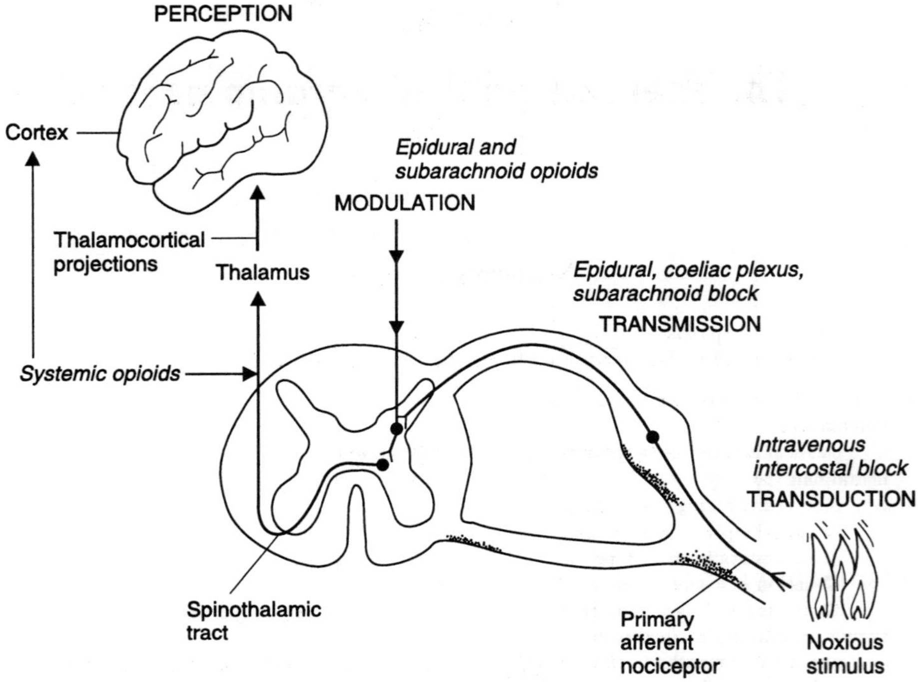

A pain pathway showing some sites of action of pharmacological intervention

Non-painful distressing conditions

- constipation, nausea, dyspnoea, decubitus ulcers

Nature of pain

- chronic pain
  - ◊ constant in site
  - ◊ area increases with time
  - ◊ severity increases with time
  - ◊ described as deep and boring, not superficial
  - ◊ awakens the patient at night

Pain relief

- during diagnosis
- during anti-tumour treatment
- advanced disease ± irreversible damage to tissue
- ensure a relatively pain free death

INADEQUATE PAIN CONTROL INCREASES SUFFERING FOR THE PATIENT AND RELATIVES, DECREASES RAPPORT AND DEMORALISES THE MEDICAL TEAM.

Management essentials

- rational use of drugs during diagnosis and treatment
- respect for the wishes of the patient
- early consideration of definitive interruption of pain pathways
- elevation of pain threshold by treatment of anxiety and depression

Pharmacological management

Drugs

- NSAIDS – paracetamol, ketorolac
- weak opioids – oxycodone, codeine phosphate
- strong opioids – morphine, methadone
- adjuvant drugs – anticonvulsants, antidepressants, steroids

Management

- specific drug for a specific type of pain
- use oral route and only use injections if
  - ◊ patient cannot swallow
  - ◊ suffers nausea and vomiting
  - ◊ is unconscious
  - ◊ unacceptable unwanted effects

Prescription

- know your pharmacology
  - ◊ rate of absorption
  - ◊ duration of action
  - ◊ potency and efficacy, equianalgesic doses by different routes
  - ◊ unwanted effects and complications
- prescribe on a regular NOT prn basis
- give each drug an adequate trial
- use drug combinations which provide additional analgesia with a reduction in unwanted effects
- treat unwanted effects
  - ◊ nausea and vomiting
  - ◊ constipation
- avoid excess sedation
- recognise the development of tolerance
- do not use placebos

Methods of drug delivery

- intravenous infusions
- subcutaneous infusions
- patient controlled analgesia (PCA)
    - ◊ spinal route
    - ◊ intrathecal
    - ◊ epidural
    - ◊ intraventricular

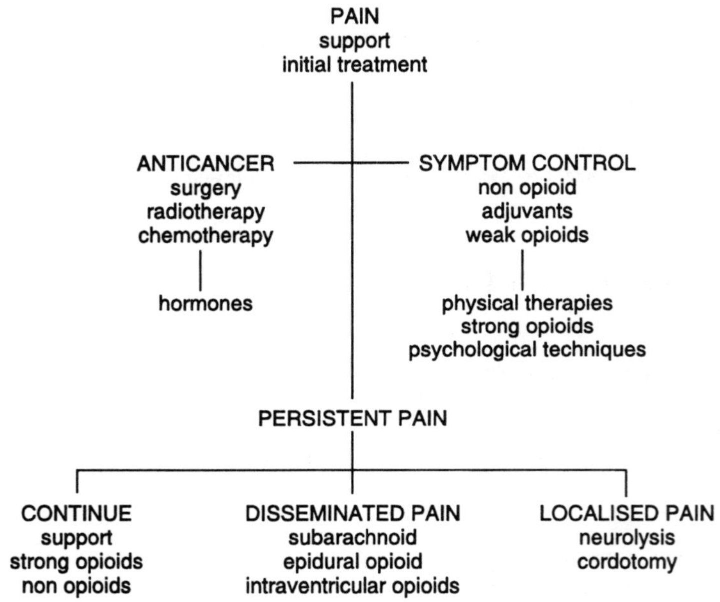

A flow diagram illustrating the steps in pain management

Non-pharmacological approaches to pain relief

- regional analgesia – epidural, intercostal, stellate ganglion block
- interruption of pain pathways – surgery or chemical (alcohol or phenol)
    - ◊ perineal pain with colostomy in situ and prepared to accept an indwelling urinary catheter
    - ◊ upper abdominal – pancreatic malignancy – coeliac plexus
    - ◊ percutaneous antero-lateral spino-thalamic tractotomy – C2 level
        - ⊖ lose contralateral pain and temperature
    - ◊ chemical hypophysectomy
        - ⊖ widespread hormone-dependent bony metastases
        - ⊖ pain relief independent from tumour progression

Chapter 16

Complications related to anaesthesia

Like any therapeutic or diagnostic intervention, anaesthesia has its complications. Some are virtually unavoidable, although their frequency can be reduced. The common complications, fortunately, are minor, but they are nevertheless important, since in many instances they are what the patient remembers most, and influence his or her subsequent attitude to surgery.

Minor complications

Vomiting

- by far the commonest minor complication of anaesthesia.
- the incidence is normally affected markedly by the following:
    - ◊ premedication – unpremedicated patients vomit only one third as often as those who receive a premedicant of any kind.
    - ◊ surgical duration – vomiting is commoner after long procedures.
    - ◊ nature of surgery – eye and ear and gynaecological operations are notorious for the frequency with which patients vomit postoperatively.
    - ◊ anaesthetic agents – some agents are much more inclined to produce vomiting, and the abandonment of cyclopropane and ether has to some extent been due to the high incidence of vomiting after their use.

Management

- ◊ apart from the avoidance of certain agents, and perhaps the omission of premedication, other factors are not under the anaesthetist's control.
- ◊ antiemetics – timing of administration is controversial, especially since some are soporifics and can prolong recovery times. Others (prochlorperazine, thiethylperazine) can produce dystonic reactions in a percentage of patients.
- ◊ metoclopramide causes the least problems but also has a lower effectiveness.
- ◊ it has to be admitted that the problem of vomiting after (general) anaesthesia is as yet unsolved.

Minor trauma

Ranges from the trivial, such as a haematoma associated with venepuncture, to the potentially significant, such as a corneal abrasion.

The following list is **not** complete:

- **Bruising** or laceration to lips and/or tongue arising as a result of the anaesthetist's manipulations, or may occur during emergence, due to the patient biting.
- **Tooth trauma**, especially when the upper anterior teeth are loose or prominent, or the patient is difficult to intubate.
- **Sore throat**, especially when throat packs have been used. It was also a very common complication of intubation.
- **Haematoma** can be avoided by the prompt application of pressure dressings after the removal of needles or cannulae. In special circumstances, e.g. when large cannulae have been used, or an

attempted cannulation has been unsuccessful, a crepe bandage should be applied for the duration of the case.

- **Infusion phlebitis** which is a chemical or physical irritation to the vein producing an inflammatory reaction, can be a very troublesome minor complication, leading to prolonged hospital stay. It is caused, for the most part, by inappropriate solutions (e.g. hypertonic dextrose), antibiotics, prolonged infusion time, and the selection of small veins for cannulation.
- **Eye trauma** is uncommon, largely due to the almost universal practice of protecting the cornea by taping the eyes shut. If the cornea is abraded, immediate application of an oily-based antibiotic ointment, such as chloramphenicol, is an effective treatment.
- **Epistaxis** may complicate transnasal intubation but nearly always settles down.
- **Granuloma of the vocal cords** may be due to intubation during anaesthesia but is rare.
- **Ulnar paresis** due to pressure on the nerve.
- temporary **paraesthesias** or **neuralgias** following local blocks, due to direct trauma to a nerve by an exploring needle or an intraneural haematoma.
- **muscle** and **joint pains**, especially in the elderly undergoing regional anaesthesia.

Major complications

The obvious major complication of anaesthesia is cardiac arrest, which may result from a wide variety of causes, usually associated with the patient's prior medical condition, or the surgery being performed. A few such events are of wholly anaesthetic origin, but although uncommon, they should be mentioned first because of their importance.

Hypoxia

- however produced, must ultimately lead to cardiac arrest, and death of the patient.
- rarely due to oxygen deprivation by failure of the gas supply.
- most often it results from an airway complication, such as accidental extubation, oesophageal intubation or disconnection of a mechanical ventilator.
- more subtle causes are
  - ◊ one-lung ventilation, due to a tracheal tube being displaced into the main bronchus after insertion
  - ◊ cuff herniation with increasing obstruction
  - ◊ pneumothorax arising as a complication of surgery or central venous line insertion.

Drug overdose

- the introduction of calibrated vaporisers outside the breathing circuit has made volatile agent overdosage rare.
- intravenous agents, especially thiopentone, are also nowadays used in lower doses, and rarely cause trouble.
- arithmetical errors in calculating the dosage of local anaesthetic agent or accidental injection into a vessel can lead to serious toxic reactions.

Drug incompatibility

- when volatile agents and adrenaline containing solutions are administered sequentially, the myocardium may first be sensitised by the volatile agent and then stimulated into an arrhythmia leading to arrest.

Anaphylaxis

- anaphylactic or anaphylactoid responses are becoming commoner, and may be life-threatening.
- onset is marked by
  - ◊ sudden hypotension
  - ◊ increased resistance to ventilation
  - ◊ cutaneous flushing
  - ◊ cyanosis
  - ◊ tachycardia.
- adrenalin is the specific treatment given intravenously in doses up to 1 mg every 3 minutes in a dilution of 1 in 10,000.
- fluid infusion and maximum oxygenation are helpful in overcoming hypotension and hypoxia. Colloids are the fluids of choice, as there is widespread capillary leak.

Aspiration of gastric contents

- regurgitation of gastric contents and aspiration of this material into the lungs during general anaesthesia when the lungs are not protected by a cuffed tracheal tube.
- vomiting may result in:
  - ◊ asphyxiation by drowning in the liquid vomitus
  - ◊ obstruction of the airway by a large chunk of undigested food
  - ◊ chemical pneumonitis which results from the effect of highly acid fluid on the tissues of the lungs and bronchi.
- the speed of onset of this acid-aspiration syndrome (named after Mendelson) depends mostly on the volume inhaled and may develop within minutes or may not be manifest for several hours.

Diagnosis

- history
- hypoxia
- wheezing and moist crackles accompanied by dyspnoea
- chest X-ray shows a pattern of widespread, discrete nodules of consolidation spreading out fan-wise from both hila, often described as a 'snowstorm'.

Treatment

Treatment is urgent and consists of:

- oxygen by appropriate means to elevate the PaO_2, often requiring intubation and mechanical ventilation.
- intravenous fluids with possible inotropic support.
- steroids are useless, and antibiotics of prophylactic value only against a complicating bacterial pneumonia.

Incidence

- once common in obstetrics, the universal practice of cricoid pressure and tracheal intubation or substitution of a regional anaesthetic technique has produced a marked decline.
- aspiration can and does occur in the post-anaesthetic period, especially if the patient is nursed supine whilst still semiconscious.

Prevention

- therapies aim to decrease both the volume and acidity of gastric contents
  - ◊ antacids
  - ◊ H_2 receptor blocking agents.

Major trauma

- nerve injury can occur to the brachial plexus or the radial nerve due to poor posturing or pressure from hard objects such as screens or retractor supports. Stirrups can also compress the common peroneal nerve against the head of the fibula.
- very occasionally, an unconscious patient can actually fall from a table or trolley due to clumsiness in handling or instability of the patient just before consciousness is lost.
- major neurological complications are exceptionally uncommon after spinal anaesthesia. Paraplegia has been reported, whilst the incidence of permanent neurological defect after epidural anaesthesia/analgesia is less than mortality following general anaesthesia (1 in 25,000–50,000)
- mortality due to surgical causes is approximately 1%, although of course there is wide variation from operation to operation.

Burns

- occur with the combination of diathermy, flammable skin preparations and anaesthetic gases.

Pneumothorax

- may result from supraclavicular brachial plexus block or injury to the pleura and lung during the insertion of a central venous line via the subclavian approach and from pulmonary barotrauma.

Malignant hyperpyrexia (refer pp 194)

- this rare condition is a genetic abnormality of muscle which is unmasked by the administration of the volatile halogenated hydrocarbons; the muscle relaxant succinylcholine is also a relatively weak trigger.
- a disturbance of normal intracellular calcium metabolism in skeletal muscle cells results in an increased utilisation of available oxygen, increased production of CO_2, resulting in oxygen desaturation, hyperventilation and tachycardia.
- temperature rise and muscle rigidity are late signs followed by acidosis and hyperkalaemia.
- even with the availability of an antidote, dantrolene, the condition has an extremely high mortality unless recognised early and energetically treated.

Succinylcholine apnoea

- prolonged apnoea following succinylcholine administration due to a congenital absence of pseudocholinesterase.
- paralysis which normally does not exceed 5 minutes after this relaxant is prolonged for up to 18 hours.
- treatment is effective artificial ventilation and sedation, and the patient comes to no harm.
- incidence of expression of the homozygous gene is 1 in 3000 to 5000 of the population.

Awareness

- the complication of general anaesthesia which is most seriously feared by patients is that they will be awake when they should be asleep.
- this has an incidence of 1%-2% of all patients undergoing general anaesthesia with muscle relaxants.
- patients may be aware for only the briefest of intervals, perhaps during intubation, but a few are paralysed and awake during the painful surgical part of the operation, and are understandably terrified by this experience.
- this may result from maladministration of anaesthesia due to an equipment malfunction (such as the vaporiser not being properly attached to the anaesthetic machine and therefore delivering the anaesthetic vapour into the atmosphere and not to the patient circuit) or miscalculation and malpreparation of intravenous drugs.
- if a patient claims to have felt or heard something during anaesthesia, the statement must be sympathetically heard and a reasonable explanation given. What the patient wants to know is whether this will **always** happen, and if reassured that the forewarned anaesthetist can take steps to prevent awareness occurring again, this will relieve their anxiety.

Chapter 17

Aspects of transplantation medicine

Organ transplantation has become an important aspect of the management of chronic end stage organ failure. Survival at one year is reliably above 60% for the recipients of hearts, livers and kidneys. Application of this technique is growing in absolute numbers, types of procedure and indication for transplantation.

For the junior physician this means exposure to increasing numbers of:

- patients considered suitable for organ donation and
- patients who are successful organ recipients presenting for non-transplantation surgery.

Beating-heart organ donation

The concept of brain death was originally described to aid the diagnosis of death in patients who clearly had no prospect of survival due to massive intracranial damage but had beating hearts and were on ventilatory support. Expertise in organ transplantation developed with the advent of better anti-rejection medication and an improving prognosis after surgery. Westernised countries now have accepted criteria for the diagnosis of death in the presence of a beating heart and subsequently allow such patients, after appropriate consent, to be referred to organ donation programs. It is important that the two processes remain distinct in the minds of the physicians involved.

Organ donation schemes

Currently it is availability of suitable organs that limits the implementation of organ donation procedures. Estimates of the numbers of patients that could benefit from transplantation by currently accepted criteria far exceed the numbers of donors. This is particularly true for renal transplantation which is held by many as the gold standard of organ replacement therapy and is now widely performed. With smaller programs (e.g. heart–lung) it is sometimes the logistics of organ retrieval which limits its applicability. In addition, despite early identification schemes, the mortality of heart and lung organ failure is such that up to 50% of those considered suitable to enter transplantation schemes die before an organ becomes available.

Improved planning and implementation, combined with increased public awareness of the issues involved will improve the number of donors available. Approaches to this include:

- consent for donation
    - ◊ opt in: (voluntary donation) with public education / awareness schemes (and possibly central registers of names)
    - ◊ opt out: (e.g. Belgium) consent is assumed by the state unless the family decide to deny permission
    - ◊ required request: (e.g. USA) here it is a legal duty of the attending physician to request retrieval
    - ◊ required discussion: where the physician must discuss the case with a transplant coordinator who will send a representative to the family if the patient is suitable.
- coordination of transplantation teams
    - ◊ national and regional coordinating bodies to identify and rank need in the recipient population
    - ◊ local (and immediate) expertise for retrieval of all organs
    - ◊ improved communications and transport (utilising national patient databases and the fastest transfers possible).

Criteria for organ donation

It is the responsibility of the retrieving surgeons to confirm donor suitability.

Absolute contraindications

- HIV, bacterial sepsis, CMV positive
- intravenous drug abuse – latent HIV infection (pre seroconversion) should be considered in high risk populations
- malignancy but not CNS primary

Relative contraindications

- serious intercurrent disease such as diabetes mellitus
- a history of cardiac arrest is NOT a contraindication

Specific criteria for individual organ donors

Kidneys

< 70 yrs old
no H_X renal disease
adequate renal perfusion
adequate urine output

Liver

< 55 yrs old
appropriate physical size
normal liver function tests
no alcohol abuse

Heart

< 50 yrs old
appropriate physical size
normal CXR and ECG
no prolonged cardiac arrest
not on high dose inotropes

Single patient heart / lung

as for heart alone plus
no lung trauma / infection
IPPV < 24 hours
$F_IO_2 < 0.4$
appropriate physical size
non smoker

Pancreas

< 50 yrs old
normal plasma amylase
no family history of diabetes

Organ maintenance

Having accepted a donor, there are a number of associated responses to brain-stem death which must be appropriately managed to ensure a viable organ at the time of donation.

The incidence of these responses is:

- diabetes insipidus 65%
- coagulopathies 40%
- hypotension 33%
- hypothermia 23%
- cardiac arrest 10%

The following management strategies are recommended:

Cardiovascular system

- raised intracranial pressure results in a Cushing response (hypertension + bradycardia)
  - ◊ β blockers such as esmolol are an effective treatment
- hypotension, in response to vasomotor centre destruction and abolition of sympathetic tone
  - ◊ maintenance of an adequate renal perfusion pressure is vital to satisfactory function of the donated kidney
  - ◊ intravenous volume loading (haematocrit 0.3 + CVP monitoring)
  - ◊ inotropic support if volume loading fails
- PCWP monitoring permits rationalisation of therapy

Respiratory system

- ventilate to maintain normocapnia
  - ◊ decreased CO_2 production may require methods to limit CO_2 removal (use of dead space)
- continue bronchial toilet
- try to avoid excessive PEEP because it activates vasopressin release
- use the lowest FiO_2 possible to maintain SaO_2 >95% and avoid pulmonary oedema

Renal function

- reduced donated organ survival if systolic BP <90 mm Hg
  - ◊ volume load and CVP
- maintain urine output >0.5 ml/kg/hr
- diabetes insipidus
  - ◊ urine output >4 ml/kg/min, osmolality <300mOsm in face of rising serum osmolality and [Na]
  - ◊ replace losses with 5% dextrose and treat with dDAVP

Metabolic and endocrine control

- abnormalities of anterior pituitary function
- cardiac function may improve with regimes that include:
  - ◊ T_3 infusions
  - ◊ cortisol replacement
  - ◊ insulin infusions to treat hyperglycaemia

Transplant recipients

As the success and incidence of transplantation has increased so it has become common to meet recipients presenting with other 'routine' medical problems. For geographical reasons they are not always able to return to the unit where their 'organ' is looked after. Usually these patients are well, many are also very knowledgeable about their condition.

The following should be considered in their management:

- what was the cause of their organ dysfunction, is it still a factor for consideration in relation to the planned surgery (e.g. lupus erythematosus) and are there associated conditions?
- what transplant follow-up programme is in place?
- current organ function and rejection status
- immunosuppressant medication and any drug or pathophysiological interactions (e.g. cyclosporin and renal failure)
- donor recipients are more prone to blood transfusion immune sensitisation (antigen exposure) and graft versus host disease
- infection – immunosuppression not only increases the risk of but also causes an abnormal response to infection

Renal allograft recipients

- potentially abnormal drug elimination by the allograft
- patients often diabetic, undergoing frequent peripheral vascular and ophthalmological procedures
- renal osteodystrophy associated with chronic renal failure and steroid administration
- paediatric recipients may have associated genetic anomalies

Cardiac allograft recipients

- disordered physiology and pharmacology of transplanted, denervated cardiac allografts
  - ◊ unusual drug responses
  - ◊ delayed heart rate response to hypoxia
- dependent on adequate preload for cardiac output

Liver allograft recipients

- altered pharmacokinetics
  - ◊ metabolism, distribution volume, protein binding
- recovery of hepatic biosynthesis
  - ◊ clotting factors, plasma proteins, glucose, urea

Chapter 18

Quality improvement

Definitions of terms

- **Quality Assurance (QA)** – monitoring the quality of service with a view to improvement. The focus is mainly on outcome and tends to be punitive
- **Quality Control (QC)** – the application of statistical techniques in an effort to identify and minimise random and non-random sources of variation
- **Quality Improvement (QI)** – the effort to improve performance. This implies measuring the level of performance and designing and implementing methods to improve it. QI looks mainly for problems within the system, not with individuals and seeks to provide individuals with ways to improve performance
- **Risk Management** – identification and minimisation of the risk to patients, staff and facilities
- **Utilisation Management** – information gathering, strategic planning and resource allocation to ensure the most cost-effective utilisation
- **Bench Marking** – the evaluating of performance against specific criteria, including competitors.

The concept of QA focuses on the outcome, or effects, of that care on consumers (both patients and surgeons). QI, on the other hand, mandates not only the measurement of levels of performance, but also the designing and implementation of methods to improve that performance. Therefore the focus is more on the system and facilities provided and not punitive to the individual. Standards, Protocols, Policies and Guidelines do not of themselves ensure quality of care, but are an integral part of the process of health care delivery. They serve to introduce a measure of control, concentrating attention on particular aspects of the system, resulting in beneficial behavioural effects. What constitutes 'quality' differs according to the observer (anaesthetists, surgeons, patients, or administrators) and the programme should accommodate their expectations.

Standards, protocols and guidelines

The Australian and New Zealand College of Anaesthetists (ANZCA) has published a range of statements and guidelines on matters varying from 'Guidelines for hospitals seeking College approval of posts for the first four years of vocational training in anaesthesia' to a 'Statement on Smoking'. Minimum facilities for safe anaesthetic practice in operating theatres, organ imaging units and the delivery suite, the anaesthesia record, monitoring facilities, use of autologous blood, specific guidelines on QA, clinical indicators in anaesthesia and a maintenance of standards programme, form the basis for departmental assessment.

Continuous QI programme

This is designed to assess both an individual's and the group's performance and working conditions, facilitating improvement, decreasing inefficiency (utilisation management) and minimising risk to both patients and staff (risk management).
A departmental QA programme may be divided into structure, process and outcome.

- the **structure** of the department takes into account both the facilities available in the way of operating and induction rooms, recovery rooms, office space, anaesthesia machines and monitoring equipment.

Organisational matters relate to leadership, numbers and training of all levels of staff; medical, nursing, technical and ancillary. Efficient deployment of available staff and appropriate supervision and training should be monitored. Recently the College has proposed a 'Maintenance of Standards Programme Guidelines' which will require provision of proof that specialists are continuing their self-education after obtaining specialist qualifications.

- the clinical **process** of delivery of anaesthesia services comprises not only the numbers of patients and proceduralists in the system, but also the nature of the services provided to them, and how those services are delivered. Utilisation management is the name given to the process of data acquisition, strategic planning and resource allocation to ensure the most cost-effective use. Attempts to identify and minimise risk to patients, staff and facilities are risk management strategies.
- **'Outcome** and satisfaction' has long been done on an informal basis through the utilisation of clinicopathological conferences, case presentations and morbidity and mortality meetings. However, hard or retrievable data were often missing and as a consequence medical audit was born.
  - ◊ **medical audit cycle:** first decide on the activity to be assessed, define what is an acceptable standard for that activity, observe the performance with reference to the standard, implement change if needed to improve performance and reassess the activity to ascertain effects.
  - ◊ **incident reporting** with a view to analysing the factors in the system which predispose to critical incident occurrences is 'case presentation' with a slightly different perspective. An incident is usually defined as any occurrence which affects or could affect the safety of the patient. Incidents may be preventable or unpreventable. The 'Australasian Incident Monitoring Study' (AIMS) is conducted on a national basis with the periodic publication of its findings.
  - ◊ anaesthesia is not therapeutic in itself. Outcomes are consequently difficult to assess, and differ depending on the observer. While the patient may be concerned most with morbidity and mortality, these are generally only crude indicators of performance. Because of this, the concept of 'clinical indicators', or 'process events', has been developed. Clinical indicators are those events requiring some corrective action on the part of the anaesthetist.

Clinical indicators

- the percentage of patients having a documented pre-anaesthesia assessment
- the percentage whose anaesthesia records comply with the minimum requirements
- the percentage of patients having a defined 'clinical event' in the recovery period. These events include but are not limited to:
  - ◊ intervention by the anaesthetist to relieve respiratory distress
  - ◊ any respiratory or cardiac arrest
  - ◊ core temperature recorded in recovery less than 35 °C
  - ◊ review by the anaesthetist in recovery to manage severe pain
  - ◊ a recovery room stay of longer than 2 hours
  - ◊ unplanned admission to an ICU facility within 24 hours
  - ◊ percentage of patients with a documented post-anaesthesia visit.

Clinical indicators may also be taken to encompass disability, discomfort or disease caused by the clinical intervention.

For any improvement programme to be effective it must have the support of all members of the department who should be made to feel that their input is important. Scheduled meetings should be held in comfort with adequate time allocated for discussion. Ideally minutes and a record of attendance should be kept. Changes proposed should be recorded, publicised and evaluated to ensure a desired effect.

MacIntosh and McCutcheon have defined seven attributes of quality which they consider require assessment:

Attributes	Questions	Activity
Safety	Is risk minimal for patient	Risk management Incident review Morbidity and mortality
Competence	Are staff appropriately trained for the service they provide	Training and supervision Certification Recertification Manpower planning
Acceptability	Are the expectations of patients, surgeons and hospital accreditors met	Evaluation by both patients and surgeons
Accessibility	Is the department able to fulfil its commitments	Anaesthesia related delays, cancellations, availability for consultation and other services
Efficiency	Are anaesthetists provided in a timely and cost effective manner	Budget information Operating room utilisation data
Appropriateness	Are services provided that should be: acute and chronic pain obstetric	Case review Bench marking against other institutions
Effectiveness	Are services delivered in the proper fashion	Patient outcomes

Further reading

ANZCA Policy Documents

MacIntosh AM, McCutcheon DJ. 'Stretching' to continuous quality improvement from quality assurance: a framework for quality management. *Canadian Journal of Quality in Health Care*, 1992; 30: 400-11.

Eagle CJ, Davies JM. Current models of 'quality' – an introduction for anaesthetists. *Canadian Journal of Anaesthesia*, 1993; 40: 851-62.

Desmonts JM (ed). Outcome after anaesthesia and surgery. *International Anesthesiology Clinics*, 1992; 6: 463-690.

Baldock GJ. Quality assurance, standards and accreditation [Editorial]. *Anaesthesia*, 1990; 45: 617-18.

Chapter 19

Safety in the operating suite

The operating room is a hazardous area for the deliverers as well the receivers of care. Surgery and Anaesthesia may be regarded as a form of 'controlled harm' where damage to the patient is part of the therapeutic process, e.g. use of diathermy to stop bleeding.

Safety is a team effort which depends on:

- the integrity of many individuals discharging their respective responsibilities
- provision of a safe therapeutic and work environment
- provision of safe, appropriately maintained equipment.

Patient safety

On the ward

Patient safety commences in the ward before departure for the OR. When admitting the patient, the resident must:

- check details of the proposed operation with the patient, the case notes and any type written correspondence
- when completing the CONSENT form check the following is present:
  - ◊ patient's name, address, date of birth and hospital ID number
  - ◊ an accurate description of the operation in language the patient understands
    - do not use abbreviations
    - use 'right' or 'left' not (R) and (L)
    - identify digits by NAME not number, e.g. right index finger not (R)1
  - ◊ Patient's signature
    - this may be used whilst the patient is unconscious as a form of identification, e.g. during administration of autologous blood
  - ◊ check the details on the operating list match those on the consent form
  - ◊ be aware of medical conditions which either predispose the patient to injury whilst in the operating theatre, e.g. rheumatoid arthritis or increase the risk to the health of theatre staff, e.g. HIV, HEP-B
  - ◊ all risks should be discussed jointly by the consultant **surgeon** and **anaesthetist** in charge of the case together with **senior theatre staff**
  - ◊ adequate time must be allowed between this discussion and the proposed start time for suitable preparations in theatre to be made.
- If there are any doubts or problems at this stage they must be clarified **before** the patient leaves the ward and **before** premedicant drugs are given.

In the operating suite

The patient in an operating theatre is entirely at the mercy of the surroundings, which are mostly not understood and can't be modified by the patient. Furthermore the patient is surrounded by potential hazards such as:

- being moved whilst unconscious
- administration of dangerous drugs which further obtund protective reflexes, e.g. gag reflex
- surgical trauma
- electrical hazards especially diathermy

Principles of patient handling

- always have regard for the maintenance of vital functions especially **airway**, **breathing** and **circulation**
- prevent pressure damage to skin and nerves where they may be trapped over bony prominences
- preserve natural joint positions whenever possible
- avoid sudden changes in posture which may lead to circulatory instability, e.g. sudden head down or head up
- reduce the risk of deep venous thrombosis by relieving pressure on the calves – support the leg with a small pillow under *tendo Achilles*
- avoiding physical injury requires sufficient, adequately trained, personnel to move the patient without risk of dropping them
- protect from extreme temperature changes – keep the patient warm.

Risk reduction during anaesthesia and surgery

Whilst many aspects of this fall within areas of specialist professional training there are some important general points which are relevant to ALL personnel who either care for, or perform procedures on semi conscious patients both within the operating theatre environment and elsewhere in the hospital.

Identification

- do not start administration of drugs which alter conscious level or perform any procedure until you have checked:
- the identity of the patient both by asking directly and confirming with reference to the identity band, chart and x-rays
- which operation is to be performed on which side to which body part and again check with the patient, the consent form and the case notes
- all necessary equipment, drugs and personnel are available

Fires and explosions

Both patients and staff are at risk of serious injury. One survey revealed 165 patients in Australia injured during a 10 year period from electrical mishaps, fires and explosions. Of these diathermy was implicated in **61%**. Almost all cases involved a fault in a piece of electrical apparatus. Detailed coverage of electrical safety in the operating theatre is outside the scope of this text but important practical points will be covered.

Diathermy

Water containing tissue can be coagulated or cut by a radio frequency current.
The magnitude of the heating effect depends on:

- power delivered (Watts)
- surface area into which this power is delivered (square metres)
- duration of application (seconds)
- Resistance of the tissues (Ohms)

The electrical energy is passed from active to passive electrodes (sometimes incorrectly referred to as earth). In bipolar diathermy, current passes from one limb of a pair of insulated forceps to the other. In monopolar diathermy current passes from the hand held active electrode, **through the patient's body**, to the passive plate. Heating occurs at **both** electrodes.

In bipolar diathermy this is desirable but with monopolar diathermy the heating effect at the passive electrode is dissipated by:

- the large surface area of the electrode plate in contact with the skin which is well vascularised and able to remove heat from under the plate.

Should the plate become partially detached from the patient, reducing the surface area in contact, current density and **heating** effect will increase proportionately. Should the plate be placed over a bony prominence or poorly perfused skin, then skin burns will result.

These mechanisms account for the vast majority of injuries caused by surgical diathermy.

Prevention of accidental diathermy burns is thus simple:

- use bipolar diathermy wherever possible
- use the minimum diathermy power for the minimum duration to accomplish the job in hand
- apply the passive electrode (earth plate) with great care to ensure maximum skin contact over a well vascularised area. Check the plate periodically during use and carefully examine the skin at the end of the case for evidence of a burn
- if the diathermy appears faulty, assume the passive electrode is partially detached and your patient is being burnt – until you can prove otherwise **do not** turn up the power level.

Electrical supply

Whilst many incidents in theatre involve electrical equipment, conventional electrocution is fortunately rare. Electrical equipment used in this environment must operate to a very high standard. Human skin is a good electrical insulator.

The risk of electrocution depends upon whether the skin is intact or breached. The latter risk will be higher if a catheter is placed directly into the heart itself.

Each scenario requires equipment designed and maintained to differing standards which can be divided into three broad categories:

- Domestic (class Z)
  - ◊ no special precautions necessary other than those which would apply to any building open to the general public. Conventional fuses, sockets and switches may be used
- Body protected (class B)
  - ◊ either the patient is unable to move away from any potential hazards (e.g. unconsciousness, electrodes attached) or there has been some breach of the skin resistance e.g. by a peripheral IV. Equipment must be designed to well defined standards and undergo periodic inspection and testing e.g. insulation testing.
- Cardiac protected (class A)
  - ◊ there is a direct electrical connection to the heart. Cardiac pacing electrodes are obvious examples but a central venous line filled with saline (an excellent conductor of electricity) amounts to the same.

Almost all electrical equipment allows a minute current to leak away to earth. If this current is greater than 10 milliamps, ventricular fibrillation can be induced. In a cardiac protected area the **sum** of **all** earth leakage currents from **all** equipment attached to the patient must be less than 10 mA.

All power for a single patient area must therefore be supplied from a common point with electrical safety devices fitted e.g. earth leakage contact breaker to monitor the leakage current.

Only perform procedures on patients using electrical apparatus in an area designated as safe for the task you are about to undertake.

Staff safety

Safety of staff in the operating theatre complex can be divided into four broad categories:

Mechanical hazards

- hoses and electrical cables positioned so that staff may trip and fall
  - ◊ keep all hoses and cables neat and tidy. Avoid long cable runs from one side of the room to the other.
  - ◊ never place a cable or hose across a walkway
- doors
  - ◊ all doors should have a window allowing one to see what is on the other side BEFORE opening
- slippery floors
  - ◊ operating theatre floors become very slippery when wet. Take care handling fluids and wipe up all spillage immediately. Many broken limbs have been caused by wet floors
- furniture
  - ◊ do not allow work areas and corridors to become cluttered with unused furniture and equipment. Return equipment to its storage position immediately after use

Pollution of the environment

Anaesthetic gases

- whilst direct physical harm from traces of anaesthetic gases has not been conclusively shown, prolonged exposure can result in headaches, fatigue and a general reduction in performance. It is prudent to avoid environmental contamination. If using anaesthetic gases, always ensure an adequate scavenging system is in use.

Organisms

- the primary organisms which may have a deleterious effect on staff are HIV, hepatitis B and C, CMV. However staff may become colonised by ANY pathogen during patient contact.
- some exposure during surgery may be unavoidable but this is greatly reduced by the use of **universal precautions** including:
  - ◊ frequent hand washing, especially before and at the end of each patient contact.
  - ◊ use of protective gloves and facial apparel (facemasks, visor, glasses)
  - ◊ safe disposal of 'sharps'
- universal precautions not only protect staff but also greatly reduce the chances of cross infection between patients.
- ensure you have been immunised against tetanus and hepatitis B.

Radiation

- stand **behind** the X-ray machine where possible
- wear a lead apron
- if frequently exposed to radiation wear a radiation monitoring badge.

Lifting and patient movement

- may easily lead to injuries to patients and back injuries to staff.
  - ◊ have enough personnel to perform the task in hand
  - ◊ use lifting and movement aids at all times e.g. patslide®
  - ◊ learn from the physiotherapist how to lift properly whilst protecting your own back.

Domestic safety

- operating theatre staff, including anaesthetists, work full time in this environment. Have a consideration for their needs:
  - ◊ respect staff locker and changing room space
  - ◊ keep noise to a minimum, especially in rest rooms
  - ◊ if you make a mess then tidy it up.

There is no 'magic' answer to safety in the operating theatre environment. Risk reduction requires **all** personnel to be aware of the risks and to make a **continuous conscientious effort** to identify and reduce risks before harm is done.

Part II

Topics Related to Resuscitation

Chapter 20

Crisis management algorithms

For use on patients breathing gas from an anaesthetic machine

- 'COVER ABCD' with tracheal tube
- 'AB COVER ABCD' with mask

Memorise and practise:

COVER

C	Circulation	* 3	establish adequacy of peripheral circulation (rate, rhythm and character of pulse). If pulseless (3%), start CPR, get help, and complete COVER as soon as possible
	Colour		note saturation; look for central cyanosis. Use pulse oximetry if possible. Test probe on own finger, if necessary, whilst proceeding with O1 and O2
O	Oxygen	2	check rotameter settings, ensure inspired mixture is not hypoxic. Adjust inspired oxygen concentration to 100% and note that only the oxygen flowmeter is operating (2%)
	Oxygen analyser	0.2	check that the oxygen analyser shows a rising oxygen concentration distal to the common gas outlet (0.2%)
V	Ventilate	20	ventilate the lungs by hand to assess circuit integrity, airway patency, compliance and air entry by 'feel', observation and auscultation; inspect capnograph trace (20%)
	Vaporiser	4	note settings and level of agents. Check all vaporiser filler and drainage ports, seatings and connections for liquid or gas leaks during pressurisation of the system. Consider the possibility of the wrong agent being in the vaporiser (4%)
E	Endo tracheal tube	14	check the tracheal tube; ensure it is patent with no leaks, kinks or obstructions. Check capnograph and oximeter for possible endobronchial placement. If necessary adjust, deflate cuff, pass a catheter, or remove and replace (14%)
	Elimination	15	eliminate the anaesthetic machine and ventilate with a self-inflating bag with 100% oxygen (from an alternative source if necessary). Retain gas monitor sampling port, but be aware of possible gas sampling or gas monitor problems (15%)
R	Review monitors	4	review all monitors in use. All monitors should have been correctly sited, checked and calibrated (e.g. oximeter, capnograph, ECG, BP, circuit pressure, NMJ)(4%)
	Review equipment	2	review all other equipment in contact with or relevant to the patient (e.g. diathermy, humidifiers, heating blankets, endoscopes, probes, prostheses, retractors etc) (2%)

* = % corrected by action.

ABCD

A	Airway	12	check patency of the unintubated airway. Consider laryngospasm (6%) or presence of foreign body (1%), or aspiration/regurgitation (5%) (total 12%)
B	Breathing	5	assess pattern, adequacy and distribution of ventilation. Consider, examine and auscultate for hypoventilation (2%), bronchospasm (2%), pulmonary oedema, lobar collapse and pneumo- or haemothorax (1%) (total 5%)
C	Circulation	14	evaluate peripheral perfusion, pulse, blood pressure, ECG and filling pressures (where possible) and any possible obstruction to venous return, raised intrathoracic pressure (e.g. inadvertent PEEP) or direct interference to (e.g. stimulation by central line) or tamponade of the heart. Note any trends on records. Bradycardia/arrythmia (5%); tachycardia / arrhythmia (2%); hypotension (5%), hypertension (1%); ischaemia (1%) (total 14%)
D	Drugs	3	review intended and consider possible unintended, drug or substance administration. Consider whether the problem may be due to an unexpected drug effect, a failure of administration (kinked cannula, extravasation) or wrong dose, route or manner of administration of an intended or 'wrong drug'. Review all possible routes of drug administration (total 3%)

Source: *Anaesthesia and Intensive Care*, 21: 579-592 (October, 1993)

COVER ABCD accounts for 95% of incidents, 3% of which are cardiac arrests. A SWIFT CHECK handles the remaining 5%. These need not be memorised but a list should be readily available in the operating room. Conditions listed under 'A' make up 4% of problems (about 1% each). The remainder (SWIFT CHECK) either contribute to cardiac arrests (e.g. vagal stimulation, bleeding, infarct) and circulatory problems or make up the residuum of 1% of incidents.

A SWIFT CHECK

A	Air embolus	hypotension, hypocarbia
	Anaphylaxis	hypotension, bronchospasm, urticaria
	Air in pleura	pneumothorax, any unexpected circulatory or respiratory deterioration
	Awareness	consider dilution of anaesthetic gases, 'resistant' patient, 'failure to deliver'
S	Surgeon/ situation	vagal stimulation, caval compression, bleeding, direct myocardial stimulation
	Sepsis	hypotension, desaturation, acidosis, hyperdynamic circulation, ARDS, rigors
W	Wound	trauma, bleeding, tamponade, pneumothorax, problems due to retractors
	Water intoxication	electrolyte disturbance, fluid overload
I	Infarct	myocardial conduction, 'ST' or rhythm problem, hypotension, poor cardiac output
	Insufflation	vagal tone, reduced venous return, pulmonary or paradoxical arterial gas embolism
F	'Fat' syndrome	desaturation and/or hypotension especially after induction and in the lithotomy position (with obese or distended abdomen), profuse bronchial secretions
	Full bladder	may cause marked haemodynamic changes and/or sympathetic stimulation
T	Trauma	consider spinal injury, undiagnosed sub- or extra-dural haematoma, bronchial or diaphragmatic injury, ruptured viscus, concealed haemorrhage, myocardial contusion
	Tourniquet down	local anaesthetic toxicity, unseen bleeding, failed block
C	Catheter/iv cannula	leaks, blocks, failure to deliver, wrong drug or label, wrong connection/ site, trauma
	Chest drain problem	tube not in or out, clamped, kinked, blocked, wrongly connected
	Cement	haemodynamic change with methylmethacrylate
H	Hyper-/ hypothermia	tachycardia and hypercarbia, poor perfusion, ECG changes
	Hypocalcaemia	consider inappropriate or inadvertent insulin administration preoperatively, fasting and β blockers, hepatic compromise and b blockers
E	Embolus	fat, thrombus, amniotic fluid; hypotension, hypocarbia, hypoxia, ECG changes
	Endocrine	hyper-/hypothyroid / adrenal medulla or cortex / pituitary / diabetes / 5-HT
C	Check	check right patient, right operation, right surgeon, correct side, correct body part
	Check	check casenotes and old notes for preoperative status, diseases, drugs and conditions
K	K^+	any electrolyte abnormality, ECG changes
	Keep	keep the patient 'asleep' until a new anaesthetic machine can be obtained (e.g. with diazepam, ketamine)

99.9% of incidents should have been identified. If the problem has not been solved, direct the available resources to its solution. Get skilled and experienced help. Work from first principles. Think 'laterally'.

Chapter 21

The medical emergency team

Mortality studies of patients suffering cardiac arrest show that although some individuals do well, the majority of patients fare very badly. Despite restoration of cardiac rhythm the prognosis for leaving hospital alive is poor. In many cases this outcome reflects the combination of serious pathology and a lack of physiological reserve and may be regarded as inevitable. However, there remain a large number of patients who suffer cardiac arrest with potentially reversible medical conditions.

Experience with victims of multiple trauma has shown that early intervention in potentially life threatening conditions improves prognosis. A Medical Emergency Team (MET) applies this approach to treat general hospital patients with life threatening conditions.

Whilst this aim of *preventing* cardiac arrest by identifying the critically ill early and targeting medical resources appropriate to their urgent needs remains yet unproven: it is appealing on logical, administrative, medical and humanitarian grounds.

The logistic requirements

- Clearly defined criteria for identification of appropriate patients
- Easy and immediate availability of the team (clear communication channels)
- Appropriate training and resources available within the team
- Period of emergency treatment/stabilisation on the ward
- Availability of senior help and resources for continued care and management decisions

Criteria for calling the MET

Certain conditions have been identified as preceding cardiac arrest:
- deterioration in respiratory function
- deterioration in mental function
- hypotension (<90 mmHg)
- uraemia.

Identification of these patterns formed the tenets for the first medical emergency team. The following list is not exhaustive but will help you to recognise patients who require urgent medical intervention, whether or not an MET exists in your hospital.

CALL FOR SENIOR ADVICE EARLY.

Specific conditions

Cardiovascular
cardiac arrest, pulmonary oedema, new arrhythmia

Shock
hypovolaemic, cardiogenic, anaphylactic & septic shock

Poisoning / trauma
drowning, carbon monoxide poisoning, severe drug overdose

Neurological
status epilepticus, uncontrollable acute psychiatric disturbance

Respiratory
severe asthmatic deterioration, respiratory failure, upper airways obstruction

Metabolic
acute diabetic emergencies

Obstetrics
amniotic fluid embolism, pre-eclampsia

Surgical
excessive bleeding or drainage

Abnormal physiology

- temperature < 35.5 or > 39.5 °C
- systolic blood pressure < 100 or > 200 mmHg
- respiration < 10 or > 30 min^{-1}
- pulse rate < 40 or > 120 min^{-1}
- urine output < 500 ml per 24 hours
- decreased or altered levels of consciousness

Abnormal pathology

- Serum K^+ < 3 or > 6 mM
- Serum Na^+ < 125 or > 155 mM
- blood sugar < 2 or > 20 mM
- arterial pH < 7.2 or > 7.55

Adapted from the pre-emergency care protocol devised by Lee A, Bishop G, Hillman KM, Daffurn K., Department of Anaesthetics & Intensive Care, Liverpool Hospital, Liverpool, NSW, Australia.

Chapter 22

Cardiopulmonary resuscitation

Ventricular fibrillation is the cause of cardiac arrest in the majority of victims and carries the better prognosis. The most important factor in producing a favourable outcome is EARLY institution of Basic Life Support (BLS) and EARLY defibrillation. Irreversible hypoxic brain damage will occur within two to four minutes if SATISFACTORY BLS is not administered.
A 'chain of survival' describes the sequence of events from patient collapse to definitive care. Each link represents a vital principle of the patient's management and if any one link is inadequate, survival rates will be poor:

- early diagnosis of cardiac arrest
- early basic CPR – buys time
- early defibrillation
- early advanced life support – on-scene paramedics

Basic life support (BLS)

Confirm loss of consciousness by shaking and shouting.
Call for help.
Place the patient on their back

- **A**irway: open the airway by tilting the head backwards and lifting the chin. Remove any debris from the mouth.
- **B**reathing: look, listen and feel for respirations. If apnoeic give two Expired Air Respirations (EAR) SLOWLY, using mouth to mouth or a pocket mask (Laerdal).
- **C**irculation: check for a major pulse (carotid, femoral). Commence External Cardiac Compression (ECC) if no pulse is palpable.

Expired air respiration

Methods

- mouth to nose –
  - ◊ resuscitation babies where the rescuer's mouth covers the victim's mouth and nose
- mouth to mouth –
  - ◊ tilt – place the palm of one hand on the top of the head, support the chin with the other hand and firmly but gently tilt the head backwards
  - ◊ blow – take a deep breath, open your mouth as widely as possible and place it over the victim's slightly open mouth, sealing the nose by pinching. Blow to inflate the victim's lungs for 2 seconds per breath, limiting the likelihood of gastric insufflation.
  - ◊ pocket mask
  - ◊ observe the victim's chest – if it does not rise, there is
    - airway obstruction
    - an inadequate seal
    - inadequate air being blown into the lungs

◊ listen and feel for exhalation – following inflation, lift your mouth from the victim's, turn your head towards the chest and with your ear about 2 cm from the victim's mouth, listen and feel the air being exhaled.

External cardiac compression

Rate

- **80-100** chest compressions should be performed every minute in an ADULT and **100-120** per minute in a CHILD
- the ratio of chest compressions to ventilations should be **15:2** for ONE rescuer, and **5:1** if TWO rescuers are present
- check the pulse every 2 cycles of Basic Life Support for at least 3 seconds
- place the patient in the recovery position if BOTH breathing and circulation return

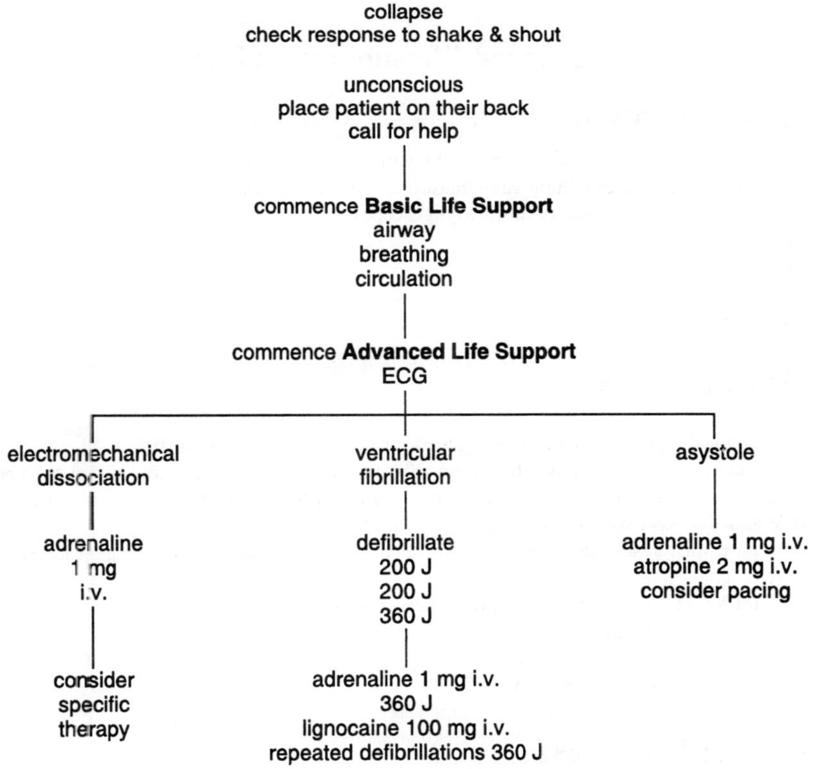

- continue Basic Life Support throughout
- give ADRENALINE every 5 minutes
- give all intravenous drugs centrally and flush in
- give double the dose via the tracheal tube if NO intravenous access

Compression site – hand position

- the lower half of the sternum for ADULTS
- the mid point of the sternum for CHILDREN

Method of compression

- place the heel of one hand on the compression point with the fingers relaxed, parallel to the ribs and slightly raised so that pressure is not exerted directly on the ribs
- the other hand is placed securely on top of the first
- all pressure is exerted through the heel of the under hand, and the body weight should act as the compressing force, such that the shoulders should be vertically over the sternum and the compressing arm kept straight

Technical factors which are important in successful compression are

- complete release of compression to allow adequate diastolic coronary perfusion
- compression must be applied over the lower HALF (**not** third) of the sternum
- the patient must be on a firm, horizontal surface
- BLS must not be interrupted for more than 10 seconds

Advanced life support (ALS)

Essential equipment

- oxygen source and method of delivery to the patient
- self inflating bag/non-rebreathing valve/mask/universal connector (15:22 mm)
- oropharyngeal airways, tracheal tube, laryngoscopes
- suction apparatus
- ECG monitor
- defibrillator
- i.v. apparatus and drugs

Defibrillation

- always familiarise yourself with the equipment prior to emergency utilisation
- use electrically conductive pads rather than jelly, to reduce the risk of arcing across the chest
- defibrillator paddles should be positioned on the victim with one electrode position beneath the right clavicle and the other over the ECG points V4 and V5
- the operator must ensure that neither he nor anyone else is touching the patient when the shock is delivered
- in resistant VF requiring repeated defibrillations consider
  - ◊ changing the paddle positions
  - ◊ changing the defibrillator
  - ◊ bretylium tosylate (see below)

Drugs in cardiac arrest

Adrenaline 1 mg i.v. or 2 mg via tracheal tube

- the most important drug because of its peripheral vasoconstrictor action (α effect) and cardiac stimulatory action (β effect)
- increases cerebral perfusion pressure by increasing mean aortic pressure thereby improving cerebral survival
- adrenaline should be repeated every 5 minutes because of its short half life

Lignocaine 100 mg i.v. or 200 mg via tracheal tube

- should be given after the 4th shock in the treatment of VF
- lignocaine is the antiarrhythmic drug of first choice to prevent recurrence of VF after successful defibrillation
  In adults the infusion regimen is
  - ◊ 4 mg/min for the first hour
  - ◊ 3 mg/min for the second hour
  - ◊ 2 mg/kg for the third hour

Sodium bicarbonate

- the metabolic acidosis which follows inadequate tissue oxygen delivery and consequent anaerobic metabolism should be treated by establishing a spontaneous circulation
- sodium bicarbonate is recommended in hyperkalaemia. If administered to correct metabolic acidosis, it should be guided by blood gas analysis. The 'base excess' (a derived figure reflecting the metabolic component of acidosis) should be used to calculate the amount of bicarbonate in mmoles required to correct the acidosis in adults, using the formula:
  - ◊ negative base excess × body weight (kg) × 0.3
- total correction is not advised and only **half** the calculated amount should be administered
- 8.4% sodium bicarbonate contains 1 mmol/ml
- the hazards of bicarbonate therapy are:
  - ◊ hyperosmolality
  - ◊ paradoxical increase of intracellular acidosis
  - ◊ shift Hb/SaO_2 dissociation curve to the left
  - ◊ alkalosis due to overcorrection
  - ◊ congestive cardiac failure

Calcium 1 g i.v. (10 ml of 10% calcium gluconate/chloride)

- calcium is only recommended in the management of electromechanical dissociation associated with:
  - ◊ hyperkalaemia
  - ◊ hypocalcaemia
  - ◊ overdose of calcium antagonists
- calcium must be used rationally because Ca^{++} ions are known to be mediators of cell death after hypoxic brain injury

Bretylium tosylate

- is the drug of choice for resistant VF
- give 10 mg/kg over 15 **minutes**
- bretylium takes 30 minutes to have effect

Post resuscitation care

- transfer to a critical care unit for monitoring
- immediate blood gas and electrolyte estimations
- continued antiarrhythmic therapy
- circumstances leading to the collapse should be clearly defined and, if possible, prevented from recurring

American Heart Association changes to guidelines

- priority to early access when initiating CPR
- increased insufflation time during mouth-to-mouth resuscitation
- placement in the recovery position
- use of barrier shields and devices for ventilation
- oesophageal obturator is not recommended
- limited use of sodium bicarbonate
- increased drug dosage for tracheal administration
- calcium infusion is not recommended

Chapter 23

Resuscitation equipment

Airway management equipment is found on the specially designated 'resuscitation carts' located in your hospital. The trolley is checked daily for correct function and completeness so that everything is ready in the event of an emergency. Be familiar with the emergency carts in your hospital and know how to check the function of the resuscitation equipment.

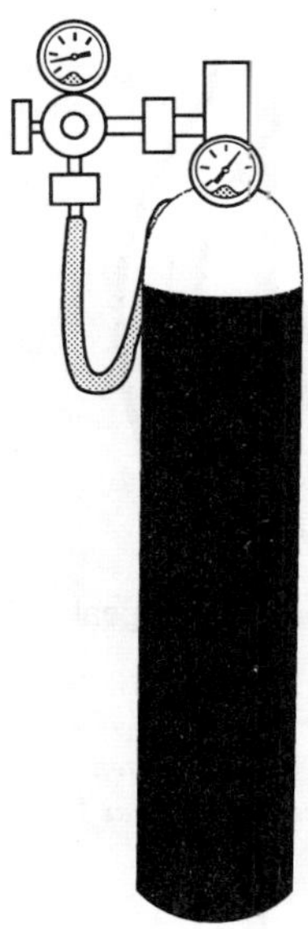

Oxygen supply

In the emergency situation, give 100% oxygen to the patient.
The gas will either be supplied from a marked wall oxygen outlet or an oxygen cylinder which is black in colour with a white shoulder (in Australia). In either case there has to be a flow meter to adjust the flowrate. The flow meter may be of a gauge or ball type. Both types are subject to inaccuracies – the gauge type will over-read the flow if there is any kink or obstruction in the delivery hose. If the ball type is 25° off the vertical, it will over read by 10%. The ball flow meters deliver flows in the range 0–15 litres/min and the flow is read against the centre of the ball.

Oxygen delivery system

It is useless having a source of oxygen but no method of giving it to the patient. The equipment used is called the patient breathing system. It may be a self-inflating bag (e.g. Laerdal, Ambu or Air-viva) or an anaesthetic type circuit.

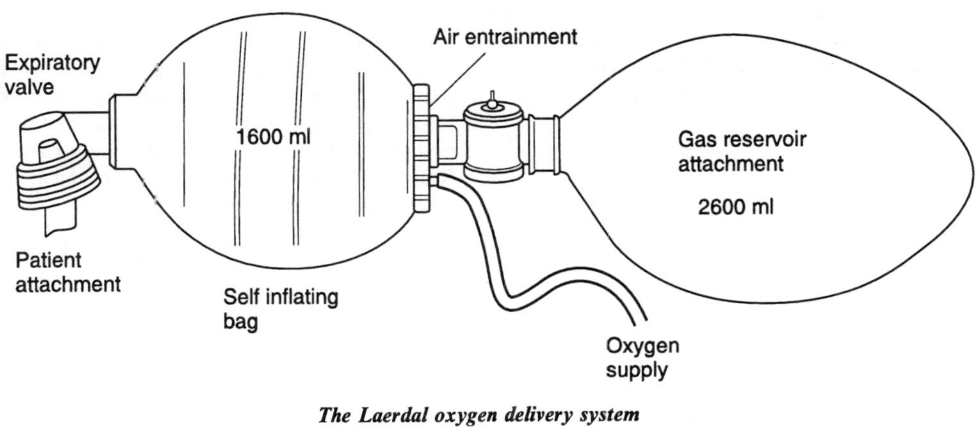

The Laerdal oxygen delivery system

rate: 12 breaths/min

tidal volume: 750 ml

oxygen flow rate: 12 litres/min

reservoir bag attached: $F_{I}O_2$ = 1.0

It is possible to deliver 100% oxygen with the reservoir bag attached, an oxygen flow rate of 10 litres/min, tidal volume of 500 ml and a lung inflation rate of 12 breaths per minute. If the reservoir bag is not attached and the same settings are used, the maximum $F_{I}O_2$ is only 0.73. With a flow rate of 15 litres/min, a tidal volume of 1000 ml and 12 breaths/min, the maximum $F_{I}O_2$ is only 0.69. The faster the breathing rate, the more air is entrained into the bag, which lowers the oxygen concentration delivered to the patient.

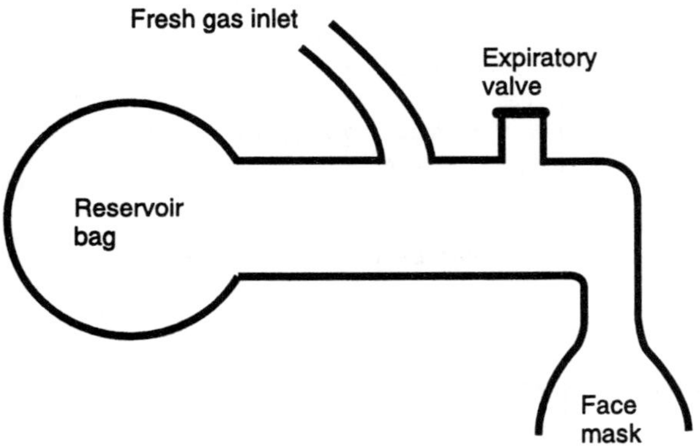

The necessary components of a simple gas delivery circuit

The anaesthetic breathing system will consist of a connection to the patient (mask or tracheal tube), an expired gas dump valve, a connection for the oxygen source and a reservoir bag. The circuit illustrated will only deliver 100% oxygen if the fresh gas flow is twice the patient's estimated minute volume.

Oropharyngeal airway

The Guedel airway is inserted into the mouth with its concave surface facing the top of the patient's head. When the bevelled tip reaches the pharynx, the airway is rotated 180° and then advanced towards the laryngeal inlet. The airway holds the tongue away from the pharyngeal wall permitting gas delivery through its central lumen towards the lungs, with the outer flange of the airway resting against the teeth.

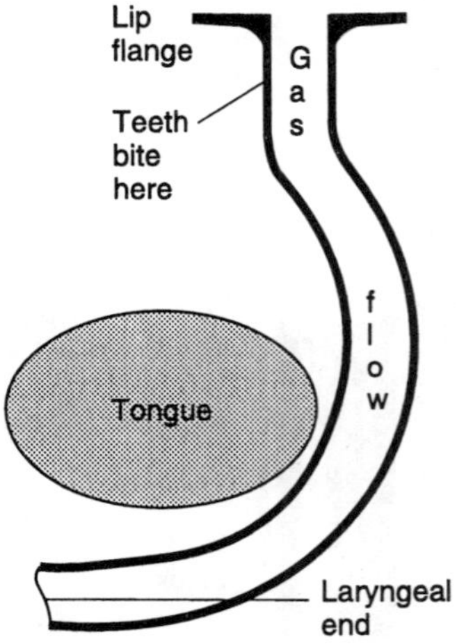

Guedel's Airway
The relationship of an orally inserted Guedel airway to the teeth, tongue and pharynx

Suction

Suction must be available and effective. It may be required to aspirate saliva, blood or vomitus from the oropharynx to permit visualisation of the vocal cords. The suction unit may be on the wall or a portable electrical, mechanical or gas powered unit. Know how to switch the suction unit on and adjust it to the maximum suction setting.

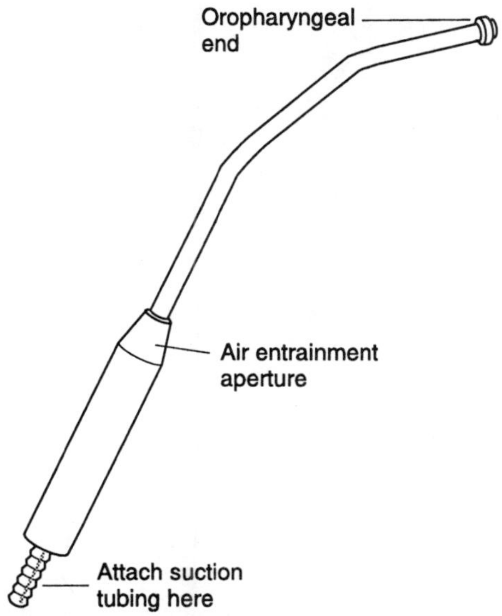

Yankauer Suction Handpiece

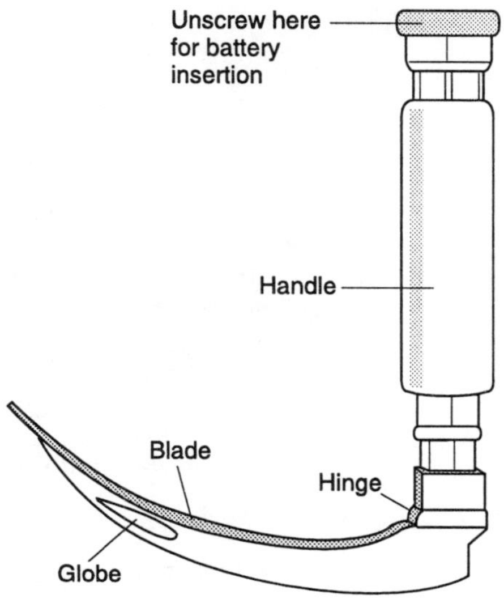

The components of an adult MacIntosh laryngoscope

The suction unit should develop a negative pressure of -500 mm Hg, aspirate 150 ml of fluid per second via suction tubing with a half inch internal diameter. A large bore rigid sucker of the Yankauer type is attached to the suction tubing to facilitate suctioning of the oropharynx.

Laryngoscope

This instrument facilitates visualisation of the larynx and there are many designs. The most commonly used one is the curved blade laryngoscope. The instrument comprises a handle and a blade. The handle houses the batteries which power the light, which is emitted approximately 2.5 cm from the tip of the laryngoscope blade. The action of opening the blade out from the handle, automatically switches on the light. If the laryngoscope fails, check that the batteries are charged, the light bulb is screwed tightly into place and that the electrical or light contact point between the blade and handle is clean.

Tracheal tube

As with laryngoscopes, there are many patterns of tracheal tube. An adult cuffed tracheal tube is illustrated.

The size of the tube is expressed as the internal diameter (ID) in millimetres and is marked on the tube. For Caucasian adults, a rough guide is a size 8.0 for a female and a size 9.0 for a male. Have available the next sizes larger and smaller than that estimated. Do NOT try to force the largest possible tracheal tube through the larynx. If the chosen tube fits tightly and there is no air leak around the tube on pulmonary inflation while the tracheal cuff is deflated, then replace the tube with a half size smaller. For children below 16 years of age, the size may be estimated according to the formula:

$$\frac{\text{age}}{4} + 4 = \text{ID}$$

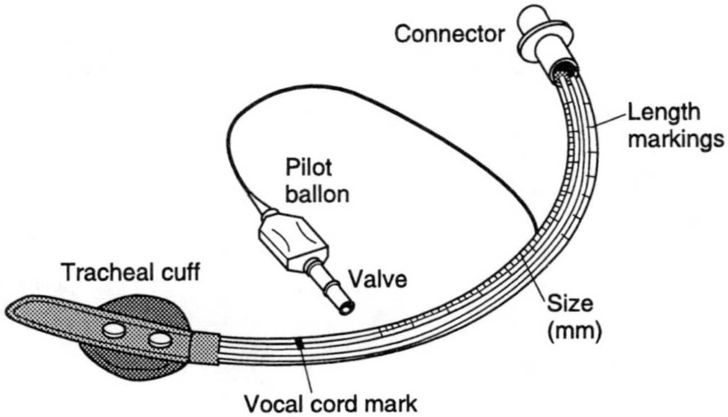

An adult, cuffed, polyvinyl chloride tracheal tube

A four year old child will require a non-cuffed tracheal tube with an estimated internal diameter of 5 mm (i.e. size 5).

The cuff is inflated within the trachea by means of a syringe attached to a one way valve and provides a seal against the tracheal mucosa, protecting the lungs from contamination from the oropharynx. The pilot balloon is connected to the cuff by a piece of fine tubing and signals to the intubator that the cuff is inflated. A radio-opaque indicator line runs down the length of the tube permitting radiological confirmation of tube position. Radiographically, the tip of the tracheal tube should lie between the clavicular heads, minimising the risk of bronchial intubation and accidental extubation. The length markings indicate the distance in centimetres from the patient's lips to the bevelled end of the tube which is inside the trachea. The correct position of the tube in the trachea is such that the top of the cuff sits just below the vocal cords. As a guideline, an estimate of the length a tracheal tube should be inserted in children under 16 years of age is given by the formula:

$$\frac{\text{age}}{2} + 12 = \text{distance in centimetres from the tube bevel to the teeth}$$

A connector inserted into the non-bevelled end of the tube is required to attach the oxygen delivery system, and is included in the packet with the tracheal tube. This male tapered connector is of standard 15 mm size and fits directly into the female 15 mm connector on a self-inflating bag.

Defibrillator

Defibrillation is an integral part of advanced life support and the resuscitator must be familiar with the equipment.

1. place electrically conductive pads over the right sternal margin and over V4,V5 ECG electrode points on the left chest wall
2. turn on the power
3. select the energy to be delivered – VT or VF 3-5 joules/kg cardioversion of atrial dysrhythmias
4. charge the paddles
5. apply the paddles firmly to the conductive pads, make sure no other part of the operator is in contact with the patient or bed
6. ask assistants to stand clear
7. push the discharge buttons on the paddles
8. check carotid pulse
9. check cardiac rhythm on the monitor

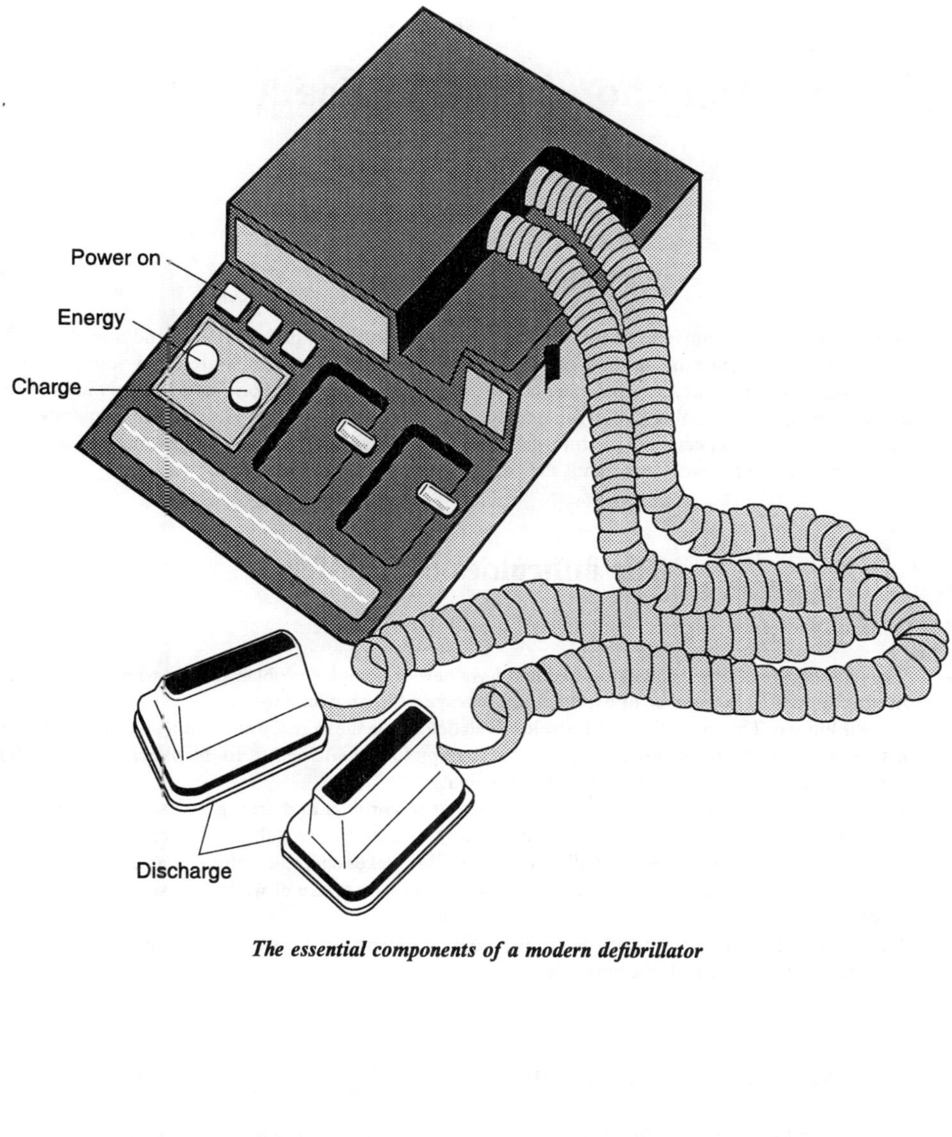

The essential components of a modern defibrillator

Chapter 24

Transport of the critically ill

Principles of transfer

Critically ill patients are transferred between sites to undergo investigations (CT scan and angiography), operation and to reach sites of specialist treatment. Whilst critically ill patients are often young trauma victims passing through an accident and emergency department, patients can originate from a wide variety of sources. There is a continual risk of organ damage during transport. *Patient* directed care demands that appropriately experienced personnel, monitoring equipment, drugs and facilities for treatment go with (or to) the patient and remain with them until they arrive in a more secure situation.

The difficulties of transfer

The following conspire to increase the potential hazard during transfer:

- The patients are often recently admitted and have new or complex problems. Even when 'stable' they are prone to a large number of expected and unexpected complications.
- Time is limited. The patient's condition alone will determine the urgency and timing of the transfer. A distinction must be made between transfer for therapy (of *definite* benefit to the patient) and transfer for investigation (of *potential* benefit to the patient).
- Resources may be stretched. There are many aspects to consider and arrangements to make prior to transfer yet the patient requires concurrent therapy to secure their stability for transfer.
- Resources from multiple agencies will be required. This makes communication complex. All elements of the transfer are dependent on each other and all must be aware of what is expected of them and when.
- Environments encountered during the transfer are *all* potentially hazardous to the patient. Limit the time exposed to these as far as possible.

Common misadventures occurring during transfer

- *Disconnections*: these can occur at any connection in any item of equipment. Equipment is commonly wrenched from the patient. ECGs, oximeter probes, iv lines, and tracheal tubes: expect anything that can be dislodged, will be.
- *Exhaustions*: All supplies are limited: electricity, inspired gas, infusions will all run out ... eventually
- *Incompatibilities*: when wanting to connect to a resource supplied by another agency (e.g. a plane/ambulance) it is not possible because the equipment standards are different (different voltage, gas connectors).
- *Failures*: not only is transfer hazardous to patients but also to equipment. It may be exposed to wind, rain or physical abuse beyond its specifications.
- *Malfunction*: cold (shivering, poor peripheral perfusion) or vibration of the transport vehicle may result in poor function of the ECG, pulse oximeter and NIBP during transfer.
- *Failed Intentions*: Transfers may involve complicated planning that does not always run smoothly, particularly when arranged through a third party. An unexpected arrival is not unknown!

Be prepared!

Discuss with senior colleagues your responsibilities regarding transfers prior to departure.
Ask about :

- location, quantity and maintenance of essential equipment, drugs and monitoring
- types of patients and problems encountered
- existing protocols and guidelines

When a transfer is requested you should first carefully assess the patient in order to:

Optimise the patient's treatment

- stabilise and monitor the patient *prior* to transfer
- it is rare for transfer to be immediately life-saving therapy
- upgrade management to ensure patient safety during transfer
- ***If in doubt: over-prepare, over-treat, and over-monitor***

Ensure continuation of the patient's current treatment

- must be adequate resources to ensure that the current level of treatment can be maintained throughout transfer.
- infusions, pumps, all medications and treatments that are needed.

Protect the patient from harm

- the critically ill are vulnerable to physical harm from the environment (particularly the cold and pressure necrosis).
- predict potential complications, practise recognition skills and plan to treat complications during the journey.

Distances and modes of transport will be defined by the geography and urgency of transfer.

Take everything you need with you

- all transfers require that patients are removed from places of relative safety through hostile environments.
- a hospital corridor is potentially dangerous to a patient critically dependent on oxygen, and safe transport demands vigilant staff and functioning monitoring equipment.
- the transporter must be completely self-sufficient.
- transfer to places such as accident and emergency, intensive therapy and operating theatre departments are made easier by the knowledge that facilities for the treatment of the critically ill are immediately available. In contrast, Radiology departments are notorious for their cramped conditions, lack of equipment and distance from experienced help. Unless absolutely certain of the facilities, make no assumptions about their adequacy for patient management.

Take extra, take spares

- ensure essential commodities such as fuel, electricity (batteries) and gas supplies
- spare equipment, check the sterility and integrity of disposables
- check drug use-by dates.

Arrange appropriate resources

Personnel

- accompanying staff must be competent in diagnosing and treating the presenting condition and those that may arise.
- this should be the most senior level available, but in reality pressure is often placed on junior staff to accompany their own sick patients.
- experienced assistance from other disciplines (nursing, paramedic and driving staff) must be available.

Monitoring

- it is often impossible to monitor a patient 'clinically' because of poor light, vibration, noise, cramped conditions and electrical interference.
- battery powered devices form the basis of a mobile intensive care unit but the performance of non invasive blood pressure (NIBP) monitors and pulse oximeters is subject to movement artefact and they are often unreliable during transfer. Direct arterial monitoring may be more satisfactory.
- remember internal batteries have a limited life.
- be vigilant! Keep the patient and monitors in your view at all times.
- all transporting staff should assume an individual and separate responsibility for the patient during transfer.

Equipment and drugs

- resuscitation needs for airway management, ventilation, drugs and circulatory support should *always* be available.
- have *a backup* for any piece of equipment or device upon which the patient's vital functions are dependent.

Intrahospital transfer example

A 70 yr old man is admitted through the A&E department. He has had an acute anterior myocardial infarction complicated by left ventricular failure and hypotension. He was very short of breath on arrival but this has improved after treatment with high flow oxygen, morphine, frusemide and a GTN (glycerol trinitrate) infusion. He is also receiving a streptokinase infusion. His CXR on arrival showed heart failure. This was a poor quality AP film and it is intended to repeat the film in the X-ray department on the way to coronary care. A&E is on the ground floor. CCU is on the 6th floor.

1. Assess the patient

Current status : RR 25, BP 100/75, HR 60 sinus rhythm and pain free.

- **Past:** What is the background? Are there other relevant conditions (e.g. diabetes)?
- **Recent past:** Is the diagnosis correct? (MI, CCF). Have other possibilities been excluded (e.g. dissecting thoracic aneurysm, pneumonia with sepsis)? What are the current complications (CCF, cardiogenic shock)?
- **Present:** Is the patient stable? Since the transfer is not urgent: has there been an adequate wait to ensure stability. (Do not leave immediately after starting new intravenous infusions if possible). Consider the patient's ABC's. Are they stable? Do you have objective evidence of his 'improvement' ? Repeat the arterial gases if possible.
- Optimise, upgrade and stabilise the patient's condition.

- **Future:** What are the complications of (i) the condition and (ii) the treatment? Consider your treatment plan for : arrhythmia (VF, VT), hypotension, further left ventricular failure (causing hypoxia), anaphylaxis (streptokinase), chest pain (angina).
- **Ensure that all continuous therapies are working well and secured against accidental removal and that equipment is available to manage common potential complications.**

2. Plan the transfer

- Personnel, route, timing. Ensure all communications have been made.
- **cancel** the X-ray (as it will not influence management and it considerably increases the hazard of the transfer).

3. Plan what to take

- Current treatment: 60 mins oxygen, infusion pumps (full batteries) and intravenous lines.
- Equipment: portable CPR kit (airway, intubation equipment, self-inflating bag and suction apparatus) and defibrillator, spare battery for pump, equipment to re-insert i.v. if drip accidentally removed.
- Drugs: resuscitation medication: atropine, adrenaline, and lignocaine, adequate quantities of GTN and streptokinase.

4. Before you leave check

- that all equipment is functioning and monitoring is secure
- that patient remains stable
- supplies are adequate for the journey; carry spares of vital equipment
- that other personnel involved are present and all know where to go and what to do
- that the patient is expected in CCU
- that the patient is warm and protected from the elements

5. On the transfer

- watch the patient
- proceed efficiently and steadily (concentrate on the patient rather than speed)
- if you become unsure of the patient's condition STOP the trolley, ask for quiet, assess ABC
- if there is a problem give immediate life-saving treatment and ***call for help,*** then proceed rapidly to the nearest backup area – either back to A&E or on to CCU.

6. Handover

- on arrival carefully transfer the patient to bed and attach to unit monitors
- assess the patient's condition relative to that prior to transfer
- handover patient's care *courteously* to the ward staff.

Consider the problems associated with (i) a journey to another hospital, (ii) the patient is Glasgow coma scale 7 (GCS7) following a head injury and is being taken for CT scan.

Problems associated with air transport

- motion sickness (in both the patient and the transferring staff)
- use the toilet before take-off (bottle or IDC for patient in flight)
- noise, vibration and motion make communication and clinical judgement very difficult
- cold
- decompress air filled spaces such as urinary catheter bags and the tracheal tube cuff should be inflated with saline
- patient access – cramped
- power for infusion devices – i.v. won't run!
- radio or electrical interference with monitoring
- show courtesy to the referring physician

Chapter 25

Shock

Untreated shock will cause the patient's demise and early recognition is fundamental to the treatment of the critically ill patient. Shocked patients often have reduced consciousness and loss of airway control (apnoea if the shock is severe) as a result of cerebral hypoperfusion and therefore the first step in the management of shock is to

ENSURE THE PATIENT HAS A PATENT AIRWAY

AND

IS BREATHING A HIGH CONCENTRATION OF INSPIRED OXYGEN.

Definition

Shock means many things to different people and confusion may arise over the meaning of this term when it is applied loosely. The pathophysiologist's definition of shock is: '*an artificial state characterised by inadequate delivery of oxygen to the tissues*'.

Since calculation of individual tissue oxygen delivery is technically demanding, this definition, whilst critical to our understanding of shock and its treatment, does not aid its recognition. There are various *clinical* syndromes of shock (described later) whose features allow rapid diagnosis of the shocked state. It is important to realise that no one particular feature of these syndromes *defines* shock (the *definition* is above). For instance, whilst the presence of hypotension is common in shock, it is not obligatory (the converse also applies: the presence of hypotension does not indicate shock must be present). Recognition of the clinical patterns of shock alerts the observer to the presence of inadequate tissue oxygen delivery. Since the individual pattern is defined by the cause of the shocked state, the physician is able to quickly direct management to
(i) treat the underlying cause and
(ii) improve tissue oxygen delivery.

The consequences of inadequate oxygen delivery

- ischaemia with organ dysfunction
- followed by infarction (permanent organ damage)
- and eventually organ death.

The aim of management is to restore perfusion of well oxygenated blood to the tissues. This reverses the ischaemia/infarction cycle. The consequence of failure to restore perfusion to an organ bed is not only progression of that organ to infarction but also the consequent release of various toxins and chemical mediators into the bloodstream from the dead tissue. These substances result in remote organ damage. The most usual expression of this secondary damage is adult respiratory distress syndrome (ARDS) which may result in *irreversible* shock and death.

Irreversible shock was described in early animal haemorrhage models of shock. It was found that if replacement of the lost blood was delayed beyond a certain point in time, the animal subsequently perished despite fully restoring the circulating blood volume.

If circulation is restored early, ischaemia is reversed, permanent organ damage is avoided and survival is increased.

Classification of shock

There are many ways of classifying shock and the following is a mechanistic method:

Hypovolaemic shock

Ventricular stroke volume is critically dependent on venous return. If the blood volume is so low that venous return is inadequate, there will be a fall in cardiac output. The venous capacitance vessels are empty.

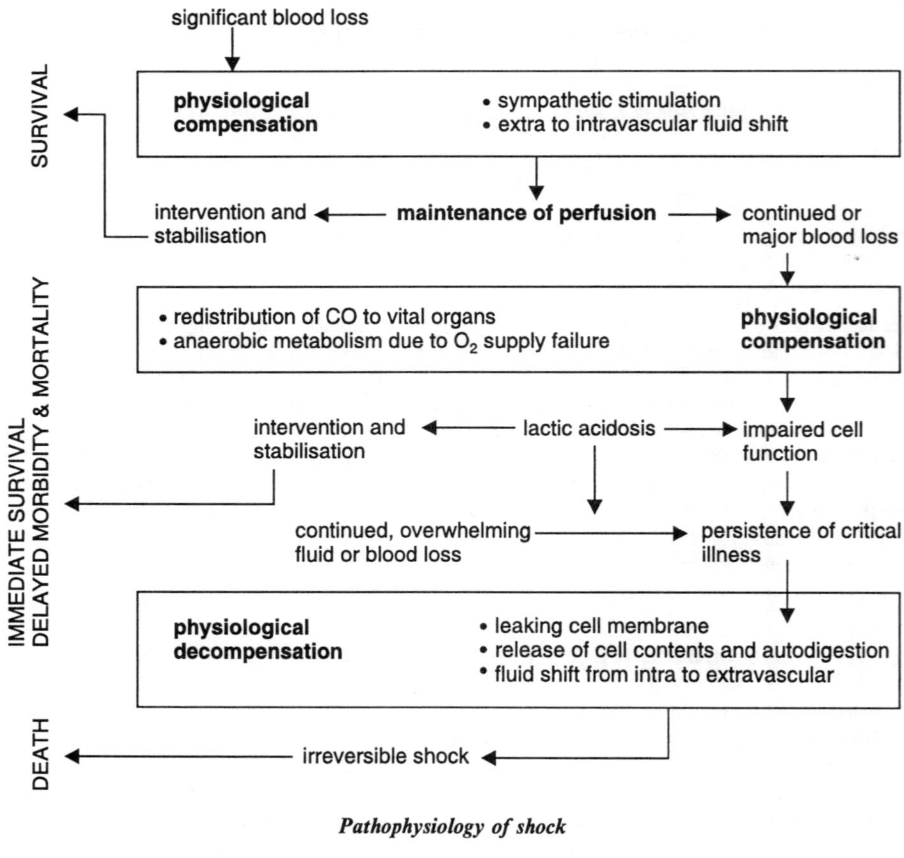

Pathophysiology of shock

Distributive shock

Venous return is not only dependent on an adequate circulating volume but also a venous pressure sufficient to direct the blood back to the heart (circulatory filling pressure). When peripheral venodilatation occurs so that the central capacitance vessels are underfilled and at low pressure, there will be a relative hypovolaemia with inadequate central distribution of circulating blood volume.

Cardiogenic shock

In this type of shock the muscle of the pump itself fails. The heart is unable to generate sufficient stroke volume to maintain an adequate cardiac output. This occurs despite adequate circulating volumes and filling pressures.

Obstructive shock

Despite a normal circulating volume and a healthy pump, the stroke volume is reduced, because the blood is physically prevented from entering or leaving the heart. This implies major specific chest pathology (pericardial tamponade, massive pulmonary embolus).

Mixed type shock

The inconsistencies in the clinical manifestations of shock result from a mixture of mechanisms. For instance, septic shock may at first be distributive due to vasodilatation, however a degree of impairment of cardiac function often rapidly complicates the picture.
The presence of hypovolaemia will significantly worsen any shocked state. ***No patient suffering from any form of shock is adequately treated if volume is unreplaced.***

Compensatory mechanisms in shock

Cardiac output = blood pressure × total peripheral resistance

Individual tissue beds autoregulate their own oxygenation (by vasodilatation for example) but the organism as a whole responds to and regulates its blood pressure. This control overrides the needs of (certain) individual tissues and maintains blood pressure by immediate changes in regional perfusion. The most important control mechanisms are the changes caused by increased sympathetic nervous system activity and circulating catecholamines (also other hormones such as angiotensin II and vasopressin).

The following all act in the acute situation to maintain oxygen delivery to the 'vital' organs (brain, lungs, heart and kidneys):

- *Tachycardia* (cardiac output = stroke volume × heart rate)
- *Splanchnic vasoconstriction*: blood flow is directed away from non vital organs (such as the skin and gut) and total peripheral resistance is raised.
- *Venoconstriction*: noradrenaline causes a 'tightening' of the venous capacitance vessels. This allows an inadequate circulating volume to generate higher filling pressures. (This is of practical importance: shock may be associated with near normal central venous pressures despite the need for continued fluid resuscitation.)
- *Fluid redistribution*: lower circulating pressures draw fluid from the extravascular and intracellular spaces to buffer losses in circulating volume. The degree of resuscitation required to restore the circulating volume usually underestimates the total body requirements for fluid, particularly saline.

Long term compensatory mechanisms (extracellular fluid volume regulation) for control of blood pressure have less relevance in the acute shock situation but are of importance in the management of the critically ill over a period of days. Consideration is given to body salt and water retention through renal mechanisms (renin-aldosterone-angiotensin axis and vasopressin). Erythropoietin stimulates bone marrow production of red cells in the weeks following shock.

Clinical features of shock syndromes

Haemorrhagic shock is the most recognisable and the best understood of the shock syndromes but it is important to recognise the similarities and differences with others.

Haemorrhagic shock

The features of 'classic' shock: pale, cold, clammy skin in association with hypotension and tachycardia are *late* signs of haemorrhage, occurring only after 30–40% of the circulating volume has been lost and when vital organ damage is imminent. Circulating volume resuscitation should be aggressive and immediate if the classic signs are present.

Grading haemorrhagic shock (70 kg male)

Haemorrhage	**Grade I**	**Grade II**	**Grade III**	**Grade IV**
% blood vol lost	up to 15 %	15 to 30%	30 to 40%	>40%
ml lost	up to 750 ml	750 to 1500 ml	1500 to 2000 ml	> 2000ml
Consequence	blood donor	needs iv fluid	needs blood	pre-terminal
Recognition				
Pulse rate	normal	normal – 100	100 – 120	140 / dysrhythmia
Systolic BP	normal	normal	reduced	< 90 mm Hg
Pulse pressure	normal	reduced	reduced	reduced
Skin perfusion	normal	pale	cold & clammy	ashen visage
Capillary refill	normal	delayed	delayed	absent
Respiratory rate	14 – 20	20 – 30	30 – 40	> 40
Mental state	mildly anxious	anxious	inappropriate	confused / lethargic
Monitoring				
Urine flow ml/hr	30 – 60	30	15	oliguria
BP	–	hourly by hand	NIBP 15 mins	arterial line
CVP	–	JVP by eye	desirable	mandatory
Resuscitation regimen				
Type	water by mouth	colloid	colloid then blood	colloid then blood
Volume	indicated by thirst	1000 ml	1000 ml plus 2 units Rcc	1000 – 1500 ml plus 4 units Rcc
Rate	–	500 fast, then 500 over an hour	1000 fast then Rcc over an hour	Fast until SBP up rpt. 'challenges'
Maintenance regimen				
125 ml 0.45% saline / 4% dextrose for every hour NBM. Add and 'backdate' this fluid to that for resuscitation				

(Rcc = red cell concentrate)

The above table shows four symptomatic shock gradings proportional to increasing severity of haemorrhage. Classical shock becomes apparent at grade III but ideally shock should be diagnosed at the grade II stage. Urine output is a sensitive and early sign of inadequate renal oxygen supply, where poor perfusion is indicated by a reduction in urine output. Exaggerated changes in blood pressure result from stress applied to patients in grade II shock revealing overt hypovolaemia – a positive posture test (30 mmHg fall in systolic blood pressure from the supine to the sitting position), decreases in blood pressure with positive pressure ventilation and excessive hypotension and sedation after appropriate opiate administration are good examples.

Conditions that modify the standard response to haemorrhage

- reduced organ system reserve (ASA ratings: ≥ III)
- age (postural hypotension)
- premorbid physical condition (athlete vs debilitated)
- medications (β blockers and antihypertensives)
- hypothermia (vasoconstriction and resistance to fluid load)
- fixed cardiac output (pacemaker, valve stenoses and CCF)

Treatment of haemorrhagic shock is not complete (or ever successful) without diagnosing and staunching the site of exsanguination. This will require a quick survey for revealed haemorrhage (stabilisation and fixation of major fractures) followed by a logical sequence of exploration for concealed haemorrhage (chest, abdomen, retroperitoneal space). Treatment will often involve surgery and therefore anaesthesia. Ideally this will be performed after resuscitation. Occasionally the bleeding is so profuse that fluid administration cannot match the rate of loss and maintain an adequate cardiac output. Under such circumstances surgery must be undertaken as soon as venous access and monitoring are established and blood is at hand.

Early intervention by the anaesthetist will increase the rate of resolution of the crisis.

Anaphylactic shock (refer p. 164)

As a reminder, the features include :

- urticarial rash
- bronchospasm
- angio-neurotic oedema

The shock is manifested as hypotension due to vaso- and venodilatation.
Treatment of the shock is to give:

- 100% oxygen
- adrenaline
- fluid

the shock is distributive and venous return is low due to relative hypovolaemia – give a fluid bolus immediately and as fast as possible (e.g. 1000 ml colloid).

Septic shock

In the initial stages of sepsis the shock is distributive in nature. Vasodilatation, pyrexia and tachycardia are all prominent. The pulse is described as bounding and the circulation is hyperdynamic. Whilst not always prominent early there is often respiratory impairment resulting in hypoxia and tachypnoea. Gram negative septicaemia (often related to surgical gastrointestinal or urological pathology) is a common precipitant although almost any severe infection may produce this syndrome.

Later, if untreated, circulating toxins cause maldistribution of fluid into interstitial spaces (peripheral and pulmonary oedema) and a negative inotropic effect. The latter is exacerbated if there is concomitant pulmonary hypertension associated with respiratory distress. Many of these patients will have had recent surgery with associated hypovolaemia with resultant cold peripheries due to inadequate cardiac output ('unresuscitated hypovolaemic shock'). Progressive renal and respiratory dysfunction if uncorrected will result in severe multi-organ failure and at this stage correction of the original infection may not reverse the shock.

Supportive management

- oxygen ± artificial ventilation
- fluid resuscitation
- inotropic support – given as an infusion which is adjusted according to the patient response measured by invasive cardiac monitoring.
  - ◊ inoconstrictors (e.g. noradrenaline) if vasodilatation is prominent
  - ◊ inodilators (e.g. adrenaline or dobutamine) if vasoconstricted
- renal protection
  - ◊ dopamine, frusemide or mannitol
- monitoring
  - ◊ arterial line, CVP, ± Swan–Ganz catheter
  - ◊ renal function
  - ◊ regular blood gas analysis to monitor hypoxia and acidosis
- early referral to intensive care

Specific therapy

Initial advanced resuscitation permits isolation of the underlying cause.

- complete clinical examination including wounds for pus
- full infection screen
  - ◊ blood, urine, sputum, 'other' cultures
  - ◊ CXR, other radiological investigations for sepsis (e.g. ultrasound)
- broad spectrum antibiotics (after cultures)
- surgical correction of underlying problem

Cardiogenic shock

When the primary problem is one of pump failure, there is usually a preceding history suggestive of ischaemic myocardial damage, but presentation after myocardial infarction can be sudden and catastrophic. Very rarely, other pathology such as an infective myocarditis may precipitate shock.

The predominant feature is one of a low cardiac output state with poor peripheral perfusion, low urine output and cold extremities, usually occurring in the presence of clinical fluid overload (raised JVP, dependent and pulmonary oedema). Hypotension will be present despite fluid overload but may not be prominent. Chronic diuretic therapy may have resulted in fluid depletion and optimal fluid management requires measurement of cardiac output, pulmonary wedge pressure (PCWP) and total peripheral resistance.

Cardiogenic shock is defined by the presence of a normal or high PCWP and a cardiac (output) index < 1.5. It cannot be diagnosed reliably in the presence of dehydration. Hypotension is always present if there is *any* dehydration.

There may not be any therapy that can cure the underlying problem of myocardial muscle failure. The following are situations where myocardial performance can be expected to improve and therefore intensive treatment is justified:

- time is required to determine myocardial recovery following
  - ◊ recent myocardial ischaemia / infarction
  - ◊ myocarditis
- myocardial ischaemia with a view to coronary artery bypass or angioplasty, thrombolytic regimes, or aortic balloon pump regimes
- sudden decompensation due to added but reversible stresses, e.g. operation, pneumonia, sepsis
- young patients suitable for heart transplantation

Treatment

The preceding should be considered as the treatment of the underlying disorder. The treatments which follow are supportive and aim to improve organ perfusion which is assessed by renal performance (urine output and urea/creatinine levels) and improvement in measured cardiovascular parameters (PCWP, cardiac index).

- Fluid status
  This will be critical. Both excessive dehydration and over distension of the heart will result in a decreased cardiac output (the down-slope of the Frank–Starling curve) and increased obstruction to ventricular ejection against a high pulmonary resistance resulting from lungs distended with fluid. Clinical evidence of fluid overload requires diuretic therapy.
- Reduce afterload
  A high calculated total peripheral resistance is common and increases the work of the heart. Vasodilatation (by infusion of glyceryl trinitrate GTN) will improve cardiac output. Inotropic support and judicious fluid challenges *after* vasodilatation are used to optimise perfusion. Drugs that cause both vasodilatation and positive inotropism ('inodilators' e.g. dobutamine and enoximone) may be used to provide this effect.
- Reduce overall work
- The agitated patient in heart failure utilises oxygen (tachypnoea, tachycardia) which is limited in supply. Rest and judicious use of small doses of sedative drugs (e.g. morphine in heart failure) may be beneficial.
- Increase cardiac muscle performance
  Inotropic medication (given by infusion) may boost the performance of the myocardium but inotropic agents also cause tachycardia (positive chronotropism) which limits their effectiveness as both left ventricular filling and coronary perfusion rely on an adequate diastolic time.

Chapter 26

Anaphylaxis

Introduction

A specific cause of severe cardiovascular collapse is the abnormal immunological response termed anaphylaxis. Many drugs and therapeutic substances have been identified as causing these reactions which have been estimated to occur in 6 out of every 10,000 hospital admissions. A 1000 bed hospital can expect as many as 60 cases per year.

Mechanism

True anaphylaxis requires that the patient be previously exposed to the substance, or to one sufficiently similar for cross-sensitivity to occur. Where severe sensitivity responses occur to substances to which the patient has no history of prior exposure, the term anaphylactoid is used. There is NO clinical difference between the two phenomena.

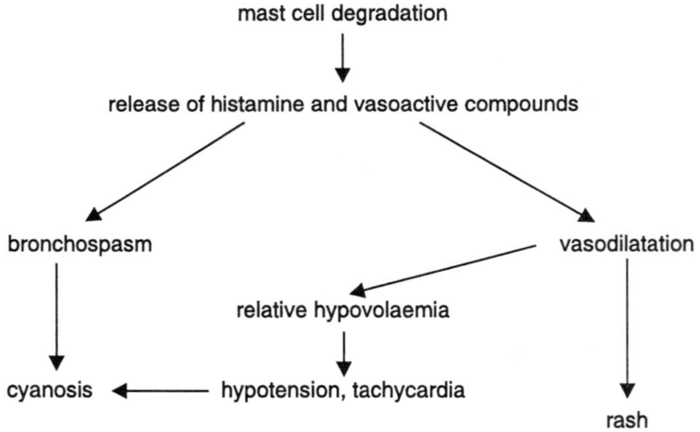

26. Anaphylaxis

It appears that the anaphylactic response results when there is an exaggeration of the 'high speed' immune pathway, in which antibody release triggers an IgE/mast cell complex to a far greater degree than normal. The outcome of these events is that the cells degranulate, releasing large amounts of histamine and other vasoactive substances. Complement may be involved, but is not thought to be central to the reaction. The above description is greatly simplified and for a more detailed explanation, it is necessary to consult the immunological literature, but in this section the emphasis is on clinical recognition and crisis management.

Diagnosis

- whenever a severe circulatory or respiratory crisis develops within a short time (seconds or minutes) of the administration of a medication or injected substance, anaphylaxis must be suspected
- the agents which may be responsible include:
  - ◊ anaesthetic induction agents, relaxants and narcotics
  - ◊ antibiotics, antivenenes, vaccines
  - ◊ contrast media
  - ◊ plasma substitutes
- but almost any drug is capable of causing the syndrome
- the presentation will be sudden and the patient will become distressed and restless. Very soon one or more of the following manifestations will appear:
  - ◊ bronchopulmonary – wheezing, dyspnoea, cyanosis
  - ◊ cardiovascular – severe hypotension, tachycardia, impalpable pulse
  - ◊ mucocutaneous – rash, erythema, oedema, angioneurotic oedema
  - ◊ rarely there is abdominal pain or gastrointestinal bleeding but these symptoms are overshadowed by the more dramatic cardio-respiratory problems
- there is NO time for investigation of this crisis and neither chest X-ray, electrocardiogram nor biochemistry are helpful in reaching a diagnosis, which is made solely on clinical grounds

Treatment

- treatment must be prompt and specific if the patient is to survive. Access to a vein is essential for the administration of drugs and fluids. Oxygen is mandatory.

Drugs

- ADRENALINE is the only drug of proven value. It should be given intravenously, in a dilution of 1:10,000 (1 mg in 10 ml). This dose (10 ml) is given every 3 minutes until the patient responds. If access to a vein is delayed the drug may be given via the tracheal tube or sublingually or even intramuscularly, but is far less effective by this latter route.
- steroids and antihistamines are USELESS in established anaphylaxis and their administration wastes valuable time which can be spent doing more constructive things.

Fluids

- intravenous fluids are helpful in restoring adequate cardiac output but should be carefully chosen and given in limited amounts.
- colloid is generally believed to be superior to crystalloid.
- if adrenaline has been given in adequate dosage, the volume of fluid required will be small and usually no more than a litre or so.

Oxygen

- oxygen must be given in HIGH concentrations, approaching 100%
- use one of the self-inflating resuscitators (Ambu, Laerdal, Air-viva) with an oxygen reservoir attached. These devices can be used on the spontaneously breathing patient and are capable of delivering suitable oxygen concentrations
- NEVER use low or fixed concentration oxygen masks on patients in this kind of difficulty
- if the patient is unconscious and obviously hypoxic, it will be necessary to intubate the larynx and probably assist ventilation
- if bronchospasm is extreme and does not respond to adrenaline, salbutamol can be introduced via the tracheal tube.

Monitoring

- the electrocardiogram (especially helpful at the stage when the blood pressure and peripheral pulses are undetectable)
- the pulse oximeter – as soon as some circulation has returned to the periphery
- an automatic non-invasive blood pressure device
- these devices should be connected to the patient as soon as time and the availability of personnel permit

Follow-up

- the outcome of timely, efficient treatment of anaphylaxis is almost always good and the great majority of patients so treated recover completely. It is then necessary to ensure steps are taken to identify the offending agent (usually more than one drug has been given) and to provide the patient with the means of warning future medical attendants of the danger.
- investigations must be delayed from 4-6 weeks because the tests to be performed will not give accurate results until such time as the immune mechanism has returned to its pre-anaphylactic state and this does not occur quickly. Subcutaneous testing with dilutions of the suspect substance is usually effective in identifying the allergen.
- when identification has been achieved, a warning bracelet or necklace should be engraved with a suitable message and worn by the patient at all times.

Part III

Good Concise Section + Relevant Information. Runs well together

Emergency Care

Chapter 27

The unconscious patient

Chronic care

In addition to the acute dangers of unconsciousness previously mentioned, additional problems arise during prolonged coma. Although principally respiratory and metabolic in origin, they can secondarily affect other systems. It is often these complications which determine the outcome of the illness and their management is vital to the survival of the patient. Some of the common problems which arise and their management are described.

Fluid and electrolytes

- injury stimulates the release of antidiuretic hormone and aldosterone, which in turn cause retention of water in excess of sodium and increased potassium loss associated with catabolism
- hyponatraemia < 130 mmol/litre, urine hypertonic with urine Na^+ > 25 mmole/litre
  - ◊ fluid restriction –1 ml/kg/hr i.v. as a dextrose/saline solution
- hypernatraemia >155 mmol/litre may arise due to
  - ◊ inadequate fluid intake
  - ◊ diabetes insipidus
  - ◊ excessive osmotic diuretic administration
  - ◊ excessive protein feeding ± glycosuria

Diabetes insipidus

- sufficient fluid given as 4% dextrose + 0.18% N saline i.v.
- lysine vasopressin nasal spray 4 hourly
- ± chlorpropamide, clofibrate, carbamazepine

Nutrition

- (consult the hospital dietitian)
- decreased energy requirements of unconsciousness and hypothermia
- increased energy requirements due to
  - ◊ the metabolic response to injury
  - ◊ hyperthermia and muscle activity (fitting, spasticity)
- first 3 days -i.v. 4% dextrose 0.18% N saline @ 100 ml/hr provides 1600 Kjoules (400cal)/day
- then nasogastric feeding as a continuous infusion to provide 3000 cal/day (i.e. 13,000 kjoules/70 kg male/day in 2.5 litres) BUT
  - ◊ the gastro-intestinal tract must be functioning
  - ◊ laryngeal protective reflexes must be present
- gastric ulceration prophylaxis
  - ◊ misoprostol if concern over gastric colonisation
  - ◊ ranitidine 150 mg 12 hourly (histamine H_2 receptor antagonist) for proven ulceration
  - ◊ gastric feeding ± mylanta 10 ml two hourly (antacid)
- total parenteral nutrition (T.P.N.) via a central venous line with peripherally administered Intralipid.

Haematological disorders

- anaemia – blood loss
- thrombocytopenia and decreased platelet aggregation
- early stage hypercoagulability with severe head injuries

Temperature control

- pyrexia exacerbates neuronal injury! The patient's core temperature is allowed to drift down to 34°C and this can be assisted by NOT heating the humidified gases, intravenous chlorpromazine (to promote vasodilatation) and active cooling.

Treatment of seizures

- clonazepam or thiopentone given slowly in a sufficient dose to terminate the seizure
- follow with phenytoin 4 mg/kg 12 hourly to achieve a therapeutic serum level of 40 to 80 mmol/l.

Prevention of injury

- the unconscious patient may not move, blink or attend to bodily functions and is therefore, unlike the conscious patient, vulnerable to injury.

For example:

◊ skin – pressure, heat, entrapment, moisture causes bedsores
◊ eyes – desiccation, abrasion, ulceration result in corneal damage
◊ mouth – moniliasis, ulceration, pharyngeal suction
◊ perineal toilet – source of infection
◊ peripheral nerves – pressure, abnormal posture
◊ foot/wrist drop – flexion deformity to limbs/spine
◊ bladder care – catheter, condom – asepsis critical
◊ bowel care – impaction, constipation, diarrhoea with enteral feeding
◊ sepsis – i.v. lines and monitoring equipment
◊ tracheal toilet – ineffectual cough and recurrent aspiration
◊ cross-infection and nosocomial infection
◊ hypostatic pneumonia

A successful outcome is as much dependent on good nursing care and physiotherapy as appropriate medical supervision of management and therefore close co-operation between all disciplines is essential.

Chapter 28

Monitoring the acute closed head injury

The special problems of closed head injury merit separate consideration. No attempt will be made here to deal with open head injuries, or those which require drainage of intracranial collections, so the ensuing discussion applies only to the non-operative management of head injury.

Even though no skull fracture or large intracranial vessel injury has occurred, damage to the brain may be such as to produce unconsciousness. Nevertheless, the prognosis for these injuries, i.e. those in which no laceration of the brain substance, and no massive contusion has taken place, should be good, provided that care is well organised and directed.

The aims of management

- Early detection of neurological deterioration
- Prevention of secondary cerebral insults
- Early treatment of concurrent medical and surgical problems

Hence immediate attention must be paid to the airway, breathing and circulation on admission, and if in doubt, the patient should be intubated. Institution of a reliable method of observation must commence immediately.

Assessment of conscious state

- the Glasgow coma scale
- the pattern of motor response to stimulation
- pupil reaction and size
- eye movements
- patterns of respiration

The Glasgow 'Coma' Scale

The Glasgow Coma Scale is now an internationally recognised system, and is reproduced below. 90% of patients with a score of 8 or less will be comatose, and a score of more than 8 is almost always associated with intact eye movements.

28. Monitoring the acute closed head injury

NAME:
Record No:

Time | Date:

COMA SCALE			Notes
	Eyes open	spontaneously	Eyes closed by swelling = C
		to speech	
		to pain	
		none	
	Best verbal response	orientated	Tracheal tube or tracheostomy = T
		confused	
		inappropriate	
		words/sounds	
		none	
	Best motor response	obey commands	Usually record the best arm response
		localise pain	
		flexion to pain	
		extension to pain	
		none	

Pupil scale (mm)	Blood pressure & Pulse rate	Temperature °C
1	240	41
2	220	40
3	200	39
4	180	38
5	160	37
6	140	36
7	120	35
8	100	34
	80	33
	60	32
	40	31
	Respiration 20	30

PUPILS			Notes
Right	size		+ = reacts
	reaction		– = no reaction
Left	size		c = eyes closed
	reaction		

LIMB MOVEMENT		Notes
ARMS	normal power	Record right (R) and left (L) seperately if there is a differance between the two sides.
	mild weakness	
	severe weakness	
	spastic flexion	
	extension	
	no response	
LEGS	normal power	
	mild weakness	
	severe weakness	
	extension	
	no response	

OBSERVATION CHART Institute of Neurological Sciences, Glasgow

28. Monitoring the acute closed head injury

Eye opening		
spontaneous	E	4
to speech		3
to pain		2
nil		1
Best Motor response		
obeys	M	6
localizes		5
withdraws		4
abnormal flexion		3
extensor response		2
nil		1
Verbal response		
orientated	V	5
confused conversation		4
inappropriate words		3
incomprehensible sounds		2
nil		1

Coma score (E + M + V) = 3 to 15

Motor response pattern

- hemiplegia
- bilateral or unilateral
- focal signs

Pupil reaction and size

- remember focal damage to globe or cranial nerves
- brainstem function
- depth of coma
- drugs – either systemic or local

Eye movements

- with head movement (oculocephalic)
- with caloric stimulation (oculovestibular)
- spontaneous

Respiratory pattern

- brainstem compression may produce disorders of:
  - ◊ respiratory pattern
  - ◊ heart rate and rhythm
  - ◊ blood pressure
    - i.e. Cushing's Triad

If observation along these lines reveals a deterioration in the patient's condition, the cause must be sought and action taken. As in all unconscious patients, it is essential to prevent hypoxia and hypocarbia, but in

the case of closed head injury, the need is so vital as to require intubation and ventilation in any patient whose Glasgow score is less than 8. Apart from hypoxia and hypercarbia, other factors which are less well understood may contribute to a rise in intracranial pressure (ICP). Such a rise is always deleterious, and many methods have been advocated in dealing with it, or preventing it, but none is as important as the preservation of blood gas homeostasis.
Measures which are advocated for the prevention/treatment of raised ICP are as follows (effectiveness of each is shown on a + / – scale)

Strategy	Effect	Comment
Posture	+++	supine
		30° head-up tilt
		head midline
		no obstruction to cerebral venous drainage
Controlled ventilation	++++	adequate sedation to suppress autonomic nervous system reflexes
Ventricular drainage	+++	aspirated acutely or 'overflow' continuous drainage
Mannitol	++++	initially, 0.25–0.5 g/kg + 0.25 g/kg 6 q6h
	+/-	later
		maintain Se Osm < 320 mosm/kg
Steroids	+/-	dexamethasone 0.1–0.25 mg/kg/dose q6h
Frusemide	+/-	0.1–1.0 mg/kg/hr continuous infusion
Barbiturates	+++	paroxysmal rises in ICP
	-	chronic intracranial hypertension
		requires extensive monitoring, there is a high incidence of complications and dubious evidence exists supporting a positive outcome

A serious additional insult is seizure activity. Even if the muscular component is controlled and the airway safeguarded during fits, there is still a substantial rise in cerebral oxygen consumption. Control of seizure activity is therefore always necessary. Acutely, thiopentone is the most effective drug (2 mg/kg), followed by midazolam in a titrated dose beginning with 1–2 mg i.v. Phenytoin is only suitable for long-term prophylaxis, and is useless in the management of active convulsions. Once this drug has been given, its administration must be controlled by serum estimations, and kept within the range of 40–80 mmol/l. Always keep in mind the possibility of hyponatraemia and pyrexia as contributing causes to seizures.

Significance of intracranial pressure level after head injury

Significance	ICP (mmHg)
normal	< 10
abnormal	> 10
further investigation	> 15
unequivocally raised	> 20
threshold for therapy	> 30
likelihood of mass	> 40

The existence of concurrent medical and (particularly) surgical problems demands attention if the head injury itself is to be managed successfully. For example, compound fractures of limbs must at the very least be immobilised, since the stimulation which otherwise occurs when the patient is moved will lead to rises in intracranial pressure. If abdominal or thoracic injuries are present they must be dealt with in the normal manner. In particular, visceral lesions which involve bleeding or perforation require urgent treatment, the priority for which takes second place only to drainage of an intracranial collection.

Chapter 29

Brain death

Sometimes the damage to the brain is such that survival is impossible although other systems may still be functioning with mechanical or pharmacological support. Cerebral death is consequent upon irreversible loss of brain function, rather than loss of cortical activity only. Death of the brain stem is a necessary and sufficient component of brain death, and brain death equates with death.

The victim's organs may, with appropriate consent, be harvested for transplantation. It is important that these opportunities of life for other patients not be denied and that expensive intensive care resources are not devoted to the futile maintenance of cardiopulmonary function in patients with no chance of cerebral recovery.

Absent cerebral function

The diagnosis of brain death requires that there is deep coma with cerebral unreceptivity and unresponsitivity. Confirmatory studies may demonstrate absence of cortical blood flow or supratentorial pulsation (ultrasound, angiography and nuclear studies). It is important to determine whether the brain is indeed dead or some other factors may be responsible for its depressed function. Some conditions may further depress an injured brain producing a deep coma-like state and must be excluded before a reliable diagnosis of brain death can be made.

These conditions are:

- drugs depressing cerebral function or muscle relaxants
- reversible metabolic or endocrine conditions
- hypothermia
- hypotension
- children have increased resistance to damage and greater potential for recovery than adults

Absent brain stem function

Reliable testing of brain stem reflexes requires a perceptive and experienced physician using adequate stimuli.

The following reflexes should be tested:

- pupillary light reflex
- corneal reflex
- oculocephalic reflex – doll's eye reflex
- oculovestibular reflex – caloric reflex
- oropharyngeal/laryngeal reflex – gag reflex
- carinal reflex – cough reflex
- respiratory apnoea reflex – absence of respiration with a $PaCO_2 > 60$ torr without hypoxia

The following findings may be confirmatory but not diagnostic:

- sustained ICP > systemic BP
- cranial skin temperature is considerably less than core temperature
- failure of the heart rate to respond to atropine

ALL of the above reflexes MUST reveal NO activity to pronounce the patient cerebrally dead. The time of death is denoted by the time the second examiner completes an examination which confirms brain stem death.

Persistent vegetative state

Persons with overwhelming damage to the cerebral hemispheres commonly pass into a chronic state of unconsciousness called the vegetative state in which the body cyclically awakens and sleeps but expresses no behavioural or cerebral metabolic evidence of possessing cognitive function or of being able to respond in a learned manner to external stimuli. Recovery from the vegetative state is possible, especially in the first few days or weeks after onset. A conservative criterion for the diagnosis of persistent vegetative state would be observed unawareness for at least 12 months, although cognitive recovery after six months is exceedingly rare in patients over 50 years of age.

The differences between brain death and the vegetative state are illustrated below:

Brain death	**Vegetative state**
irrecoverable brain damage	
no brain stem function	no cortical function (neocortical necrosis or white matter disconnection)
no respiration	spontaneous respiration
no brain stem reflexes	some brain stem reflexes
heart stops in days	may live weeks, months or years

A physician's determination that a patient is unlikely to regain consciousness is the usual prelude to deliberations about withdrawing or withholding life support. Once this issue has been raised, its legal and ethical dimensions must be considered.

Further reading

Hicks, RG. Torda, TA. Cerebral death. *Anaesthesia and Intensive Care*, 1979; 7: 169–173.
Jennett, B. (1981). Brain death. *British Journal of Anaesthesia*, 1981; 53: 1110–1119.
President's commission for the study of ethical problems in medicine, biomedical and behavioural research. Guidelines for the determination of death. *Critical Care Medicine*, 1982; 10: 62–65.

Chapter 30

Acute spinal injury

Introduction

- the annual incidence of spinal cord injury is 15–20 per million population.
- commonest causes of spinal injury are
  - ◊ road traffic accidents
  - ◊ domestic and industrial accidents
  - ◊ sporting injuries
  - ◊ assaults or self-harm
- any unconscious or intoxicated trauma patient must be considered at risk of spinal injury until proven otherwise.
- adequate immobilisation of the entire spine and avoidance of inadvertent manipulation are essential.

Pathophysiology

- corticospinal tract controls ipsilateral motor function and is tested by voluntary muscle contractions or involuntary response to pain.
- spinothalamic tract controls contralateral pain and temperature sensation. Posterior columns control ipsilateral proprioception tested for by vibration or joint position sense.
- autonomic injury leads to loss of bladder control, anal tone and priapism.
- reflexes may initially be reduced or absent, then subsequently increased below the level of a cord lesion.
- a complete spinal cord lesion is suspected in the absence of any sensory or motor function.
- an incomplete lesion may be followed by some recovery. Sacral sparing with preserved perianal or perineal sensation and reflexes may be the only initial sign.
- spinal shock is a transient dysfunction characterised by initial flaccidity and arreflexia, that is either replaced by restoration of function or the appearance of spasticity after days to weeks.
- neurogenic shock is hypotension with bradycardia associated with a cervical or high thoracic spinal cord injury, caused by damage to descending sympathetic nerves and loss of vasomotor tone.

Clinical features

- in conscious patients, ask about local pain, tenderness on palpation and associated limb weakness or sensory loss
- palpate for areas of tenderness, swelling or deformity, examining the entire spine by log-rolling the patient with suitable in-line cervical immobilisation.
- assess for limb weakness, reflex loss, sensory deficit and loss of saddle area sensation and anal tone.
- suspect a cervical cord lesion in any patient with respiratory difficulty, abdominal breathing, flaccid areflexia, hypotension with bradycardia and priapism.

Myotomes		Dermatomes		Reflex	
C5	shoulder abduction	**C5**	outer, upper arm		
C6,C7	shoulder adduction	**C6**	outer forearm		
C5,C6	elbow flexion	**C7**	middle finger		
C7	elbow extension	**C8**	inner forearm		
C6	pronation & supination	**T1**	inner, upper arm		
(C6),C7	wrist flexion	**T4**	nipple		
C6,(C7)	wrist extension	**T10**	umbilicus		
C8	finger flexion			**C5(C6)**	biceps
C7	finger extension			**(C5)C6**	supinator
T1	intrinsic hand muscles			**(C6) C7,C8**	triceps
L1,L2	hip flexion	**L3**	medial lower thigh & knee	**L3,L4**	knee
S1	hip extension	**L4**	medial calf	**L5,S1**	ankle
L5	knee flexion	**L5**	lateral calf		
L3,L4	knee extension	**S1**	lateral border foot & sole		
L5	ankle dorsiflexion				
S1	ankle plantar flexion				

Treatment

- total spinal immobilisation including semi-rigid cervical collar, head secured with tape and sandbags or on a spine board, thoracic and lumbar spine protection.
- hypoventilation requires urgent airway control by tracheal intubation and must if possible be performed by a skilled operator.
- restoration of circulatory volume looking for sources of blood loss in the presence of hypotension before diagnosing neurogenic shock.
- radiology:
    - ◊ lateral cervical spine as part of 'Trauma Series' X-rays in all multiple injury patients along with CXR and pelvis X-ray, once the resuscitation phase is underway (see Multiple Injuries, Chapter 31)
    - ◊ all seven cervical vertebrae and C7/T1 junction must be visualised
    - ◊ open-mouth and AP cervical spine views may be performed subsequently
    - ◊ thoracic and lumbar spine according to mechanism of injury and clinical findings
- early referral to orthopaedic, neurosurgical or spinal injury specialist
- spinal cord damage may be reduced by intravenous steroids such as high dose methyl prednisolone but their use is controversial.

Chapter 31

The patient with multiple injuries

Young adults in developed countries are more likely to die (or be severely disabled) as a result of major trauma than any other cause. Death as a result of trauma occurs during one of three periods:

- **Immediate**: the *primary insult* is so massive that it is incompatible with life. Such victims perish at the scene.
- **Intermediate**: the victim dies within the first few hours of the injury, mainly due to the primary insult but often hastened by *secondary insults*, such as cardiorespiratory arrest due to hypoxia resulting from airway obstruction as a result of unconsciousness associated with head injury or death due to hypovolaemia from blood loss after major pelvic and lower limb fractures. *Secondary insults* are often preventable if expert medical attention is given early.
- **Late**: this occurs weeks (or even longer) after the event and is most commonly the result of thromboembolism, sepsis or therapeutic withdrawal in the face of massive, irreversible neurological damage.

Trauma investigators refer to the '***golden hour***' as being the first hour after *injury* (timing does *not* start on arrival in hospital) when survival can be improved by preventing secondary insults with aggressive medical and surgical intervention.
Some surveys have found that up to half of those dying after trauma do so in the presence of untreated, potentially reversible conditions.

Philosophy of trauma management

- Deliver expert care to the patient as early as possible :
  - ◊ educate the public in first aid
  - ◊ form medic/paramedic teams to respond to emergency calls
  - ◊ form a coordinated regional policy for major and minor disaster management with a designated trauma centre(s)
- Assess all patients' condition rapidly and accurately.
- Determine the priorities for treatment using protocols.
- Provide emergency treatment to the patient(s) to resuscitate and stabilise the condition.
  - ◊ perform this on the basis of established priorities
  - ◊ use no drugs during the resuscitation phase except as part of a cardiopulmonary resuscitation regimen.
  - ◊ do no further harm
- Determine if a patient's needs are likely to exceed a facility's capabilities.
- Once the patient has been fully assessed and is stable, emergency treatment may be discontinued and definitive treatment arranged.
- Transfer the patient to an establishment with expertise to manage the patient's problems as early as possible.

Trauma centres are hospitals with resources to provide complete care to the victim of trauma. The minimum resident specialties are:

- accident and emergency
- anaesthesiology
- diagnostic radiology (CT)
- general, orthopaedic, thoracic and neuro- surgery

USA experience shows that survival is improved by treatment in a designated trauma centre. Because of their high cost, provision of these services is largely determined by population density and they are rare outside major cities. Where treatment is best provided will depend on balancing the distances involved against the patient's needs. In the rural community the patient is likely to be stabilised and given emergency treatment at a local hospital and then transferred to a trauma centre for definitive care. In the city, where distances are shorter, a local hospital may be bypassed in favour of the trauma centre.
A similar dilemma exists by the roadside: '*scoop and run*' (depart the scene as soon as possible) or '*wait and play*' (delay departure whilst resuscitation starts at the scene). An excessive delay at the scene may contribute to a bad outcome.
If the journey contemplated is long, the minimum requirements are

- a secure airway
- stable respiration
- commencement of resuscitation
- clinical assessment of all the major injuries

Assessment priorities

When assessing a trauma victim, the process used is different from the comprehensive techniques of classical history taking. Due to the serious nature of the patient's injuries information gathering must not hinder the process of treatment.

- The physician must learn a problem orientated approach, and actively seek evidence of life threatening processes and immediately treat them.
- Assessment is continuous, and the most serious problems are sought first.
- A process of ***continual reassessment*** will not only monitor the effectiveness of their treatment but also generate a detailed and comprehensive view of the patient's condition as different and progressively less threatening pathologies are identified.

A logical sequence of treatment priorities for each victim must be rapidly established based on information from the following sources:

- mechanism of injury (MOI)
- injuries present
- vital signs
- emergency investigations
- urgent investigations

The sequence of treatment phases is:

Primary survey: ABC

A – airway maintenance with cervical spine control

B – breathing and ventilation

- ◊ high flow O_2 therapy with ventilatory assistance as required
- ◊ therapeutic intervention in major thoracic trauma (chest drain)

C – circulation and haemorrhage control including

- ◊ insertion of large bore intravenous cannulae in each antecubital fossa and blood sampling (FBC, U & E, crossmatch)
- ◊ central venous access
- ◊ splint major fractures and apply pressure to bleeding points

D – disability: assess neurological status:
- ◊ **A**lert
- ◊ responds to **V**oice
- ◊ responds to **P**ain
- ◊ **U**nresponsive

E – exposure: completely undress the patient

Resuscitation phase

- replacement of lost vascular volume with warmed crystalloid fluids and blood
- control of haemorrhage
- continual reassessment of ABC
- placement of urinary catheter and nasogastric tube unless contraindicated

Secondary survey

This must not start until the primary survey is complete and resuscitation started
- look, feel, listen: evaluate the body in regions
- head to toe comprehensive examination
- carefully assess the history of the injury and the patient's past history
- continually re-evaluate the patient's progress and injuries
- special procedures (e.g. diagnostic peritoneal lavage) as indicated
- obtain CXR, lateral cervical spine X-ray (and other less important X-rays as indicated)
- rectal examination

Definitive care phase

- stabilisation in preparation for transfer
- management of all the injuries of the patient in a logical order

Triage

This is an ongoing process which organises the treatment priorities for a group of patients. It is based upon initial assessment of individual needs.
Two situations exist:
- The number of patients and the severity of their injuries do not exceed the treatment facility – the most severely injured are treated first.
- The number and severity of injuries exceed the capabilities of the unit – those with the greatest chance of survival, the least expenditure of time, equipment and supplies are managed first.

ABCs in multiple trauma

The importance and conduct of basic resuscitation in the management of trauma is no different from that performed elsewhere. Select simple techniques first, their inadequacy or otherwise indicating the need for alternative management.

Management priorities

Injury to the head and neck

Airway management

In the unconscious patient with a suspected cervical cord injury, the neck should be maintained in a neutral position. Emphasis is placed upon prevention of neurological damage by inadvertent neck movement during airway manipulations. The potential for neurological damage to the cervical cord is highest in patients with the most difficult airway problems (maxillofacial trauma) and those who may have most to gain from intubation (unconscious, head injured patients). In addition to difficulties caused by these factors *always assume that the stomach is full* and take steps to prevent aspiration of the stomach contents.

Neck injury *(refer p. 177)*

- spinal immobilisation is either:
  - ◊ a hard cervical collar with head taped to spinal board with sandbags either side or
  - ◊ manual in-line immobilisation (an assistant to fix the head).
- ATLS considers nasotracheal intubation is appropriate in the *breathing* patient with possible neck injury who requires intubation, but it is permissible to proceed with orotracheal intubation whilst stabilising the neck. If the view at laryngoscopy is inadequate *the neck should not be moved* and an alternative method should be chosen.

Maxillofacial trauma

- (full stomach) intubation choices are
  - ◊ rapid sequence induction
    - most dangerous: be prepared to perform emergency cricothyroidotomy, use with cricoid pressure
  - ◊ awake intubation
    - usually using a fibreoptic bronchoscope – difficult in the presence of oral debris
  - ◊ emergency / urgent / semi-elective surgical cricothyroidotomy safest option if someone with adequate expertise is present
- assume damage to the neck in all unconscious patients with significant injury above the clavicle
- only a specialist neurosurgeon, radiologist or orthopaedic surgeon should pronounce the neck normal from the lateral neck X-ray.

Head injury

This subject is covered more extensively in Chapter 28. Significant head injury is suspected from the MOI (index of suspicion), patient alertness (primary survey), repeated neurological testing (Glasgow Coma Scale – secondary survey), close inspection of the head (skull depression, CSF oto- and rhinorrhoea) and the presence of fracture on skull X-ray.

Thoracic trauma

Chest trauma results in death in about 25% of trauma cases. Many of these patients reach hospital alive. The majority of chest injuries (85%) can be managed by simple techniques (high inspired O_2, insertion of chest drains and supported ventilation) without the need for surgery and are therefore often managed at the trauma site or local hospital before transfer.

Clinical evaluation of chest trauma

- cyanosis (only present if circulating haemoglobin is high enough)
- tachypnoea and respiratory distress
- position of the trachea (deviated in tension pneumothorax)
- chest movement (especially uneven)
- auscultation and percussion in zones

The need for oxygen therapy

The fundamental feature of chest trauma is hypoxia due to disruption of the functional integrity of the respiratory apparatus. Even when the primary clinical condition is not immediately apparent oxygenation is improved and time 'bought' by administration of high flow (F_IO_2 > 85%) oxygen via a mask, valve and reservoir apparatus.

OXYGEN THERAPY SHOULD ALWAYS BE THE FIRST MANOEUVRE WHEN TREATING RESPIRATORY INSUFFICIENCY

Immediately life threatening chest injuries

The following injuries, if untreated, will result in death of the patient and should be identified and corrected during the primary survey:

- airway obstruction.
- tension pneumothorax
  - ◊ clinical diagnosis (suspect if unexplained hypotension not responding to fluid replacement and tracheal deviation)
  - ◊ decompression is by needle aspiration in the 2nd intercostal space, mid-clavicular line. Leave the needle in place
  - ◊ definitive treatment is subsequent chest drain insertion.
- open pneumothorax (sucking chest wound).
  - ◊ if the thoracic cavity is opened to atmospheric pressure with a hole larger than the trachea, air will be preferentially sucked into the chest cavity via the chest wall defect during inspiration
  - ◊ treatment is to seal the defect with an occlusive dressing followed by later drainage and definitive repair.
- Massive haemothorax
  - ◊ diagnosis: shock, absent breath sounds and a stony dull percussion note on one side of the chest
  - ◊ treatment: *rapid* resuscitation with i.v. fluid followed by type specific blood along with *simultaneous* insertion of a large (#38 F) chest drain in the midaxillary line at the level of the nipple for decompression
  - ◊ continuing loss >200 ml/hr : exploratory surgery is indicated.
- Flail chest
  - ◊ paradoxical movement of the chest wall can occur when large contiguous sections of ribs are fractured
  - ◊ always associated with underlying pulmonary contusion
  - ◊ treatment is supportive with high dose oxygen and often requires a period of artificial ventilation.
- Cardiac tamponade
  - ◊ usually results from a *penetrating* thoracic injury but also consider following blunt chest trauma where there are cardiac complexes without cardiac output
  - ◊ even small amounts of fluid within the pericardial sac cause disruption to cardiac function in such a way that *supra*normal venous filling pressures are required for adequate cardiac output
  - ◊ signs of shock, absent heart sounds and raised venous pressure are difficult to elicit in the emergency room especially after significant haemorrhage
  - ◊ echocardiography will diagnose this condition with confidence
  - ◊ the diagnosis will be made after diagnostic pericardiocentesis in a patient with chest trauma who has otherwise been adequately resuscitated but who remains shocked. Aspiration of only a few mls of pericardial fluid will cause immediate improvement in the patient's condition.

Other potential chest injuries to seek in the secondary survey

- pulmonary contusion
- myocardial contusion
- traumatic diaphragmatic hernia
- tracheobronchial disruption
- oesophageal disruption

Abdominal trauma

- prime site of concealed haemorrhage

In the acute phase of trauma management it is important to recognise those patients who will benefit from early exploratory laparotomy. It is of less importance to diagnose the specific abdominal injury.

Diagnosing abdominal injury

- **History:** blunt injury requires a high index of suspicion with regard to the degree and pattern of force to elicit the diagnosis of a disrupted viscus.
- **Inspection:** log roll the patient to visualise front to back to appreciate the route of a penetrating injury. Flank haematoma represents retroperitoneal bleeding from a pelvic fracture.
- **Palpation:** look for signs of unequivocal peritonism.
- **Percussion:** to elicit the rebound tenderness of *peritonism.*
- Rectal and vaginal examination must not be omitted.
- **Special tests:** CXR (air under diaphragm), nasogastric tube (blood aspirate or tip in chest on CXR).

Diagnostic peritoneal lavage (DPL)

- indications:
  - ◊ difficulty with the abdominal examination
    - ⊖ equivocal findings – with pain due to other injuries
    - ⊖ unreliable findings – intoxication, head injury or paraplegia
  - ◊ unexplained hypotension or blood loss.
- criteria for laparotomy after DPL
  - ◊ > 5ml blood (rbc count > 100,000 mm^{-3}) or enteric contents
  - ◊ lavage fluid exiting from chest tube or urinary catheter

Indications for early laparotomy

- blunt trauma
  - ◊ unequivocal peritoneal irritation
  - ◊ positive diagnostic peritoneal lavage (see above)
  - ◊ evidence of ruptured viscus (X-ray contrast studies)
- penetrating trauma
  - ◊ the nature of the wound and high incidence of visceral and vascular injury justifies a low threshold for intervention.
    - ⊖ gunshot wounds (all)
    - ⊖ stab wounds: selective laparotomy depending on the MOI (weapon, site and angle of entry) and the anatomy involved.
    - ⊖ lower chest wounds: penetrating chest injuries often involve the abdomen when entry is below the nipple (anteriorly) or the inferior tip of the scapula (posteriorly) (visceral damage occurs with 60% of gunshot wounds and 20% of stab wounds), but flank (20%) and back (10%) woundings have a lower incidence of visceral injury.

Haemorrhage from pelvic fractures

- mortality from major pelvic fractures is high.
- diagnosis: X-ray, clinical evidence of pelvic disruption (bony fragments felt on anal or vaginal examination) or systematic pelvic compression.
- management: resuscitation using crystalloid fluid and blood followed by exclusion of any other sites as the cause of ongoing blood loss.
  - ◊ a pneumatic antishock garment will stabilise most venous bleeding followed by later external fixation of the fractures.
  - ◊ peritoneal lavage catheter should be inserted above the umbilicus to avoid confounding contamination of peritoneal fluid by blood originating from pelvic fractures.
  - ◊ persistent bleeding is diagnosed by pelvic vessel arteriography and treated by embolisation of bleeding points.

Extremity trauma

With the exception of time spent immobilising major fracture sites to control pain and haemorrhage, most attention will be spent on the extremities in the secondary survey. It is particularly important to reduce and splint open fractures which otherwise remain a site of exsanguination. A tally of major limb fractures will give an estimate of revealed blood loss (important in searching for concealed loss).
Examination should be comprehensive with particular attention paid to limb threatening complications:

- interruption to the neurovascular bundle
- compartment syndrome

Wounds should be decontaminated, tetanus prophylaxis and antibiotic given.

Trauma in pregnancy

- foetal well being depends on maternal care
- signs of maternal shock may be reduced by the physiologically increased intravascular volume associated with pregnancy and the diversion of blood away from the uterus
- resuscitation and monitoring should occur with the patient lying on her side, or supine with a wedge placed under her right hip to prevent aortocaval compression
- high potential for foetal distress; foetal monitoring should be with a foetal heart monitor
- vaginal bleeding should alert the physician to the need for urgent obstetric assessment of the mother and foetus.

Paediatric trauma

Paediatric injuries are managed identically to those that occur in adults, however the patient's size and altered physiology must be taken into account during resuscitation. Multiple trauma has implications for future developmental potential in children and careful management in the initial hours will lessen the physical, psychological and social impact of the injury.

Pattern of injury

- blunt trauma is common, with falls and motor vehicle accidents accounting for over 80% of Western paediatric injuries. Children represent a small target resulting in concentration of forces and intense application of energy
- multiple organ injuries are common because the child's skeleton is incompletely calcified and although resilient to applied stress there is a higher prevalence of underlying internal organ damage (pulmonary contusion is more common than rib fracture).

Venous access

- preferred siting of venous infusions:
  - ◊ percutaneous
  - ◊ internal jugular vein
  - ◊ cutdown on
    - great saphenous at the ankle
    - median cephalic at elbow
    - main cephalic higher in the arm
  - ◊ Long bone intraosseous infusion (never distal to a fracture)
    - anterior tibial plateau
    - inferior third of femur

Fluid resuscitation

Normal blood volume is approximately 80ml/kg and shock may only become clinically manifest once 25% of the blood volume has been lost

- signs: tachycardia, hypotension on tilt test, lethargy and reduced consciousness, cold extremities with decreased capillary refill
- resuscitation commences with 20 ml/kg haemaccel solution given up to three times followed by 10 ml/kg packed red cells if clinically indicated
- children requiring this degree of resuscitation should be investigated urgently for a site of concealed haemorrhage.

Head injury

- children < 3 years have worse outcomes from severe head injury than older children and should be managed aggressively with particular attention to preventing secondary brain injury from hypoxia and hypovolaemia.
- infants may become hypotensive due to blood loss from a scalp injury or underlying extradural haematoma, especially with skull fracture.
- bulging fontanelle or sutural diastasis indicate raised intracranial pressure and severe head injury.
- intracranial pressure monitoring should be used in patients with severe head injury or those undergoing surgery for other conditions.

Chapter 32

Acute poisoning

A poison is any substance that causes harm to an organism. Poisons can be of animal, mineral or vegetable origin. The term 'acute poisoning' should replace the term 'drug overdose', with its pejorative connotations.

Poisoning may be

- accidental
  - ◊ small child
  - ◊ adolescent seeking unusual experience
  - ◊ iatrogenic – miscalculated or inappropriate therapy
- deliberate (self poisoning)

Acute poisoning is always an emergency. It may present an opportunity to assist the patient to find stronger coping mechanisms. The medical practitioner should not eschew this opportunity.

Diagnosis

- assess ABC first
- has anything been ingested?
- how much has been ingested?
- when was it ingested?
- is it important?

High index of suspicion

think of poisoning if :

- drowsiness, hypoventilation, hypotension
- convulsions
- hyperventilation
- haematemesis
- ulcerated mouth
- extrapyramidal signs
- hallucinations

Course of management

- most recover with observation
- serious poisoning requires intensive supportive therapy
- few require essential antidotes
- initial resuscitation THEN specific treatment of the poisoning

Identification of the poison(s)

- **ask the victim while still conscious**
- ask ambulance officers, relatives
- check for any notes, empty bottles (note: often a number of bottles arrive with the patient, which may or may not be related to the ingested drug)
- avoid self-contamination
  - ◊ clothing, skin with organophosphorous insecticides
  - ◊ mouth (mouth to mask or mouth to nose ventilation)
  - ◊ exhaled breath (carbon monoxide, poison gas)
- urine and stomach contents may be analysed to screen for paracetamol and benzodiazepines
- specific blood levels can be obtained if the drug is known, but screening for drugs is usually limited to urine, as protein causes too much interference with analysis
- dry chemistry has enabled a rapid and accurate assessment of theophylline levels allowing appropriate early institution of charcoal haemoperfusion.

Differential diagnosis of an altered conscious state

- acute poisoning
- intracranial disease – alcohol and extradural
- metabolic disturbance
  - ◊ hyponatremia
  - ◊ hypo/hyperglycaemia
- hypothermia
  - ◊ often associated with poisoning because of
    - exposure
    - vasodilatation
    - central nervous system depression
    - decreased basal metabolic rate

Prevention (advice to patients/parents)

- identify, dispose of unwanted poisons and storage of poisonous substances in a locked cupboard
  - ◊ in original containers
- use non-poisonous alternatives
- insist on 'child proof' packaging of medicines
- protect yourself against environmental hazards – protective clothing, masks with insecticide sprays, painting, cleaning oven

First aid

- remain with the victim
- call for help
- seek advice from
  - ◊ Poisons Information Centre
  - ◊ Hospital Emergency Department
  - ◊ Ambulance service
  - ◊ the victim's local medical practitioner

Basic life support

- the initial conscious state may change rapidly
- the first four things to worry about are:
  - the airway
  - the airway
  - the airway
  - the airway

then

- ◊ breathing – pattern, rate, depth
- ◊ circulation

Advanced life support

The 'V.I.P.' approach is a functional method of dealing with overdose:

- Ventilate
  - ◊ protect the airway,
  - ◊ assist ventilation if there is an altered conscious state
- Infuse
  - ◊ establish intravenous access
  - ◊ volume load
  - ◊ inotropic support may be needed
- Pump
  - ◊ assess circulatory status, and follow CPR protocol
- V.I.P. – the 'very important pause'
  - ◊ reassess,
  - ◊ evaluate the success of current management
  - ◊ identify the underlying problems

Specific therapy

Management of acute poisoning involves initial assessment and resuscitation of the patient, then actions directed at the poison itself. There are four main approaches:

- decrease absorption of poison
- increase excretion of poison
- altered metabolism of the poison
- administer specific antidote(s)

It is helpful to identify poisons for which there are specific antidotes or methods of treatment, as early intervention may be life-saving.

Decrease absorption

- identify sources of exposure
  - ◊ skin
  - ◊ gastrointestinal tract
  - ◊ eyes
  - ◊ lungs
  - ◊ parenteral (needlestick)

- remove clothing and wash skin (avoid contact to self)
  - ◊ topical exposure (organophosphorous insecticides)
  - ◊ *do not give water to drink*
    - may increase absorption
    - increases danger of aspiration
  - ◊ activated charcoal
    - palatable if mixed with a cola drink
    - 50g immediately, then 50g four-hourly
    - has replaced Ipecac as the first line treatment of most acute poisonings.

Increase excretion

- emesis (induced vomiting) – controversial therapy
  - ◊ 6% syrup of ipecacuanha 1–2 ml/kg
  - ◊ contraindicated
    - if unconscious, drowsy, fitting
    - if the following has been swallowed:
      acids
      caustic alkalis (e.g. household cleaners)
      petroleum products (kerosene)
      camphor or strychnine (cause convulsions)
      small disk batteries
- gastric lavage
  - ◊ needs a controlled environment with full resuscitation facilities by someone who is properly trained in airway management.
  - ◊ within 1 hour of ingestion.
- faecuresis – induced diarrhoea – doubtful value
- diuresis – potentially dangerous and of limited value, and is no longer recommended
- haemodialysis/charcoal haemoperfusion – restricted to specific substances

Altered metabolism of the poison

- competitive inhibition of metabolism reducing the production of toxic metabolites – e.g. ethyl alcohol administration for methanol overdose
  - ◊ also requires emergency charcoal haemoperfusion
  - ◊ if the blood methanol level is greater than 500mg/l or
  - ◊ the minimal lethal dose of 30 ml has been ingested and acidosis, visual or mental disturbances are present

Specific antidote

A number of specific and non-specific antidotes exist. In some cases, it is better to provide supportive therapy only. In others, the specific antidote may be life-saving, but must be given within a specified time period of acute exposure to a poison.

Examples include:

- digoxin-binding antibodies (Fab fragments)
- N-acetyl-cysteine for paracetamol
- glucagon for β-blockers
- vitamin K, FFP for warfarin
- protamine for heparin

- naloxone for opioids
- flumazenil for benzodiazepines
- pralidoxime for organophosphorous insecticides
- physostigmine for central anticholinergic syndrome
- sodium thiosulphate for cyanide
- benztropine for extrapyramidal side effects
- glucose for insulin

Relative efficacy of haemodialysis

Effective	Relatively ineffective	Ineffective
alcohols chloral hydrate salicylates phenobarbitone theophylline antibiotics inorganic phosphates	meprobamate phenytoin lithium glutethimide methaqualone procaineamide	digoxin amphetamines tricyclics phenothiazines chloroquine paraquat butyrophenones

Central anticholinergic syndrome

Drug group	Example
antidepressants	tricyclic antidepressants
antipsychotics	thioridazine
antihistamines	promethazine
antiparkinsonian	beztropine
belladonna alkaloids	scopolamine
ophthalmic preparations	atropine 1%
antispasmodics	propantheline
proprietary preparations	
toxic plants	morning glory

Drugs removed by exchange transfusion

- antihistamines
- heavy metals
- alcohols
- barbiturates
- quinine

Part IV

Topics

Related to

Emergency Care of Recreational Injury

Chapter 33

Abnormalities of thermal regulation

Basic physiology

Thermoregulation is a balance between

Heat GAIN	Heat LOSS
Endogenous	Environmental
Environmental	Conduction
	Convection
	Radiation
	Evaporation.

Heat GAIN

- basal metabolism (40 cal/meter^2/hour)
- heat production
  - ◊ muscle tone/muscle activity (shivering)
  - ◊ sympathetic activity (neural, circulating catecholamines – uncoupled oxidative phosphorylation)
  - ◊ hormones – thyroxine – slow adaptation
- environmental
  - ◊ absorption of heat energy from surroundings

Heat LOSS

- Conduction / Convection 15%
  - ◊ conduction to air is not efficient
  - ◊ conduction to water is extremely efficient
- Radiation 60%
- Evaporation (sweating) 25%

Fanning is efficient if used with evaporation of water.

Evaporation of 1 gram water provides heat loss of 0.58 cal (1 cal = 1 Kcal = 4.184 Kilojoules). Therefore, evaporation of the normal adult insensible water losses (600ml/day) results in a daily heat loss of 350 cal.

Sweating is the only physiological method of heat loss when environmental temperature exceeds body temperature. The maximum achievable heat loss by this mechanism is supposedly 2000 cal/hour (4 litres/hour).

Humans are designed to lose heat efficiently, NOT to conserve heat.

Normal rectal temperature

[up to 40] °C	Hard exercise
[39]	Emotion/moderate exercise
[38]	Some normal adults, many active children
[37]	Usual normal range.
[36]	
[35]	Early morning, cold weather.

Normal temperature is increased by up to 0.5°C at time of ovulation

Body temperature

- core – rectal, auditory meatus, (most accurate central venous blood temp)
- average body temperature: [(0.7 * CORE) + (0.3 * SURFACE)]
- distribution of body temperature depends on surface perfusion.

Temperature regulation is a **dominant** mechanism and will over-ride other reflexes i.e. a centrally heated individual with depletion of blood volume will vasodilate and sweat until further depletion produces a shock state.

Neural control of thermoregulation is via
- hypothalamic center acting as a thermostat. ('factory preset' to 36 –37°C)
- skin receptors
- local mechanisms

Thermoregulation during anaesthesia

- All general anaesthetics produce a linear dose-dependent decrease in core temperature (3°C/ % isoflurane)
- in adults nonshivering thermogenesis has minimal effect but in infants the activation of brown fat energy stores doubles the metabolic rate which may result in heat stress and hypoglycaemia
- general anaesthesia also impairs sweating and active vasodilation
- deviations within 4°C of normal are accurately sensed during anaesthesia but the thermoregulatory response is not triggered

Hypothermia

Why

- patient uncovered, environment 20°C
- anaesthesia causes vasodilatation
- lungs ventilated with dry, cold gases
- skin prepared with cold antiseptic
- heat loss from evaporation from surgical incision

Pattern

- rapid phase of cooling (1°C in 30 min) due to redistribution of heat from the core to the surface
- the slow, linear decrease due to heat loss exceeding heat production (1°C/hr) and stabilises after 3–4 hours
- thermoregulatory vasoconstriction of peripheral tissues maintains core temperature but peripheral heat loss (energy) continues

Effects

- 2–3°C of hypothermia provides marked protection against tissue ischaemia and hypoxaemia but has complications
    - ◊ prolonged drug action
    - ◊ coagulopathy
    - ◊ negative nitrogen balance (decrease wound healing, increase muscle wasting)
    - ◊ shivering
    - ◊ increased stress response to surgery, increasing catabolism

Monitoring

- skin surface temperature is not clinically meaningful and does not confirm a putative diagnosis of malignant hyperthermia
- central temperature measurement may be rectal, oesophageal, nasopharyngeal, urinary bladder

Prevention

- limit heat loss by
    - ◊ warm operating environment
    - ◊ covering the patient (90% of heat lost from skin surface) decreases heat loss by 30%
    - ◊ Bair Hugger® – forced air transfer of heat increases mean body temperature by 1.5°C/hr
    - ◊ warm i.v. fluids – 1 litre of fluid at ambient temperature decreases mean body temperature by 0.25°C
    - ◊ heat-and-moisture exchangers and humidifiers prevent tracheal damage but do not prevent hypothermia

Shivering

- complications
    - ◊ 200–500% increase in metabolic rate
    - ◊ increased intracranial and intraocular pressures
    - ◊ increased pain
- shivering can be prevented by maintaining normothermia
- shivering associated with regional anaesthesia is a response to hypothermia and heat redistribution and demonstrates the typical waxing and waning pattern of cold hypothermia
- shivering can be suppressed with i.v. pethidine or clonidine

Environmental hypothermia

Introduction

Hypothermia is a condition in which there is a body core temperature ≤35°C
Hypothermia is common and its onset is insidious.
It results from any situation in which heat loss exceeds heat production:

- immersion in cold water
- inadequate protection from cold environment, especially when combined with high altitude, wind, moisture and physical exhaustion (the 'wind chill' factor)
- immobilisation and exposure to cold; the unconscious, the young, the elderly, the seriously ill, the drugged, the seriously injured including major burns and spinal cord injuries.

Hypothermia should be expected in any first aid situation where a victim has been immersed or immobilised.

Prevention (advice to the public)

On land

- education and training
- adequate protection by appropriate clothing
- physical activity
- adequate food and water intake
- adequate shelter
- avoiding exhaustion.

In water

- wearing a life jacket
- wearing as much clothing as possible, especially over the head
- keeping still
  - ◊ exercise hastens cooling in water ≤20°C
  - ◊ treading water will increase the rate of cooling 30% faster than keeping still in a life jacket
  - ◊ swim only if certain of reaching safety
  - ◊ adopting a Heat Escape Lessening Posture (HELP) if a flotation device is available.

Recognition

- initially non-specific with abnormal behaviour and a deterioration in mental and physical performance
- the victim is cold to touch and pale.
- ≤30°C there is a risk of cardiac dysrhythmias which may progress to cardiac arrest
- if unconscious, respiration and pulse may be difficult to detect and the victim may be wrongly diagnosed as dead
- resuscitation must be continued until the victim is rewarmed
  - ◊ hypothermia protects the brain from oxygen deprivation and full recovery has been reported following prolonged and profound hypothermia, particularly in children
- the clinical picture may be complicated by the cause of the unconsciousness from other causes (drug overdose, exposure, medical or surgical conditions)

Management

- if unconscious, maintain care of the Airway, Breathing and Circulation
- check for local cold injury
- do not elevate the head if cerebral perfusion pressure is low
- prevention of further body cooling
- slow rewarming
  - ◊ as a rough 'rule of thumb', rewarming should not exceed 1°C per hour
  - ◊ if a warming blanket is used it should be less than 3°C above skin temperature to prevent skin burns
- **Do not give alcohol**.
  - ◊ it impairs shivering (heat production)
  - ◊ dilates blood vessels (heat loss)
  - ◊ alters the victim's conscious state
- inotropic support with dopamine and adrenaline have both been shown to be effective in the presence of profound hypothermia.

Hyperthermia

Causes

- malfunction of thermostat itself
- bacterial/viral pyrogens
- tissue injury/breakdown
- excessive external gain plus inadequate loss – as in 'fun runs'
- excessive production plus inadequate loss
- dehydration.

AT OVER 41°C – CELLS BEGIN TO DIE

Artificial cooling is **only** effective if heat loss exceeds heat production and can be potentially **harmful.**

- Vasoconstriction will increase peripheral vascular resistance and may result in:
  - ◊ hypertension (increase afterload)
  - ◊ left ventricular decompensation
  - ◊ pulmonary vascular congestion
  - ◊ pulmonary oedema
- Increased heat production (shivering) increases oxygen consumption by up to 500%.

Cooling

- fanning alone
  - ◊ inefficient and can result in increased core temperature
- fanning with evaporation – more useful
- application of ice-packs
- cooling mattress
- lavage with cold water
  - ◊ gastric
  - ◊ peritoneal
  - ◊ rectal
- drugs (aspirin).

With surface cooling vasoconstriction simply prevents heat conduction to the surface and ***core temperature may increase!***

Shivering uses energy and may maintain temperature, therefore additional measures may be required:

- chlorpromazine ± thiopentone may be given to alter the central response and produce vasodilatation.
- artificial cooling in the conscious individual will produce normal reflexes, which include the severe discomfort associated with the sensation of cold and sedation may be required for the person's comfort.

Malignant hyperthermia

- malignant hyperthermia (MH) is due to abnormal skeletal muscle cell Ca^{++} metabolism and is not an abnormality of temperature control per se but results in heat production which outstrips heat loss mechanisms
- incidence 1:250,000 anaesthetics, but 1:60,000 if suxamethonium is used and has a fulminant mortality of 10%
- characterised by marked temperature elevation, muscle rigidity, oxygen consumption and carbon dioxide production
- 50% autosomal dominant, 3% associated with a myopathy, 20% multifactorial
- in vitro testing of biopsied muscle to halothane and caffeine
- triggers – volatile agents, suxamethonium,
- treatment – give O_2, dantrolene sodium i.v., bicarbonate, cooling, antidysrhythmics

Heat stroke

Precipitating factors

- environmental
  - ◊ air temperature
  - ◊ radiant heat
  - ◊ humidity
- excessive or unaccustomed activity
- dehydration
- heavy dark clothing
- infection
- extremes of age
- drug

First aid management

- rapid and effective cooling
  - ◊ remove clothing
  - ◊ ice packs, air conditioning, ice water bath
- correct hypovolaemia and electrolyte imbalance
  - ◊ use electrolyte supplemented drinks

Hospital management

- oxygen ± IPPV
- invasive CVS monitoring in the elderly
- anticonvulsants
- watch for hypoglycaemia
- cease cooling at a core temperature of 39°C

Avoidance in endurance sport

- observe for exhaustion, dehydration, salt depletion, hypothermia (water sports) and hyperthermia (athletics)
- pre-event acclimatisation
- complete event before 10.30 a.m. and in cooler months
- never participate after recent viral illness

Chapter 34

Envenomation

Envenomation is acute poisoning due to exposure to biological toxins and results in a broad range of symptoms, ranging from mild acute illness to death.

Pressure immobilisation

This technique is recommended for the treatment of land and sea snake bite and the majority of other bites and stings.

It is NOT used for envenomation by:

- red back spider, scorpions, centipedes.
- venomous fish – stone fish, bullrout, stingrays.

Snake venom is transported from the site of envenomation (bite) via the lymphatics to the bloodstream. Animal research has shown that pressure applied over the bitten area markedly retards venom spread. Some inactivation of venom and venom components occurs when the injected venom remains in the vicinity of the injured site. Furthermore, lymph production and transport is considerably decreased with immobilisation.

The pressure immobilisation technique

- first – apply firm local pressure over the site of envenomation
- then, apply a firm bandage to the affected limb, preferably crepe:
  - ◊ initially around the limb over the bitten area and then down to the fingers/toes, returning to cover as much of the limb as possible. Apply as tightly as for a sprained ankle.
- splint or otherwise immobilise the limb
- keep the victim at rest and do not remove clothes unnecessarily
- bring transport to the victim if possible
  - ◊ muscle movement in the affected limb facilitates lymph production and spread of venom.

Precursors for management

- 70% of bites are to the limbs
- if the bandage and splints are applied correctly, there will be no discomfort and they can be left on for many hours. There is time to reach help in all but the most unusual circumstances.
- if a crepe bandage is not available, improvise by using any material that can be torn into wide strips.
- when alone, the victim should apply pressure to the bitten area and proceed to seek help.

Most deaths are preventable if the rescuer

- keeps the victim under constant observation
- gives basic life support if indicated
- applies pressure immobilisation
- seeks prompt medical care.

Cause of death with snake bite

- geographical isolation
- inadequate observation
- massive sudden envenomation – venous strike
- wrong antivenom given
- correct antivenom – INADEQUATE quantity.

Snake bite

- 120 snake species in Australia, 20 of which are venomous
- 200 antivenom administrations per year
- snake bite mortality, 5 patients per year
- untreated effective taipan bite has 100% mortality
- untreated tiger snake bite has a 45% mortality

Snake venom

contains varying amounts of

- neurotoxins
  - ◊ cause pre-synaptic blockade preventing acetylcholine recycling
- coagulants
  - ◊ prothrombin is converted to thrombin resulting in a secondary afibrinogenaemia
- haemolysins
  - ◊ cause platelet lysis and disseminated intravascular coagulopathy
- rhabdomyolysins
- enzymes – hyaluronidase, phospholipase A, myotoxins, cytotoxins

Snake identification

- snake markings and their recall are unreliable
- snakes are mostly nocturnal
- Enzyme Linked Immuno-sorbent Assay (ELISA)
  - ◊ produces accurate venom identification using washings from the bite, blood or urine in 40 minutes

Antivenom

- a real or suspected snake bite is SERIOUS
- antivenom is indicated with
  - ◊ regional lymph node tenderness
  - ◊ systemic envenomation
- polyvalent antivenom is safer than the WRONG specific monovalent antivenom

Signs and symptoms of snake bite

- bite
  - ◊ scratch marks, multiple punctures, may be painless, little local reaction
- envenomation
  - ◊ headache, nausea, abdominal pain, regional lymph node tenderness
- late signs
  - ◊ ptosis, double vision, dysarthria, dysphagia, muscle weakness
- advanced signs
  - ◊ semi-comatose, ventilatory failure, haemorrhage, renal failure

Laboratory investigations

- urine – myoglobin, venom detection
- blood – cross-match, coagulation profile, creatinine, urea, electrolytes
- ECG

First aid

- pressure immobilisation
- DO NOT WASH, CUT OR APPLY A TOURNIQUET
- reassure, safe transport, alert hospital

Hospital management

- assessment of Airway, Breathing and Circulation
- history, signs of envenomation and ELISA diagnosis
- LEAVE bandage and splint for as long as possible
- diluted specific antivenom infusion over 30 minutes
- give additional doses for ongoing envenomation before transfusion
- supportive therapy
  - ◊ plasma volume expansion
  - ◊ correct coagulopathy
  - ◊ acute renal failure protocol
  - ◊ tetanus prophylaxis ± antibiotics

Sequelae

- most recover completely
- equine immunoglobulin sensitivity
- isolated neurological or ophthalmological symptoms remain for months
- major organ failure retards recovery and is proportional to the degree of envenomation

Pitfalls of management

- fang marks may not be visible
- rapid bandage release may give massive systemic envenomation
- slightest doubt regarding snake identity, use polyvalent antivenom
- early paralysis may be missed if victim is asleep
- be prepared for anaphylaxis and acute renal failure

Coelenterate envenomation

Portuguese man-o'-war, hair jellyfish, hydroids, coral

Symptoms and sign of envenomation

- pain of varying severity
- weals from blue bottles are white in the centre with beading effect and with hair jellyfish, the weals are irregular and white with red zigzag lines
- burning and itching
- nausea, headache, vomiting
- abdominal pain and joint pains.

First aid

- rescue and restrain the victim from rubbing the stung area
- monitor Airway, Breathing and Circulation and commence resuscitation if necessary
- remove tentacles using water and apply ice to relieve pain – review after 10–15 minutes and if pain persists, re-apply ice
- seek medical help, if pain is not relieved by ice or other symptoms develop.

Box jellyfish, irukandji, jimble, fire jelly fish

Symptoms and signs of envenomation

- immediate severe pain
- irrational behaviour
- cessation of breathing
- frosted ladder pattern is characteristic
- cardiovascular collapse.

First aid

- rescue and restrain the victim
- douse the sting area with vinegar
  - ◊ vinegar prevents further stinging (tissue damage) but does NOT relieve pain, nor reverse the effects of the venom
- do not leave the victim, even if conscious
  - ◊ observe the victim's conscious state, airway, breathing and circulation – commence resuscitation if necessary. This takes priority
- apply pressure immobilisation over as much of the vinegar treated sting area as possible but NOT the untreated area
- send for ambulance, medical assistance and box jellyfish antivenom
- keep the victim still to lessen absorption of venom and immobilise bandaged limbs with splints
- apply ice to relieve pain and review after 10–15 minutes

If vinegar is not available:
- apply pressure immobilisation only ABOVE the sting
- pull off any adherent tentacles with fingers – the skin of the rescuer's fingers is too thick to permit penetration of nematocysts.

Mollusc envenomation

Blue-ringed octopus, cone shell

Symptoms and signs

- cone shell – severe pain
- blue-ringed octopus – may be painless
- numbness of lips and tongue
- progressive weakness of muscles of respiration leading to cessation of breathing.

Management

- stay with the victim
- observe for signs of breathing difficulty
- commence expired air resuscitation – may have to be continued for up to 8 hours
- apply pressure immobilisation and keep victim still

Fish envenomation

Stonefish, bullrout, stingray, cobblers

Symptoms and signs

- intense pain
- swelling
- grey/blue discoloration
- sometimes an open wound
- irrational behaviour and panic

Management

- to relieve pain, place the stung hand or foot in water as warm as the victim can tolerate taking care not to burn the patient
- the pain may require local anaesthetic infiltration for relief
- antivenom is available
- do NOT apply pressure immobilisation as this will result in tissue destruction.

Stingrays

- most wounds occur on the lower limbs but trunckal wounding may be associated with penetrative damage to internal organs
- wounds require thorough cleansing and tetanus prophylaxis
- two deaths have been reported following penetration of the heart

Arthropod envenomations

Bees, wasps, ants

Symptoms and signs

- painful red swelling – the sting may be visible
- allergic symptoms
    - ◊ itchy rash
    - ◊ puffy eyelids
    - ◊ wheezing and difficulty in breathing

First aid

- do not pull the bee's sting out with finger and thumb because this may cause further injection of venom from the gland attached to the sting. Brush or scrape the bee sting off sideways with a finger nail or a knife blade.
- apply ice compress to relieve pain
- if the victim has a history or any signs of allergy:
    - ◊ apply pressure immobilisation
    - ◊ seek urgent medical care

Spiders

Funnel web (atrax Robustus)

- large and aggressive, male venom 5 times more toxic than female
- venom contains
    - ◊ atraxotoxin which causes acetylcholine release
    - ◊ hyaluronidase
    - ◊ gamma aminobutyric acid

Symptoms and signs

- immediate fasciculation in bite vacinity
- general fasciculation, salivation and lachrymation
- hypertension, tachycardia and dysrhythmias
- hypoventilation and coma
- later – pulmonary oedema

First aid

- apply pressure immobilisation, and transport to hospital
- keep the victim at rest and under constant observation
- commence CPR as necessary.
- antivenom is available and should be used if any respiratory difficulty
- atropine, midazolam

Red back spider, scorpions and centipedes

- female is venomous
- related to the black widow and katipo spiders
- non-aggressive, 22% of bites to genitalia
- serious in the young, frail or elderly

Symptoms and signs

- immediate pain at bite site
- sweating, nausea and headache
- abdominal pain, pyrexia, hypertension

First aid

- apply an ice compress to lessen the pain
- antivenom is available
- pressure immobilisation is not used because the venom acts slowly and any attempt to retard its movement tends to increase local pain.

Ticks

Symptoms and signs

- local irritation
- lethargy, muscle weakness (especially in children), unsteady gait
- diplopia, dysphagia
- symptoms develop over several days

Tick removal

- do not squeeze the tick, because even gentle traction may precipitate further release of venom
- slide the open blades of a pair of sharp, pointed tweezers, one on each side of the tick, and lever it outwards
- check the ears, the waist line, the groin, axilla and hair for other ticks
- a severe allergic reaction and cardio-respiratory collapse can occur
    - ◊ give basic life support and antivenom

Chapter 35

Effects of altitude

High altitude is usually > 3000 metres. A spectrum of illness due to hypobaric hypoxia ranges from acute mountain sickness to high altitude cerebral oedema, high altitude pulmonary oedema and high altitude retinal haemorrhage. Other problems related to a mountain environment include hypothermia, frostbite, trauma, lightning injury, ultraviolet keratitis, dehydration and venous thrombo-embolism.

Pathophysiology

- hypoxia in the setting of too rapid ascent in unacclimatised persons
- poor ventilatory response with inadequate ventilation and failure of salt and water homeostasis with fluid retention
- pulmonary vasoconstriction and pulmonary hypertension
- cerebral hypoxia and vasodilatation
- generalised capillary fragility

Acute mountain sickness (AMS)

- predisposed to by exertion, dehydration, alcohol, sedative drugs and continued rapid ascent.
- symptoms: headache, insomnia, anorexia, nausea, dizziness and dyspnoea.
- usually benign: responds to stopping for 24 hours or further acclimatisation or descent. Supplemental oxygen, simple analgesics and acetazolamide (also used for prophylaxis) may help.

High altitude cerebral oedema (HACE)

- life-threatening – affects 1–2% people > 3,500 metres
- progressive neurological deterioration with altered mental status, ataxia, stupor, coma, even death.
- mandates immediate descent, supplemental oxygen, acetazolamide and steroids may help (dexamethasone).
- new, lightweight, portable hyperbaric pressure bags.

High altitude pulmonary oedema (HAPE)

- affects up to 15% people > 3,000 metres.
- develops as progression of AMS or appears rapidly as an isolated respiratory disorder. Causes cough, fever, cyanosis, tachypnoea and tachycardia.
- pink, frothy sputum and haemoptysis, dyspnoea.
- mandates immediate descent, supplemental oxygen, frusemide, IPPV. Recent reports of nifedipine as a pulmonary vasodilator.
- portable hyperbaric pressure bags limited by claustrophobia and inability to lie flat.

High altitude retinal haemorrhage (HARH)

- relatively common and benign.
- small, flame-shaped retinal haemorrhages.
- descent recommended if central, macular vision affected, but otherwise self limiting, disappearing within weeks.

Chapter 36

Decompression illness

Introduction

Over 150 deaths in professional and recreational divers reported in Australasia between 1980–1989 due to drowning, pulmonary barotrauma and air embolism. Chronic lung disease, history of pneumothorax and obstructive lung disease particularly asthma should disqualify potential divers. Traditional classification of decompression illness has been end-organ based:

- barotrauma to air-containing cavities
  - ◊ ears, sinuses
  - ◊ equipment – mask compression
  - ◊ pulmonary
    - pneumothorax
    - surgical emphysema
    - pneumomediastinum
- cerebral arterial gas embolism (CAGE)
- decompression sickness
  - ◊ mild
    - musculoskeletal pain
    - cutaneous
    - lymphatic
  - ◊ serious
    - neurological
    - cardiopulmonary
    - audiovestibular

An alternative classification is temporal and descriptive:

- evolution
  - ◊ progressive
  - ◊ static
  - ◊ spontaneously improving
  - ◊ relapsing
- manifestation
  - ◊ pain: musculoskeletal, girdle
  - ◊ neurological, audiovestibular, cardiopulmonary, cutaneous lymphatic, constitutional
- additional information
  - ◊ presence of barotrauma
  - ◊ inert gas burden
  - ◊ response to treatment
  - ◊ investigations

Pathophysiology

- barotrauma refers to tissue injury resulting from a gas-filled body space failing to equalise its internal pressure to corresponding changes in ambient pressure.
- decompression sickness refers to liberation of inert gas from solution forming bubbles, with vascular or lymphatic obstruction and activation of inflammatory mediators.

Clinical

- symptoms can occur during, immediately after, within hours and up to two days following a dive.
- joint pains, fatigue, rashes, chest pain, dyspnoea, motor and sensory losses, labyrinthine disturbance, deafness, fits, confusion or coma may occur.
- tension pneumothorax and cardiac dysrhythmias may be immediately life-threatening.

Treatment

- oxygen
- pneumothorax drainage
- intravenous rehydration and mild analgesia (do not give opiates)
- every patient within 48 hours of a dive developing any symptoms or signs however bizarre or vague should be discussed with a specialist in diving medicine
- immediate recompression in a hyperbaric chamber is definitive, even if after a delay of several days.

Chapter 37

Submersion injury

Over 300 deaths by drowning in Australia in 1989, with age peaks at 0–4 years and 15–24 years. Alcohol, drugs, inadequate supervision, recreational accidents, acute illness or injury e.g. myocardial infarct, seizure, head or neck injury all contribute. Hypothermia is often associated.

Pathophysiology

- 10% do not aspirate water (dry drowning), but asphyxiate from laryngospasm and glottic closure.
- differences between seawater and freshwater drownings are largely academic as both result in surfactant destruction and hypoxia due to
  - ◊ atelectasis
  - ◊ ventilation – perfusion mismatch
  - ◊ alveolar–capillary membrane breakdown.
  - ◊ aspiration of bacteria and particulate matter e.g. sand and vomit.
- noncardiogenic pulmonary oedema follows from direct lung injury, surfactant loss, contamination and cerebral hypoxia.
- metabolic and respiratory acidosis, electrolyte imbalances or blood volume changes are seldom significant.

Treatment

Prehospital

- rapid, cautious removal from water with spinal injury precautions
- airway cleared, and ventilation assisted as necessary
- supplemental oxygen in all cases
- immediate basic CPR commenced on all patients with cardiac arrest
- prior postural drainage is unnecessary
- all victims transported to hospital, including those asymptomatic at scene but with a definite period of immersion.

Inhospital

Arrested patients

- tracheal intubation, FiO_2 1.0, IPPV, standard CPR protocol
- remember possibility of cervical spine injury, hypothermia
- continued support for the near-drowned, hypothermic child because of the higher chance of a successful outcome

Unconscious patients, respiratory failure or post-arrest

- supportive treatment including mechanical ventilation with PEEP, intensive monitoring, serum electrolytes, blood sugar, blood gases and serial CXR.
- nasogastric tube, urinary catheter and 12 lead ECG.

Conscious patients

- supplemental oxygen, repeated chest examination for wheeze or crepitations, investigations as above.
- look for the precipitating illness or injury
- clinical deterioration may necessitate tracheal intubation, bronchoscopy and physiotherapy
- antibiotics and steroids are NOT used prophylactically
- all patients are observed for a minimum of 6 hours as delayed symptoms may appear after initial recovery
- conscious and alert patients should all survive neurologically intact, as will the majority of initially obtunded patients with a purposeful response to pain.

Chapter 38

Electrical and lightning injuries

Electrical injuries

A successful outcome requires
- immediate treatment of life threatening sequelae
- thorough assessment of the circumstances of the injury once the victim is stabilised
- monitoring for major complications, once recovery has begun

There are 3 phases of management
- immediate threat to cardiac performance as a consequence of electric current
- intermediate management involves the treatment of burns, trauma, neurological sequelae and ongoing cardio-respiratory support
- long term surveillance and rehabilitation

Immediate phase

Unconscious patient

- ensure an electrical injury is the cause of unconsciousness and that the rescuer will not be similarly injured
- treat cardiac arrest in the usual manner – the most likely cardiac action is ventricular fibrillation

Ambulatory patient

- 12 lead ECG – look for conduction defects

Intermediate phase

History

- likely current pathway and likely organs and muscle mass involved
- voltage involved and method of application to the body
- collateral evidence of premorbid physical and psychological state

Examination

- cardio-respiratory function
- locate entry and exit burns and other burns if high voltage (> 1000V)
- special senses function if in the current pathway
- associated trauma – intracranial, intrathoracic, intra-abdominal

Investigations

- ECG
- CXR ± CT scan of current path
- full blood examination, liver function tests and cardiac isoenzymes
- urine – myoglobin

Management

- severely injured (any burns, cardio-respiratory dysfunction or myoglobinuria)
    - ◊ admit to ICU
    - ◊ physical cooling of burns – thoracic and abdominal muscle burns and intestinal ischaemia
    - ◊ large volume fluid replacement to maintain urine output > 1ml/kg/hr and monitor myoglobin levels
    - ◊ insert a urinary catheter and nasogastric tube
    - ◊ hourly re-examination for compartmental compression syndromes and perform fasciotomies if limb perfusion is threatened
    - ◊ do not give steroids, antibiotics or blood unless Hb < 8 g/dl
- apparently well patient (positive history without ECG change or other overt signs on presentation)
    - ◊ admit to coronary care for 6 hours monitoring – if ECG unchanged, urine negative for myoglobin and no other complaints – discharge
    - ◊ new symptoms are treated on their merits

Long term surveillance

- Significant sequelae may develop, usually proportional to the magnitude of the injury
    - ◊ special senses – electric cataract
    - ◊ neurological – rarely myelopathies, autonomic neuropathy may occur
    - ◊ psychological – post electric shock syndrome does not correlate well with initial injury severity
        - lassitude, fatigue, memory loss, depression, loss of concentration ability and finer cognitive function

Lightning injuries

Presentation

Cardio-respiratory arrest

- treat as per CPR protocol and dysrhythmia management
- prevention of secondary hypoxic insults
- intensive care admission – outcome variable

Intact cardio-respiratory function

- outcome good
- monitor as per electrical injury patients for 24 hours

Associated injuries

- keraunoparalysis
    - ◊ limbs in current pathway appear cold, pulseless and blue or mottled – similar to a compartment syndrome but compartment pressures are normal
    - ◊ resolves in minutes to hours
- special senses
    - ◊ ruptured tympanic membrane
    - ◊ ocular damage – punctate keratitis, retinal detachment, pupillary damage
    - ◊ mouth and nose – due to current passage through portals of entry
- neurological
    - ◊ intracranial bleeding often involving brain stem and cerebellum
- covert trauma
    - ◊ pulmonary and intra-abdominal blast injury
    - ◊ pulmonary barotrauma

- burns – small full thickness entry and exit burn

Long term sequelae

- ECG abnormalities resolve with time
- myelopathic changes can occur many months after the injury and can localise
- psychological sequelae are common after lightning injury

Reference

Andrews CJ, Darveniza M, Mackerras D. Lightning injuries: A review of clinical aspects, pathophysiology and treatment. *Advances in Trauma*, 1989; 4: 241–289.

Appendices

Appendix I

Being a 'street-wise' houseman

The scene

A young intern approaches the ward nurse after surgery and asks 'What is this surgeon's normal post-operative regime for fluid management?', to be greeted with 'Don't they teach you anything at university?'. It is often not what you do, but how you go about it that makes the difference.

The first day

Most hospitals have an orientation programme for new staff. Make sure you get to this programme. There is vital information collected together – it is what the hospital feels you need to know. Do not expect to remember everything – the information load is too great. Keep clear, concise and simple notes regarding whom to contact at a later date for clarification, and make a point of defining the questions you want answered. Some things (like signing on, tax forms, ID badges) need to be done straight away. Some things can wait. Try to get to know your colleagues, even if you find the whole scene overwhelming. They are the people you will be doing business with later that year, and possibly in future years. Initially, you will get most help from them, because they understand what you are going through better than anyone else.

By the end of the day you will feel exhausted and confused. This is normal. You have gone from a free thinking environment to a rigid organisation where people are categorised by their job. That is, by what they do, rather than who they are. Most of you will be rejecting this notion, but will have to find ways to live within it. It is often helpful to make a point of learning the names of the people you will be working with – the bedside nurses, the wardsmen, the social worker, the physiotherapist. If you don't know what to talk about, ask them about their job, what it entails, how you can help them make it easier. Take this thought with you as you move from the orientation programme to the ward.

The first weekend

By this stage you should be exhausted. Plan to take a day off and really unwind on the Saturday. But keep Sunday free if at all possible to revise the notes you made during the orientation programme. Get it all clear in your mind at this point – it will save you hours of confusion and frustration later. Read the hospital Resident's manual if there is one. It usually represents hours of work by large numbers of your peers, written specifically to help you. Respect their effort by making one of your own.

Date and time

In the early 1970s, there was a consensus conference held in Geneva, at which agreement was reached that all hospital times would be in military format (24 hour clock, hh:mm – 21:30 for 9.30 p.m.), and all hospital dates would be in dd-mmm-yy format (e.g. 01 Aug 90).

On call at night

It is a good idea to check with the wards you are covering between 22:00 and 23:00, asking if there are any little problems that need sorting out. Ask specifically about night sedation and i.v. fluid orders. Then check to make sure that all post-operative patients have adequate analgesia ordered and that the regime chosen is working, and that all pre-operative patients have sedation if they desire it. While the anaesthetist will have checked with the patient about sedation, several hours will have elapsed since the visit, and circumstances may have changed. This can be done by telephone, which then gives a list of jobs to do. It is better to seek out work at 22:00, than to be rung by an aggressive night nurse at 01:00 with a complaint about something that could have been sorted out hours before.

'Hospital street laws'

1. The admission of ignorance is the first step on the path to wisdom.
   If you don't know how things work, ask. The ward staff know the specialist's routine. More senior medical staff can advise about investigation/management. Most specialists don't mind being asked to talk about their specialty, but become annoyed when fundamental ignorance is displayed. Try to revise what you know about their field before you start asking their opinion.

2. The seeking of knowledge is the second step on the path to wisdom.
   Your medical degree is a licence to learn from your peers, while caring for patients who put their trust in you. Post-graduate medical education is your responsibility, and yours alone. While others may take the trouble to help you on the path, they are not required to do so. You should respect their efforts and attend any post-graduate sessions arranged. Use the library regularly for both journal scanning and electronic searches of the literature.

3. The most respected and knowledgeable doctors are usually humble.
   'First there is ignorance, then arrogance, then despair. Afterwards comes enlightenment and humility.'

4. There is always a secondary gain.
   Even when things go wrong, seek out the causes and look at the sequence of actions and the logical consequences of those actions. In so doing, benefits may be found. For example, if a patient in your care dies and a post-mortem has been arranged – make it a point of honour to attend. In this way you ensure that a copy of the report comes to you, and that you have the best possible understanding of the reason for that person's death.

Appendix II

Essay writing in examinations

The most frequent criticism by examiners of student essay answers is failure to answer the **SET question.** Essay technique is vital to success if the student's knowledge is insufficient to comprehensively answer the question or if the student wishes to achieve high marks as a means of gaining 'value' for 'time spent in preparation' for the exam.

Why does a student who is told that this section of the book is **mandatory reading**, either skim through it or ignore it, and then continue to perform below capability? I assume the reason for this behaviour is that this kind of information is boring, bears no relation to the clinical subject matter and the student thinks he has heard it all before!!

These brief notes intend to encourage the student to apply the same self discipline to their essay writing as they apply to their study.

Let's start with the basics:

Read the instructions

THREE questions in **ONE and a HALF** hours! That's thirty minutes per question!!

Divide your time up equally – e.g. the exam commences at, say, 3 p.m.. You should write on your paper as a constant reminder: **3.30 4.00 4.30.**

This makes considerable sense because it is much easier to get the first 30% of the marks for a question, than the last 30% (i.e.70–100%). Logically three equally answered questions have a higher chance of success than one brilliant and two poor answers, especially if the student has only left five minutes to scramble an illegible, illogical and irrelevant answer to the last question attempted.

Read the question

During the time allocated to read the question before the commencement of writing, jot your immediate, instinctive thoughts at the side of the question paper. It wastes time and disturbs your rhythm, if later you have to recall a thought that came to your mind at the beginning of the exam, which, during the actual writing of your answer, seems impossible to retrieve.

Read ALL the questions

Even if you can 'do' the first three questions, the fourth may give the first three some perspective. For instance, there are unlikely to be two questions out of four on CPR, and even if you think that is the case, the emphasis may well be different in the two questions, and more apparent only after reading ALL the questions.

Do not rewrite the question

This practice is a ludicrous waste of time and a hang over from antiquated methods of primary school teaching. It gains no marks and wastes the student's time that should be allocated to producing a factual answer.

How to write an essay plan

First – what type of question is it?

COMPARE:	look for similarities and differences
CONTRAST:	set in opposition to facilitate demonstration of the differences
CRITICIZE:	give your judgement and support it by weighing the evidence
DEFINE:	give a precise meaning
DESCRIBE:	give a detailed account of
DISCUSS:	investigate by argument, presenting **both** sides giving reasons, pros and cons
EVALUATE:	make an appraisal of the worth of something
EXPLAIN:	make plain, interpret, account for
ILLUSTRATE:	make clear by concrete examples or diagram
INTERPRET:	expound the meaning of
JUSTIFY:	show adequate grounds for decisions
LIST:	catalogue by groups or classes with minimal explanation
OUTLINE:	give the main features or general principles
RELATE:	show how things are connected to each other and how they affect each other
REVIEW:	make a survey, examine critically
STATE:	present in clear, brief form
SUMMARIZE:	give a concise account of the chief points
TRACE:	follow the development of a topic

Second – pick out the key words

e.g.: *'What are the clinical and biochemical abnormalities which may be present in a patient suffering from 10% dehydration due to diarrhoea?'*

key words: clinical abnormalities
biochemical abnormalities
10%
dehydration
diarrhoea

Each line listed above could form the basis of the essay, albeit in a more logical order and not with equal weighting.

Any **numbers or demographic** data (age, sex, weight) are included in the question for a significant reason. If the question includes words that are underlined or highlighted, they must be given importance and ignoring those words means **FAILURE.**

Third – construct a plan

Using the above example:

- 10% dehydration – definition, shock
- diarrhoea – composition, ECF
- clinical
    - ◊ rate (*history*) × amount (*10%*) × type (*ECF*)
    - ◊ symptoms
        - thirst, confusion
    - ◊ signs
        - skin, urine, mucosa, BP, PR
- biochemical
    - ◊ diarrhoea loss
        - water + electrolytes
    - ◊ shock
        - acid/base + electrolytes
    - ◊ compensation
        - water retention
        - ADH
        - electrolytes
        - acidosis + (respiratory)
        - fluid shifts – ICF-ECF-IV
    - ◊ effect of treatment
        - N saline
        - 5% dextrose
        - K^+
    - ◊ expected serum electrolytes and acid/base

Obviously the student cannot write about all of this in detail in thirty minutes and must emphasise the latter two subject headings and not get bogged down in one aspect – for example: producing a general dissertation on shock.

Write your plan at the beginning of the essay paper **instead** of copying the question!

If a point won't come to your mind immediately, leave a space in your plan or put an *. Do not let this situation become irritating and disturb your concentration. Later as the essay begins to flow, these minor facts will load into your cerebral RAM, rather than remaining in your cerebral ROM. Often, these points are minor and unlikely to make any major difference to your final performance, particularly if a close marking system is used by the examiner.

If the question is **a 'discuss'**-type – do NOT present a summary, essay plan or a diagram. Write your main points in a discussion form without any padding!

If the question is divided into two parts, try to allocate equal time to both parts, unless you recognise one part of the question as obviously being of less importance.

The student must habitually refer to the question during his answer. For example, statements like 'relating the clinical findings to the biochemical abnormalities in the patient dehydrated due to diarrhoea ....', show the examiner that the student is trying to answer the specific set question, and not giving a general answer on dehydration – it also helps to keep the student on track.

Introductions and conclusions

If you want to use this form of essay technique during an exam, then the introduction must be organised and full of fact. Generalised statements like 'the biochemical abnormalities of dehydration are typical', not only don't make sense and are often wrong, but also contain absolutely NO information. An examiner then struggles to maintain interest in the rest of your answer. A conclusion is perhaps useful in discussion questions to show the examiner that the student can weigh the facts and arrive at a balanced opinion.

Do not change the question

If the question refers to diarrhoea, then this is what the examiners wa [illegible] discussion on peritonitis, which although it may be vaguely relatec [illegible] referred to in the question. It is even worse if the student starts disc [illegible] dehydration!

Do not explain medical terms to the exar [illegible]

'Oliguria, or a decrease in urine output...' – this type of statement wa [illegible] but it ignores the reason for learning the language of medicine. Th [illegible] familiar with the term 'oliguria' and may find it irritating or insulting [illegible] define such a term in his essay.

Do not write 'motherhood' statements

'CPR is sometimes necessary to save lives' – this sort of statem [illegible] provokes the response 'so what' from the examiner. 'Oxygen is es [illegible] may be true, but is more the type of statement that one expects from a child at school, rather than a university student about to sit his or her MBBS finals.

Abbreviations

There is no place for personalised abbreviations in your essay unless you define their meaning. 'this is measured by HPLC' may mean little to someone not familiar with the technology. Common medical abbreviations, in context with the question and your answer may be acceptable, such as BP, CVP and K^{+}.

Writing legibly

Writing essays is a means of demonstrating to the examiner that the student has enough knowledge on the subject asked to deserve a pass, or better. The student fails if this information cannot be processed by the examiner. If the examiner has to struggle to distinguish words, the benefit of the doubt will not necessarily be given to the student, especially if it is a discussion question where the student's argument may rest on a negative or positive statement – 'I wouldn't give isoprenaline to these patients' could be written 'I would give .....'. The opposite meaning is easily construed if the writing is illegible. If the student has poor handwriting then space out the words and write on every **second** line and the student must definitely write on only **one side** of the page.

Conclusion

Following these simple guidelines will improve exam performance considerably allowing learned knowledge to be presented in such a way that the examiner finds it easy to award pass marks or better – good luck is no longer critical to success, but may still be advantageous!!

Appendix III

Operating suite discussion guide and record of achievement

Guidance for students

This booklet indicates **minimum** learning objectives and practical skills which should be mastered whilst in the operating room during anaesthesia. You should also allocate time to the anaesthetic assessment clinic, the intensive care unit, pain clinic, the recovery room and the surgical wards. Learning objectives are given in the form of a question as it might appear in an examination. The student should use these questions as guides for informal tutorials during quiet discussion in the operating room with the anaesthetic staff.

Some topics are purely for discussion (indicated by ☺). Others are practical tasks (indicated by ☑). You are expected to document your attempts at practical procedures. *Mere completion of the task is not enough.* The student should be **capable of performing** and understanding the task.

If the task has been acquired during other attachments e.g. intravenous cannulation, do not repeat the process. Spend time efficiently practising skills and discussing topics which you feel are the most difficult. Introductory texts and reference materials are listed on the following pages.

Guidance for tutors

Rather than list endless 'objectives', example questions are given. It is hoped that these will form the basis of discussion topics. The questions are not intended to limit what is taught. However a student who can discuss the topics in an informed way will have developed a 'core of knowledge' around which future learning may be based.

There are areas in the text where a signature is required. We do not want you to sign for every procedure. Rather we want your opinion as to whether the student has grasped the **fundamentals** relevant to the section and an understanding of the topic.

At your discretion, you may suggest a student need not complete a practical section if they already possess the required skills e.g. intravenous cannulation.

If a student finds a topic difficult, please expand the questions and suggested practical experience as necessary. We are more interested in the student learning skills than recording a given number of attempts.

Each student is required to record a preoperative assessment on less than one A4 page and indicate how the patient's medical condition may be optimised. Please choose a suitable patient for the student, i.e. one who has concurrent medical conditions which may predispose to anaesthetic problems. The aim here is to assist the final year medical student in integrating his or her knowledge in an efficient and practical way.

Teaching resource materials

The following resource materials should be used to answer specific questions.

- Lecture Notes on Anaesthetics – JN Lunn (Blackwell, 1991, 4th edition)
- Textbook of Anaesthesia – AR Aitkinhead & G Smith (Churchill Livingstone)
- Techniques of Regional Anaesthesia – DB Scott (Appleton and Lange, 1991)
- Cardiopulmonary Resuscitation – Australian Resuscitation Council booklet.
- Euthanasia: Should We Kill the Dying – B Pollard (Little Hills Press, 1989)

This part of the book is designed as a guide to learning. It is intended to provide a structure for tutorial discussion. Not all the questions carry equal weight. Some questions require reference to a textbook or your lecture notes. The more of the record you complete, the more you will learn and the more YOU will have achieved. Completion of every question is not compulsory or even expected, but the questions do define examinable material.

Section index

Task completion index

1 Care of the unconscious patient

During this section you should learn how to safely care for an unconscious patient, recognise respiratory insufficiency and intervene effectively until more experienced help arrives.

1. Airway and oxygenation

☺ Describe available techniques for the administration of oxygen to the upper airway in both the operating room and on the ward. What are the advantages and disadvantages of each technique?

☑ Administer oxygen from an anaesthetic face mask to an awake patient whilst maintaining verbal contact.

Proposed operative procedure	Age	Weight	Respiratory rate	Oxygen flow rate (l/min)
1				
2				
3				

☺ Which factors may make maintenance of a clear airway difficult by patient position alone?

☑ Maintain a clear airway by means of jaw, head and neck position in an unconscious patient. Practise in both supine and lateral positions.

Attempt	Age	Weight	Operation performed
1 Supine			
2 Supine			
3 Supine			
4 Supine			
5 Supine			
6 Lateral			
7 Lateral			
8 Lateral			

2. Bag and mask

☺ How does an oropharyngeal airway work?

What damage can it do to a patient?

What alternative airways are available?

☑ Insert an oropharyngeal airway into an unconscious patient.

Attempt	Age	ASA	Airway type	Airway size
1				
2				
3				
4				
5				

III. Operating suite discussion guide and record of achievement

☺ Describe 'bag and mask ventilation'.

☺ Using equipment readily available in your hospital, compare a 'bag-valve-mask resuscitator' (Mapleson C circuit) with an Air Viva, Laerdal or Ambu Bag.

☑ Ventilate an unconscious apnoeic patient using a 'bag and mask'. VERY IMPORTANT !!!!!

Attempt	Age	ASA	Proposed operation
1			
2			
3			
4			
5			
6			
7			
8			
9			
10			
11			
12			

Tutor's Signature...

3. The laryngeal mask airway

☺ What is a laryngeal mask airway? Describe some hazards associated with its use.

☑ Practise insertion of a laryngeal mask airway in anaesthetised patients.

Attempt	Age	Weight	Proposed operation
1			
2			
3			
4			
5			

4. Tracheal intubation

☺ List the indications for tracheal intubation.

1...

2...

3...

4...

☺ Describe the characteristic components of a tracheal tube? How is it connected to a breathing circuit?

III. Operating suite discussion guide and record of achievement

☺ What are the anatomical relations of a tracheal tube cuff correctly placed in the trachea?
List clinical and radiological findings indicating endobronchial intubation.

☺ Discuss three methods used to confirm the correct placement of a tracheal tube.

1.

2.

3.

Which is the most reliable?

☺ What equipment is required to perform tracheal intubation? Complete the following words:

1.	L	4.	Sy
2.	T	5.	C
3.	I	6.	Su

List airway management equipment you might need to have available when attending the scene of a serious road traffic accident.

1.

2.

3.

4.

5.

6.

7.

8.

III. Operating suite discussion guide and record of achievement

☑ Demonstrate the passage of a tracheal tube and confirm its correct placement.

Attempt	Age	ASA	Tube type	Tube size	Proposed operation
1					
2					
3					
4					
5					
6					
7					
8					
9					
10					

Tutor's Signature..

☺ A patient presents for urgent surgery who has not been fasted preoperatively. How may the risk of pulmonary aspiration in such a patient be reduced?

☺ Which pharmacological agents may be used to enhance patient safety in this clinical situation?

How do they work?

☑ Practise the administration of cricoid pressure (Sellick's manoeuvre).

Attempt	Age	Weight	Clinical condition
1			
2			
3			
4			
5			

5. Assessment of the difficult airway

☺ How may possible difficulty in tracheal intubation be assessed at the bedside? Describe a scheme for grading ease of intubation.

III. Operating suite discussion guide and record of achievement

☑ Assess the ease of intubation in 3 patients preoperatively. Were your findings verified at laryngoscopy?

Attempt	Age	Weight	Mallampati	Cormack & Lehane
1				
2				
3				

Tutor's Signature...

6. Artificial ventilation

☺ What is meant by the terms:

	Definition	Normal values (70 kg adult male)
minute volume		
tidal volume		
respiratory rate		
PEEP		
CMV		
IMV		
CPAP		

☺ List indications for artificial ventilation of the lungs.

How would you distinguish pulmonary failure from respiratory muscle failure?

☺ What is the role of the physiotherapist in the care of the ventilated patient?

☺ List problems associated with prolonged artificial ventilation. What techniques are available for prevention?

☑ List the alarms incorporated into a ventilator on the Intensive Care Unit. What will you do if the ventilator stops ventilating the patient?

Tutor's Signature...

7. Positioning

☺ What is the fundamental difference between vomiting and regurgitation?

What factors predispose towards regurgitation in an unconscious or semi-conscious patient?

☺ Which peripheral nerves are vulnerable to damage by incorrect patient positioning?

☑ Place an unconscious postoperative patient in a safe position for return to the recovery room. Don't forget to give O_2 and support the airway.

Attempt	Age	Weight	Position description
1			
2			
3			
4			
5			

☺ Describe the required characteristics of the suction equipment.

☺ What damage may be done to a patient with suction equipment?

☑ Set up a suction system and postoperatively suction the airway of the unconscious patient.

Attempt	Age	Weight	Machine type	Sucker type	Max pressure
1					
2					
3					
4					
5					

☺ 'Every unconscious patient should have a nasogastric tube.' Discuss this statement. Describe four indications for nasogastric tube insertion.

III. Operating suite discussion guide and record of achievement

☺ In what incorrect positions can a nasogastric tube be placed?

How do you confirm correct placement?

☑ Either place or witness the positioning of a nasogastric tube in a patient.

Attempt	Age	Weight	Placement purpose
1			
2			

Tutor's Signature..

NOTES

2 Intravenous therapy

On completing this section you should be able to gain venous access and prescribe fluid therapy effectively.

1. Venepuncture

☺ What is a Luer lock?

☺ Describe the 'universal safety precautions' which should be employed by the operator when performing venepuncture.

☺ Which bottle does a blood sample go in for full blood count?

What are the requirements for labelling blood samples for cross match?

Why is the strict observation of these requirements important?

☺ Record the blood tests performed on 3 patients. Were these appropriate?

Patient Δ	Hb	U & Es	LFTs	Others	Comment

Tutor's Signature...

2. Intravenous fluids

☺ Describe the features of an intravenous giving set which is designed to minimise air embolism.

What are the special considerations of giving i.v. fluids to small children?

☺ Describe precautions which should be taken when making additions to intravenous fluids.

Where can you obtain information regarding compatibility of additives?

☺ What is a pressure infusion device?

When would it be used?

How might misuse lead to a patient's sudden death?

III. Operating suite discussion guide and record of achievement

☑ Examine intravenous solution composition and establish an infusion.

Fluid	Cal/L	Osmolality	Note the fluid composition
N Saline			
5% D			
4% & N/5			
Haemaccel			
Hartmann's			

Where appropriate include blood warming apparatus.

Tutor's Signature..

3. Intravenous cannulation

☺ Describe the characteristics of an intravenous cannula suitable for blood transfusion.

☺ List, in order of preference, suitable anatomical sites for intravenous cannulation.

1.

2.

3.

4.

☺ When would you use local anaesthesia prior to intravenous cannulation?

What methods of anaesthetising the skin are available?

☑ Place an intravenous cannula in a patient, suitable for crystalloid administration.

Attempt	Age	Weight	Cannulation site
1			
2			
3			
4			
5			

Tutor's Signature..

4. Blood transfusion

☺ List the data recorded on the label of a bag of blood.

What preservatives are added to blood for transfusion?

What problems might arise because of blood transfusion during a ruptured aortic aneurysm? (massive transfusion)

early:

late:

☺ Describe the treatment of a 'blood transfusion reaction'.

☑ With a medically qualified colleague, check a unit of blood for patient administration.

Sex	Age	Weight	Patient's blood volume	Volume blood given	Blood group

Tutor's Signature..

3 Resuscitation

You have already received tuition in basic and advanced life support. This section will consolidate your knowledge and teach you how to apply it during the management of life-threatening situations.

1. CPR

☺ Describe to your tutor how you would perform cardiopulmonary resuscitation or basic life support in both adults and children.

☺ What is the main difference between basic and advanced life support?

☺ Describe the immediate treatment of VF (ventricular fibrillation), asystole, EMD (electromechanical disassociation).

☺ The following conditions may lead to cardiac arrest. What difference does the cause make to your management of the patient?

- Myocardial infarction
- Electrocution and lightning strike
- Drowning
- Acute poisoning
- Hypovolaemia
- Respiratory failure

Tutor's Signature..

2. Allergic reactions

☺ Describe the clinical symptoms and signs associated with an acute allergic reaction.

Outline your management.

☺ List, in order of importance, drugs used to treat an acute allergic reaction.

III. Operating suite discussion guide and record of achievement

☺ A patient has survived an acute drug reaction. What further investigations are necessary?

☺ What will you tell the patient after an acute drug reaction?

Tutor's Signature...

3. Hypovolaemic shock

☺ Describe the clinical signs and symptoms of hypovolaemic shock.

☺ What fluids will you prescribe for a 50 year old male patient who has fallen downstairs, is bleeding internally, has a pulse of 120 and blood pressure of 80/60?

What clinical and laboratory findings will modify your prescription?

☺ What is renal protection? How might it work?

☺ Describe the anatomy of the great veins of the thoracic inlet.

What routes can be used to gain central venous access?

☑ Watch the insertion of a central venous cannula. List possible acute and long term complications.

☑ Watch the insertion of an arterial cannula.

☺ Discuss the place of intra-arterial and central venous pressure monitoring during resuscitation.

Tutor's Signature...

4. 'Septic shock'

☺ Describe circulatory changes occurring during 'systemic inflammatory response syndrome' (i.e. septic shock) (SIRS).

III. Operating suite discussion guide and record of achievement

☑ List three clinical situations in which SIRS is likely to occur.

1.

2.

3.

☺ What are 'third space' losses?

Which intravenous fluids are appropriate in this condition? Why?

☑ Review an ICU patient with your tutor.

Record

number of infusions

infusion composition

rates of administration

monitoring

respiratory

cardiovascular

renal

biochemical

III. Operating suite discussion guide and record of achievement

☺ How has this been optimised?

☺ What is meant by ‘oxygen flux’?

Tutor’s Signature..

4 Pain relief

Pain is common and its management in hospital is often inadequate. In this section you will learn some of the analgesic techniques available and gain sufficient knowledge to make decisions as to what is appropriate for your patients.

1. Drugs and acute pain

☺ Review the clinical pharmacokinetics of commonly used opiates.

☺ Discuss the advantages and disadvantages of morphine, pethidine and fentanyl.

Drug	Clinical T½	Vd	Elimination	Routes of administration
morphine				
pethidine				
fentanyl				

☺ What unwanted effects are common to all opiate drugs?

☺ Which non-opiate analgesics are available in your hospital?

Discuss the place of non-steroidal analgesics (NSAIDs) in the management of acute and chronic pain.

☺ Describe the time course of acute pain following surgery.

☺ Describe the monitoring required to allow the safe use of potent analgesics in the ward environment.

☺ Write below an analgesic prescription for an 80 year old, 50 kg woman who has had her fractured neck of femur repaired today.

III. Operating suite discussion guide and record of achievement

☑ Study the administrative steps involved in the completion of the dangerous drug book.

Tutor's Signature..

2. Chronic pain relief

☺ Outline the differences between acute and chronic pain.

☺ How may emotional factors influence pain perception?

☺ Compare the drug treatment of cancer versus non-cancer pain.

☺ What is causalgia or reflex sympathetic dystrophy? How may it be treated?

☺ List the classes of drug which have a place in the management of chronic pain?

☺ Why is rehabilitation from chronic pain required?

Tutor's Signature..

3. Specialised analgesic techniques

☺ Describe the advantages and disadvantages of patient controlled analgesia (PCA).

III. Operating suite discussion guide and record of achievement

☑ Write a PCA prescription for a 50 kg woman following laparotomy.

☑ Watch the preparation and attachment of PCA to a patient.

☺ Outline the mechanism of action of epidural and intrathecal opiates.

What are the benefits and risks of this form of treatment?

☺ A patient has received epidural morphine in the operating room.

Write out below your observation instructions for the nursing staff in the patient's ward.

☺ Subcutaneous infusion of opiate is gaining popularity as a very effective means of drug administration.

What are its advantages and disadvantages?

☑ Witness the setting up of an analgesic/anaesthetic drug infusion. What is PCA sedation?

☺ What neurosurgical treatments may be of use in the treatment of chronic pain?

III. Operating suite discussion guide and record of achievement

☺ Acupuncture is effective in the relief of some types of chronic pain. What current theories are used to explain the underlying mechanism?

☺ How can drug therapy modulate acupuncture analgesia?

Tutor's Signature...

NOTES

5 Local anaesthesia

Local anaesthesia is practised by both specialists and general practitioners. In this section you will learn how to perform a selection of blocks safely and manage common complications.

1. Drugs

☺ Describe the mode of action of local anaesthetic drugs.

What factors influence speed of onset?

☺ Local anaesthetic drugs can cause cardiovascular and central nervous system toxicity. Describe the symptoms and signs and progression of toxicity in each system.

List the equipment and drugs required for treatment.

☺ In physiological terms what happens during a faint?

Why is this relevant to the safe practice of local anaesthesia?

☺ Why are vasopressors added to local anaesthetics?

How may vasopressors cause problems during anaesthesia?

III. Operating suite discussion guide and record of achievement

☺ List the commonly available local anaesthetic agents.

Drug	Concentration	mg/ml	Max safe dose plain	Max safe + adrenaline	Uses
lignocaine	1%				
	5% heavy				
	10% spray				
bupivacaine	0.125%				
	0.25%				
	0.5% heavy				
prilocaine	1.0%				

What volume of 1% lignocaine with 1:200,000 adrenaline may be used in infiltration anaesthesia in a 70 kg man?

☺ What is the strength in g/ml of:

1:1000 Adrenaline ....

1:200,000 Adrenaline ....

Tutor's Signature..

2. Intravenous regional anaesthesia (IVRA) or Bier's Block

☺ List equipment required to perform IVRA.

What complications may occur and how may this affect the patient?

☺ If acute toxicity develops, how is it treated?

☑ Either witness or perform IVRA on two occasions

Attempt	Age	ASA	Proposed surgery
1			
2			

Tutor's Signature..

3. Femoral nerve block

☺ Describe the anatomy of the femoral nerve in the inguinal region.

What tissues are innervated by this nerve?

What are the indications for this block?

What is a '3-in-1' block?

☑ Witness or perform 2 femoral nerve blocks.

Attempt	Age	Weight	Clinical condition
1			
2			

Tutor's Signature...

4. Digital nerve block

☺ Describe the anatomy of the digital nerves in the fingers.

What is an end artery?

☺ What particular safeguards are important with this block?

☑ Perform two digital nerve blocks.

Attempt	Age	Weight	Clinical condition
1			
2			

Tutor's Signature...

(Experience gained in the emergency department may be included)

5. Spinal and epidural anaesthesia

☺ What are the advantages of spinal and epidural anaesthesia over general anaesthesia?

List the absolute contraindications to central nerve block.

1.

2.

3.

4.

☺ Describe the anatomy of the sympathetic efferent system.

What unwanted effects may accompany lumbar puncture?

How could a spinal anaesthetic performed in the lumbar region lead to a Horner's syndrome?

☺ What is post dural puncture headache (PDPH) and how may it treated?

☑ Witness two spinal anaesthetics being performed. VERY IMPORTANT !!

Attempt	Age	Weight	Needle type	Needle size	Anaesthetic & volume	Vertebral level inserted
1						
2						

☺ Compare and contrast epidural and spinal anaesthesia.

III. Operating suite discussion guide and record of achievement

☺ Draw a cross section through the vertebral column and overlying tissues. Indicate the location of the epidural and sub-arachnoid spaces.

What are the cephalad and caudal anatomical limits of the lumbar epidural space?

cephalad...

caudad...

☺ A patient returns to the ward with an epidural catheter in situ.
What steps should you take to ensure patient safety?

☑ Witness 3 lumbar or thoracic epidurals being performed.
If you get a chance, watch a caudal epidural – note the differences:

Epidural region	Age	Weight	Clinical condition

Tutor's Signature...

6. Analgesia during labour

☺ What analgesic techniques are available to a woman in labour?

1.

2.

3.

4.

5.

6.

III. Operating suite discussion guide and record of achievement

- ☺ What are the effects of central nerve block on the mother and her baby?
- ☺ What safeguards should be applied to a woman labouring under epidural analgesia?
- ☺ What is Mendleson's syndrome?

How may it be averted?

Tutor's Signature...

NOTES

6 Preoperative assessment

All doctors must be able to assess the risks of anaesthesia and surgery so that they can provide appropriate advice to their patient and family.

In this section you will learn how to detect those patients likely to experience problems and how to optimise their management.

1. General condition

☺ What is the ASA grading system?

1.

2.

3.

4.

5.

E

What is the mortality associated with each grade?

☺ Why is a history of previous anaesthesia important?

☺ How might the state of a patient's preoperative nutrition affect the course of anaesthesia and surgery?

2. Cardiorespiratory health

☺ Describe a rapid assessment of the extent of a patient's cardiorespiratory reserve.

III. Operating suite discussion guide and record of achievement

☺ How may lung disease be optimised preoperatively?

How should a patient with asthma be managed perioperatively?

☺ How may cardiac disease be optimised prior to surgery?

What is the significance of 'mild heart failure' to anaesthetists?

☺ Many drugs used in hypertension and cardiac disease interact with anaesthetic agents. Describe some of these.

☺ A man aged 50 yr presents for elective cholecystectomy with a past history of 'heart attack' 6 weeks ago. Write notes on how you would proceed.

Tutor's Signature..

3. Common metabolic problems

☺ Describe the preoperative management of a patient with insulin dependent diabetes mellitus scheduled for small bowel resection.

☺ Mature onset diabetes mellitus is very common in the elderly. How should their diabetic medications be managed preoperatively?

III. Operating suite discussion guide and record of achievement

☺ Describe the relevance of thyroid disease to anaesthesia.

☺ A patient presents for surgery with obstructive jaundice. Discuss their perioperative fluid and drug management.

☺ Mild chronic renal impairment is very common in the elderly surgical population.

Discuss the prevention of acute renal failure in these patients.

Tutor's Signature...

4. Familial conditions relevant to anaesthesia

☺ What is the significance of a history of severe muscle pain after exercise or previous anaesthesia?

☺ What is the relevance of myasthenia gravis to anaesthesia?

☺ Muscular dystrophies and myopathies are rare but they are very important to anaesthetists. Why?

☺ What is Malignant Hyperpyrexia. How may it present during anaesthesia?

☺ How would you treat acute porphyria?

☺ Discuss the effects of pseudocholinesterase deficiency. Which drugs should be used with caution in these patients?

Tutor's Signature...

5. The assessment case history

☑ You, personally, should assess a patient prior to surgery, either on the ward or in the anaesthetic outpatient clinic. Suitable patients are those scheduled for vascular, urological or eye surgery and fixation of a fractured neck of femur. On **one** sheet of A4 paper, describe the relevant history and physical findings, indicate which preoperative investigations you would order and suggest a possible premedication and method of anaesthesia.

NOTES

7 Monitoring

This section introduces various methods of monitoring patient well-being. These techniques are being applied more frequently in the ward environment.

You will evaluate the benefits and problems of interpretation associated with each type of monitor and how the monitor might be usefully employed.

1. Cardiovascular monitoring

☺ Describe the assessment of the adequacy of respiration and the circulation without electrical monitoring apparatus.

What are the clinical signs of cardiovascular collapse?

☺ What does a 3 lead ECG monitor tell you?

What does it not tell you?

☺ Draw the ECG appearances of

atrial fibrillation

ventricular tachycardia

and ventricular ectopics.

How would you manage these arrhythmias in the immediate postoperative period?

☑ Attach 3 ECG electrodes to each patient using the CM_5 placement and then draw one pQRS complex in the box below for each lead configuration

Sex	Age	Weight	Lead I	Lead II	Lead III	Swap R & L

III. Operating suite discussion guide and record of achievement

☺ What is meant by the term NIBP?

What factors can give rise to false readings?

☺ Attach an NIBP monitor to 3 patients and record their blood pressure.
Measure pressure using a manual sphygmomanometer on the other arm.
Was there a difference and if so, why do you think this occurs?

Sex	Age	Weight	Systolic NIBP	Diastolic NIBP	Mean NIBP	Sphyg (R)	Sphyg (L)

Tutor's Signature...

2. Respiratory monitoring

☺ How does a pulse oximeter detect hypoxia?

When might misleading readings occur?

☺ Describe the difference between PaO2 and SaO2?

What is the graphical relationship between them?

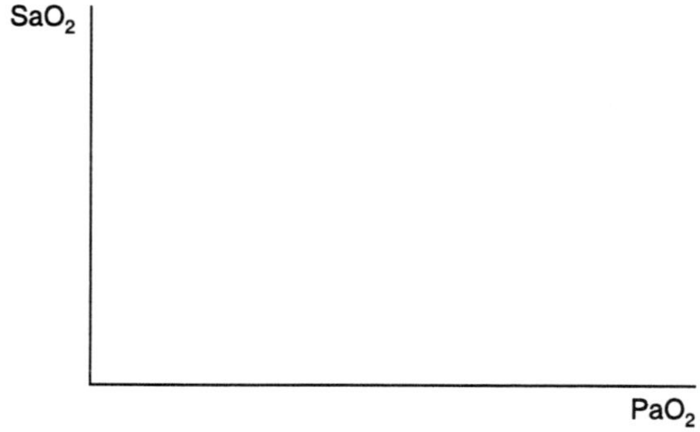

III. Operating suite discussion guide and record of achievement

☺ Outline the difference between an oxygen analyser and a pulse oximeter.

Why do we need both on an anaesthetic machine?

☺ Attach a pulse oximeter to 3 patients about to undergo anaesthesia.
Did the saturation fall during induction. If so why?

Attempt	Age	Weight	Record SaO_2 (%) every 30 sec for 4 min							
1										
2										
3										

☺ Discuss the diagnostic value of a blood gas profile. What is a buffer?

☺ What is meant by the term compensated metabolic acidosis?

☑ Perform blood gas analysis on 3 patients, using radial stab with local anaesthesia or by taking samples from an indwelling arterial line.
Record and interpret the analysis.

Site	Age	Weight	pH	$PaCO_2$	PaO_2	HCO_3	BE	Diagnosis

☺ What is capnography?
Draw and label the waveform obtained from a capnograph during normal quiet respiration.

☺ How would the capnograph appear with the following:

oesophageal intubation

endobronchial intubation

asthma large pulmonary embolus

☑ Set up a capnograph and establish patient monitoring. Ask your tutor to adjust the gas flows and observe what happens to the E_TCO_2

Aspiration Site	Age	Weight	Fresh gas flow	Record E_TCO_2 every 15 min				

Tutor's Signature..

NOTES

8 Anaesthesia

In this section you will discover some of the art and science of anaesthesia and a little about the drugs we use. Whilst it is not intended to teach you how to do it, if you find it interesting ...

1. The process of anaesthesia

☺ Look in detail at an anaesthetic chart. What is the purpose of recording this information?

Follow the progress of a patient from the ward to the operating room, observe their operation, help recover the patient and return the patient to the ward.

With your tutor, or another anaesthetist, study an anaesthetic machine and follow the oxygen supply from the wall outlet to the patient.

☺ Discuss the aims of premedication. Which drugs are used and why?

'Shadow' one of the anaesthetists you have contact with as they perform their premedication round for one list. How is patient reassurance achieved?

Tutor's Signature..

2. Induction, maintenance and recovery

☺ What is meant by depth of anaesthesia? At which times during anaesthesia is the patient most vulnerable?

☺ Which pieces of equipment must be available prior to the induction of anaesthesia or administration of sedative drugs?

☑ Make a list of the drugs you see being used for the induction and maintenance of general anaesthesia. Discuss with your anaesthetic colleague what each drug does and why they used it.

Generic	Proprietary	Drug class	Use

III. Operating suite discussion guide and record of achievement

☺ What are emergence phenomena?

Should a doctor have a 'chaperone' whilst administering sedation to a patient?

☺ What do you think is the most important aspect of care in the recovery room?

☑ Help to recover patients following general anaesthesia under the guidance of the recovery room nursing staff.

Wound site	Age	Weight	Complications (vomiting, hypoxia, pain)

☺ A patient has been described as atopic and gives a history of multiple allergic reactions. How does this affect the choice of anaesthetic agent?

☺ The three most commonly used volatile agents are Halothane, Sevoflurane and Isoflurane. Discuss factors which influence the choice of one agent over another.

Recovery Sister's Signature...

3. The patient who does not wake up

A patient does not wake up as expected or becomes unrousable after return to the ward. Describe your management.

What investigations would you order?

III. Operating suite discussion guide and record of achievement

☺ Which sedative drugs may be 'reversed' by specific antagonists?

☺ What is CO_2 narcosis?

How might it develop postoperatively?

☺ The concept of brain death should be familiar to all doctors but intensivists deal with this most frequently. Discuss this topic with an intensivist in your hospital.

☺ What is the procedure for the declaration of someone 'brain dead'?

☺ What is a 'beating-heart donor'?

☺ If you suspect a patient suitable as an organ donor, how should you proceed?

Intensivist's Signature..

NOTES

Self assessment

A very important skill to learn is self evaluation of what you are good at and not so good at. The aim of this assessment is for you to evaluate your strengths and weaknesses before the final exam.

Please mark on the visual analogue scales how you think you rate in each of these areas. In addition please add any comments below the line.

Knowledge:

Total ignorance ________________________________ Know more than my tutor

Understanding:

None ________________________________ Better than my tutor

Practical Skills:

None ________________________________ Can intubate a mosquito

Addendum

This course has attempted to provide an environment for the student to gain an education – it is not intended to be solely a teaching programme. Acquiring knowledge is supposed to be fun. Some of the questions in this book are intentionally provocative and some of the answers will not be definitive.

We hope that the intellectual and dextrous skills required to deliver anaesthesia have been demonstrated and that you now have some insight into the quality of care anaesthetists deliver to their patients.

Appendix IV

Drug dose compendium

compiled by

Dr. Frank Shann

with

**Drs Alan Duncan, Warwick Butt, Robert Henning,
Michael South and James Tibballs**

at

**The Intensive Care Unit
Royal Children's Hospital
Parkville, Victoria 3052, AUSTRALIA**

Considerable care has been taken to ensure that the information in this section is accurate, but the user is advised to check the doses carefully. The authors are not responsible for any errors in publication.

DRUGS – listed by generic name

1/100=1%=10mg/ml, 1/1000=1mg/ml, 1/10000=0.1mg/ml

Acarbose. 1-4mg/kg/dose (max 200mg) 8H oral with food.

Acebutolol. 4-8mg/kg/dose (max 400mg) 8-24H oral.

Acemetacin. 1.2mg/kg/dose (max 60mg) 8-12H oral.

Acetaminophen. see paracetamol.

Acetazolamide. 2-7.5mg/kg/dose (max 350mg) 8H oral.

Acetyl sulfisoxazole. 1.16g = 1.0g sulphafurazole (qv).

Acetylcysteine. Paracetamol poisoning (irrespective of time elapsed): 150 mg/kg in 5%D IV over 15 min, then 10 mg/kg/hr for 72hr (longer if still encephalopathic); monitor serum potassium.
Give if paracetamol >1000umol/l (150μg/ml) at 4hr, >500 μmol/ml 8hr, >250μmol/ml 12hr. Meconium ileus equivalent: 5ml/dose (NOT/kg) of 20% solution 8H oral. CF: 4-8mg/kg/dose 8H oral.

Acetylcysteine 5% + hypromellose 0.35% eye drops.
1-2 drops/eye 6-8H.

Acetylsalicylic acid. see aspirin.

Acipimox. 5mg/kg/dose (max 250mg) 8-12H oral.

Acitretin. 0.5-1.5mg/kg (max 75mg) daily oral.

Aclarubicin. 60mg/m^2/day for 3-5 days by IV infusion, then 25-100mg/m^2 infusion every 3-4wk (usual total dose 300-600mg/m^2). Lower doses in combination regimens.

Acrivastine. 0.15mg/kg/dose (max 8mg) 8H oral.

Acrosoxacin. 3mg/kg/dose (max 150mg) 8H oral.

IV. Drug dose compendium

ACTH (Corticotrophin). 1unit/kg (max 40u) IM daily.

Activated charcoal. see charcoal.

Acyclovir. Cutaneous herpes: 250mg/m^2/dose 8H IV over 1hr.
Herpes encephalitis, varicella or EB virus: 500 mg/m^2/dose 8H IV over 1hr; neonate 10mg/kg/dose IV over 1hr daily (<30wk gestation), 18H (30-32wk), 12H (1st wk life), 8H (2-12 wk).
Genital herpes (NOT/kg): 200mg/dose oral x5/day for 10 days, then 200mg/dose x2-3/day for 6mo if required.
Zoster (NOT/kg): 400mg/dose (<2yr) or 800mg/dose (> =2yr) oral x5/day for 7 days.

Adenosine. 0.05mg/kg (max 3mg) stat rapid IV push, incr by 0.05mg/kg (max 3mg) every 2min to max 0.25mg/kg (max 12mg).

Adrenaline. Croup: 1% (L isomer) or 2.25% (racemic) 0.05 ml/kg/dose diluted to 4ml by inhalation or 1 in 1000 0.5ml/kg/dose (max 5ml) by inhalation.
Cardiac arrest: 0.1 ml/kg of 1 in 10,000 IV or intracardiac or via tracheal tube (up to 1 ml/kg/dose if no response).
Anaphylaxis: 0.05-0.1 ml/kg/dose of 1:10,000 intravenously.
SC: 0.01mg/kg (0.01 ml/kg of 1 in 1000), x 3 doses 20min apart if required.

Agar. see paraffin (and phenolphthalein) and agar.

Albendazole. 400mg/dose (NOT/kg) 12H for 3 days.
Enterobiasis: 400mg (NOT/kg) once, repeat in 2-4wk.

Albumin. 20%: 2-5ml/kg IV. 5%: 10-20ml/kg.

Albuterol. see salbutamol.

Alclometasone, cream or ung 0.05%.
Apply 8-12H.

Alcuronium. ICU: 0.3mg/kg IV prn. OR : 0.3mg/kg IV stat, then 0.05mg/kg/dose.

Aldesleukin (synthetic interleukin-2).
see interleukin-2.

Alfacalcidol. 0.05µg/kg (max 1µg) daily oral or IV, adjusted according to response.

Alfentanil. 10µg/kg IV or IM stat, then 5µg/kg prn. OR (ventilated): 30-50µg/kg IV over 5min, then 15µg/kg prn or 0.5-1µg/kg/min.
ICU: 50-100 µg/kg IV over 10min, then 0.5-4µg/kg/min.

Alfuzosin. 0.05mg/kg/dose (max 2.5mg) 6-12H oral.

Alginic acid (Gaviscon). Infants: 1-2g powder with feed 4H.
1-12yr: liquid 5-10ml, or granules ½ sachet after meals.
>12yr: liquid 10-20ml, or granules 1 sachet after meals.

Alglucerase. Initially 60u/kg IV over 2hr every 1-4wk according to response, reducing every 3-6 month.

Allopurinol. Gout: 2-12mg/kg/dose (max 600mg) daily oral. Cancer therapy: 2.5-5mg/kg/dose (max 200mg) 6H.

Allyloestrenol. Adult: 5mg/dose (NOT/kg) 8H (threat abortion), 12-24H (habit abortion), 3-6H (premature labour) oral.

Alprazolam. 0.005-0.02mg/kg/dose (adult 0.25-1mg) 8H oral.

Alprenolol. 1-4mg/kg/dose (max 200mg) 6-12H oral.

IV. Drug dose compendium

Alprostadil (prostaglandin E1, PGE1).
0.01-0.1μg/kg /min (10-100ng/kg/min).
To maintain PDA with 0.01 μg/kg/min (10ng/kg/min): <16kg put 30μg/kg in 50ml saline, run at 1ml/hr;
>16kg put 500μg in 830/Wt ml saline, run at 1ml/hr (e.g. 20kg child, 500μg in 41.5ml saline at 1ml/hr).
Pulmonary vasodilatation with 0.1μg/kg/min (100ng/kg/min) put 500μg in 83/Wt ml saline and run at 1ml/hr (5.0 μg/kg/min nitroglycerine = 2.0 μg/g/min, nitroprusside = 0.1 μg/kg/min PGE1 approx).

Alteplase (tissue plasminogen activator).
0.2mg/kg (max 10mg) over 2min,
then 1mg/kg (max 50mg) for 1hr,
then 0.5mg/kg (max 25mg/hr) for 2hr IV (keep fibrinogen >100mg/dl).
Local IA infusion: 0.05mg/kg/hr for 4-8hr.

Altretamine. 150-300mg/m^2 daily oral.

Aluminium acetate, solution 13% (Burrow's lotion).
For wet compresses, or daily to molluscum contagiosum.

Aluminium chloride hexahydrate, lotion 20%.
Daily at night for 1wk, then x1-2/wk.

Aluminium hydroxide. 5-50mg/kg/dose (adult 0.5-1g) 6-8H oral.
Gel (64mg/ml) 0.1ml/kg/dose 6H oral.

Aluminium hydroxide 40mg/ml, magnesium hydroxide 40mg/ml, simethicone 4mg/ml (Mylanta).
0.2-0.4 ml/kg/dose (adult 10-20ml) 4-6H oral. ICU: 0.5ml/kg /dose 3H oral if gastric pH <5.

Alverine. 1-2mg/kg/dose (max 120mg) 8H oral.

Amantadine. 2mg/kg/dose (max 100mg) 12-24H oral.
Flu A prophylaxis: 100mg daily (5-9yr), 100mg 12H (> 9yr).

Amcinonide 0.1% lotion, cream, ointment.
Apply 8-12H.

Amethocaine, eye drops 0.5%, 1%.
1-2 drops.

Amikacin. Single daily dose IV or IM: 7.5mg/kg (<30wk gestation), 10mg/kg (30-35wk gestation), 15mg/kg (1st wk life), 22.5mg/kg (2+ wk), 18mg/kg (>10yr).
Trough <5mg/l.

Amiloride. 0.2mg/kg/dose (max 5mg) 12H oral.

Aminobenzoate. 60mg/kg/dose (max 3g) 6H oral.

Aminocaproic acid. 100mg/kg (max 5g) stat, then 30 mg/kg/hr (max 1.25g/hr) until bleeding stops (max 18 g/m^2/day) oral or IV. Prophylaxis: 70mg/kg/dose 6H.

Aminoglutethimide. Adult: 250mg (NOT/kg) daily oral, incr over 4wk to 250mg 6H.

Aminophylline (100mg aminophylline = 80mg theophylline).
Load: 10mg/kg (max 500mg) IV over 1hr. Maintenance: 1st wk life 2.5mg/kg/dose 12H; 2nd wk life 4 mg/kg/dose 12H; 3wk-12mo (0.12 x age in wk) + 3mg/kg /dose 8H; 1-9yr 1.1mg/kg/hr (55mg/kg in 50ml at 1ml/hr), or 6mg/kg/dose IV over 1hr 6H; 10-16yr or adult smoker 0.7mg/kg/hr (<35kg 35mg/kg in 50ml at 1ml/hr; >35kg 25mg/ml at 0.028ml/kg/hr), or 4mg/kg/dose IV over 1hr 6H; adult non-smoker 0.5mg/kg/hr (25mg/ml at 0.02 ml/kg/hr), or 3mg/kg/dose IV over 1hr 6H; elderly 0.3 mg/kg/hr (15mg/kg in 50ml at 1ml/hr), or 2mg/kg/dose IV over 1hr 6H. Monitor theophylline level: 60-80μmol/l (neonate), 60-110 (asthma) (x0.18=μg/ml).

5-Aminosalicylic acid. see mesalazine.

IV. Drug dose compendium

Amiodarone. IV: 25μg/kg/min for 4hr, then 5-15μg/kg/min (max 1.2g/24hr).
Oral: 4mg/kg/dose (max 200mg) 8H 1 wk, 12H 1 wk, then 12-24H.
After starting tablets, taper IV infusion over 5 days. Reduce dose of digoxin and warfarin.

Amitriptyline. usually 0.5-1.0mg/kg/dose (max 100mg) 8H oral. Enuresis: 1.0-1.5mg/kg nocte.

Amlodipine. 0.05-0.2mg/kg (adult 2.5-10mg) daily oral.

Amodiaquine. Treatment: 10mg/kg daily for 3 days oral. Prophylaxis: 5mg/kg once a wk.

Amoxapine. 0.5-2mg/kg/dose (max 100mg) 8H oral.

Amoxicillin. see amoxycillin.

Amoxycillin. 10-20mg/kg/dose 8H IV, IM or oral.
Severe infection: 50mg/kg/dose (max 2g) IV 12H (1st wk life), 6H (2-4 wk), 3H or constant infusion (4+ wk).

Amoxycillin and clavulanic acid.
dose as for amoxycillin.

Amphetamine. see dexamphetamine.

Amphotericin B. Test dose 0.1mg/kg IV over 6hr, then 0.5-1.0mg/kg IV over 6hr daily; total dose 30-35mg/kg over 4-8wk.
Oral (NOT/kg): 100mg 6H treatment, 50mg 6H prophylaxis.
Bladder washout: 25μg/ml. Cream or ointment 3%: apply 6-12H.

Amphotericin, liposomal. 1mg/kg daily IV over 1hr, incr over 2-4 days to 2-3mg/kg daily.
Total dose typically 20-60mg/kg over 2-4wk.

Ampicillin. 15-25mg/kg/dose 6H IV, IM or oral. Severe infection: 50mg/kg/dose (max 2g) IV 12H (1st wk life), 6H (2-4 wk), 3H or constant infusion (4+ wk).

Ampicillin 1g + sulbactam 0.5g.
20-40mg/kg/dose (max 2g) of ampicillin 6H IM or IV over 30min.

Amrinone. <4wk old: 4mg/kg IV over 15 min, then 3-5 μg/kg/min. >4wk old: 1-3mg/kg IV over 30min, then 5-15μg/kg/min.

Amsacrine. 450-600mg/m^2 IV over 2hr daily for 3-5 days.

Amylobarbitone. 0.3-1mg/kg/dose 8-12H, or 2-4mg/kg at night, oral.

Anistreplase. Adult: 30u (NOT/kg) IV over 5min.

Anthraquinone. see Sennoside.

Antithrombin III. No. IU = (desired – actual level) x Wt / 1.4.

Antithymocyte (lymphocyte) globulin.
see immunoglobulin, lymphocyte.

Antivenom to jellyfish (box), snakes (black, brown, death adder, sea, taipan, tiger) spiders (funnel-web) and ticks.
Dose depends on amount of venom injected, not size of patient. Higher doses needed for multiple bites, severe symptoms or delayed administration.
Give adrenaline 0.005mg/kg (0.005ml/kg of 1 in 1000) SC. Initial dose antivenom usually 1-2 amp diluted 1/10 in Hartmann's solution IV over 30min. Monitor PT, PTT, fibrinogen, platelets. Give antivenom repeatedly if symptoms or coagulopathy persist.

Antivenom, red back spider. 1amp IM, may repeat in 2hr.
Severe envenomation: 2 amp diluted 1/10 in Hartmann's solution IV over 30min.

Antivenom, stonefish. 1000u (2ml) per puncture IM.
Severe envenomation: 1000u/puncture diluted 1/10 in Hartmann's solution IV over 30min.

Apraclonidine, 1% eye drops. 1-2 drops/eye 12H.

Aprobarbital. 1-3 mg/kg oral at night.

Aprostadil. see prostaglandin E1.

IV. Drug dose compendium

Aprotinin (1kiu = 140ng = 0.00056epu).
Shock: 10,000 kiu/kg (max 1,000,000kiu) IV over 1hr, then 1,000 kiu/kg/hr (max 50,000kiu/hr). Haemorrhage prophylaxis: 4,000kiu/kg slow IV, then 2,000kiu/kg/dose 6H. obstetric haemorrhage (NOT/kg): 1,000,000kiu over 30min, then 200,000kiu/hr.

Aqueous cream; pure, buffered or with 5% or 10% olive oil or peanut oil.
A base for other ingredients, or before cold compresses.

Arginine HCl. mg/kg = BE x 70 (give ½ this) IV over 2hr.

Ascorbic acid. Scurvy: 100mg/dose (NOT/kg) 8H oral 10 days.
Urine acidification: 10-30mg/kg/dose 6H.

Asparaginase-L. Test 2-50u intradermal.
Typical dose 6000u/m^2 every 3rd day x 9 doses IV over 4hr, IM or SC.

Aspirin. 10-15mg/kg/dose (adult 300-600mg) 4-6H oral. Antiplatelet: 2-5mg/kg daily.
Kawasaki: 25mg/kg/dose 6H 14 days (monitor levels), then 4mg/kg daily.
Arthritis: 25mg/kg/dose (max 2g) 6H for 3 days, then 15-20 mg/kg/dose 6H. Salicylate level (arthritis) 0.7-2.0 mmol/l (x13.81 = mg/100ml).

Astemizole. 0.2mg/kg (max 10mg) daily oral.

Atenolol. Oral: 1-2mg/kg/dose (max 100mg) 12-24H. IV: 0.05mg/kg every 5min till response (max 4 doses), then 0.1-0.2 mg/kg/dose (max 10mg) over 10min 12-24H.

Atracurium. 0.3-0.6mg/kg stat, then 5-10μg/kg/min IV.

Atropine. 0.02mg/kg (max 0.6mg) IV or IM, then 0.01 mg/kg/dose 4-6H.
Organophosphate poisoning: 0.05 mg/kg IV, then 0.02-0.05mg/kg/dose every 15-60min until atropinized (continue 12-24 hr).
Colic: RCH mixture (12 μg/ml) 2.5-5ml oral before feeds (max 15ml/day).
See also Colic Mixture, and diphenoxylate and atropine.

Auranofin. Adult: 6-9mg (NOT/kg) daily oral.

Aurothioglucose. 0.25mg/kg wkly IM, incr to 1mg/kg (max 40mg) weekly for 20wk, then every 1-4wk.

Azapropazone. 10mg/kg/dose (max 600mg) 12H oral.
Acute gout: day 1 6H, day 2 8H, then 12H.

Azatadine. 0.02-0.04mg/kg/dose (max 2mg) 12H oral.

Azathioprine. 25-75mg/m^2 (approx 1-3mg/kg) daily.

Azelaic acid (micronised). 20% cream applied 12H.

Azidothymidine (AZT). see zidovudine.

Azithromycin. 10mg/kg/dose (max 500mg) day 1, then 5 mg/kg/dose (max 250mg) days 2-5 oral.

Azlocillin. 40mg/kg/dose 8H IV.
Severe infection: 100mg/kg /dose (max 5g) IV 12H (1st wk life), 8H or constant infusion (2+ wk).

Aztreonam. 30mg/kg/dose 8H. Severe infection: 50mg/kg /dose 12H (1st wk life), 8H (2-4 wk), 6H or constant infusion (4+ wk) IV.

Bacampicillin. 15-25mg/kg/dose 8-12H oral.

Bacillus Calmette-Guerin (BCG) vaccine (CSL).
Live. Intradermal (1mg/ml): 0.075ml (<3mo) or 0.1ml (>3mo) once.
Percutaneous (60mg/ml suspension): 1 drop on skin, inoculated with Heaf apparatus, once.

Bacillus Calmette-Guerin (BCG) suspension, about 5 x 10^8 cfu/vial.
Adult: 1 vial (OncoTICE) or 3 vials (ImmuCyst) left in bladder for 2hr each wk for 6wks, then at 3, 6, 12, 18 and 24mo.

Bacitracin 400u/g + neomycin 5mg/g + polymyxin B 5000u/g (Neosporin). Ointment or eye ointment: apply x2-5/day. Powder: apply 6-12H (skin infections), every few days (burns). Eye drops: see gramicidin.

Baclofen. 0.1mg/kg/dose 8H oral, incr by 0.1 mg/kg/dose every 3 days. Effective dose about 0.5 mg/kg/dose 8H (max 1mg/kg/dose 8H). Intrathecal infusion: 2-20µg/kg (max 1000µg) per day.

Bambuterol. 0.2-0.4mg/kg (max 20mg) daily at night oral.

BCG vaccine. see Bacillus Calmette-Guerin vaccine.

Beclomethasone. Rotacap or aerosol (NOT/kg): 100-200µg (<8yr), 150-500µg (>8yr) x2-4/day.

Beclomethasone dipropionate, nasal. Aerosol or pump (50µg/spray): 1spray 12H (<12yr), 2spray 12H (>12yr).

Benazepril. Usually 0.2mg/kg/dose (max 10mg) oral daily.

Bendroflumethiazide. see bendrofluazide.

Bendrofluazide. 0.1-0.2mg/kg (max 10mg) daily oral.

Benorylate. 30mg/kg/dose (max 1.5g) 8H oral.

Benperidol. 5-15µg/kg/dose (max 1.5mg) 12-24H oral.

Benserazide. see levodopa and benserazide.

Benzhexol. 0.02-0.3mg/kg (max 15mg) daily oral.

Benzocaine, topical 1%-20%. Usually applied 4-6H.

Benzoic acid 6% + salicylic acid 3%, ointment (Whitfield's). Apply 12H.

Benzonatate. Adult: 100mg/dose (NOT/kg) 4-8H oral.

Benzoyl peroxide, liquid or gel 2.5%-10%. Apply x1-3/day.

Benzphetamine. 0.5-1mg/kg/dose (max 50mg) 8-24H oral.

Benzquinamide. IM: 1mg/kg (max 50mg) stat and repeat in 1hr if needed, then 3-4H prn. IV over 1min: 0.5mg/kg (max 25mg) once.

Benzthiazide. 0.5-2mg/kg/dose (max 100mg) 12-24H oral.

Benztropine. 0.02mg/kg stat IM or IV, may repeat in 15min. 0.02-0.1mg/kg/dose (max 6mg) 12-24H oral.

Benzylpenicilloyl polylysine. see penicilloyl polylysine.

Benzyl benzoate, lotion 25% Scabies: apply from neck down after a hot bath, remove in bath after 24hr; repeat after 5 days.
Lice: apply to infected region, wash off after 24hr; repeat after 7 days.

Benzylpenicillin. see penicillin G.

Bepridil. 4-8mg/kg (max 400mg) daily oral.

Beractant (bovine surfactant, Survanta). 4ml/kg intratracheal 4 times in 48hr (each dose in 4 parts: head and body inclined down with head to right, body down head left, body up head right, body up head left).

Betacarotene. Porphyria: 1-5mg/kg daily oral.

Betahistine. 0.15-0.3mg/kg/dose (max 16mg) 8H oral.

Betamethasone. 0.01-0.2mg/kg daily oral. Betamethasone has no mineralocorticoid action,
1mg = 25mg hydrocortisone in glucocorticoid action.

Betamethasone; gel 0.05%; cream, lotion or ointment, 0.02%, 0.05%, 0.1%. Apply sparingly 12-24H.

Betamethasone acetate 3mg/ml with betamethasone sodium phosphate 3.9mg/ml (Celestone Chronodose). Adult: 0.25-2ml (NOT/kg) intramuscular, intra-articular, or intra-lesional injection.

IV. Drug dose compendium

Betaxolol. 0.2-0.8mg/kg (max 40mg) daily oral.
Eye drops 0.25%-0.5%: 1-2 drops per eye 12H.

Bethanecol. Oral: 0.2-1mg/kg/dose (max 50mg) 6-8H. SC: 0.05-0.1 mg/kg/dose (max 5mg) 6-8H.

Bezafibrate. 4mg/kg/dose (max 200mg) 8H oral with food.

Bicarbonate. Under 5kg: dose (mmol) = BE x Wt/4 slow IV.
Over 5kg: dose (mmol) = BE x Wt/6 slow IV. These doses correct half the base deficit.

Bifonazole 1% cream. Apply daily for 2-4wk.

Biperiden. 0.02-0.1mg/kg/dose (max 4mg) 6-12H oral.

Bisacodyl. NOT/kg: $<$12mo 2.5mg PR, 1-5yr 5mg PR or 5-10mg oral, $>$5yr 10mg PR or 10-20mg oral.

Bismuth subcitrate. see tripotassium dicitratobismuthate.

Bisoprolol. 0.1-0.4mg/kg (max 20mg) daily oral.

Bitolterol. Respiratory solution (0.2%): 1ml/dose diluted to 4ml 3-6H (mild), 2ml/dose diluted to 4ml 1-2H (moderate), undiluted constant (severe, in ICU). Aerosol 370μg/puff: 1-2 puff 4-6H.

Bleomycin. 10-20u/m^2 IM, SC or IV over 15min x1-2/wk. Max total dose 250u/m^2.

Blood products. See albumin, cryoprecipitate, factor 8, fresh frozen plasma, packed cells, platelets, prothrombinex and whole blood.

Bretylium. 5-10mg/kg IV over 1hr, then 5-30μg/kg/min.

Bromazepam. 0.05-0.25mg/kg/dose 8H oral.

Bromocriptine. 0.025mg/kg/dose (max 1.25mg) 8-12H, incr wkly to 0.05-0.2mg/kg/dose (max 2.5-10mg) 6-12H oral. Inhibit lactation: 2.5mg/dose(NOT/kg) 12H.

Brompheniramine. 0.1-0.2mg/kg/dose (max 10mg) 6-8H oral, SC, IM or slow IV.

Buclizine. 0.25-1.0mg/kg/dose (max 50mg) 8-24H oral.

Budesonide. Metered dose inhaler (NOT/kg): $<$12yr 50-200μg 6-12H, reducing to 100-200μg 12H; $>$12yr 100-600μg 6-12H, reducing to 100-400μg 12H. Nebuliser (NOT/kg): $<$12yr 0.5-1mg 12H, reducing to 0.25-0.5mg 12H; $>$12yr 1-2mg 12H, reducing to 0.5-1mg 12H. Nasal spray or aerosol (NOT/kg):100-200μg/nostril daily.

Bumetanide. 25μg/kg (max 1mg) daily oral, may incr to 8-12H.

Bupivacaine. Max dose: 2mg/kg (0.4ml/kg of 0.5%). With adrenaline: max dose: 2mg/kg

Buprenorphine. 3-9μg/kg/dose (max 600μg) 6-8H sublingual, IM or slow IV.

Bupropion. 2-3mg/kg/dose (max 150mg) 8-12H oral.

Buserelin (gonadorelin analogue). Adult. Intranasal: 100 μg/dose (NOT/kg) 4H, or 150μg (NOT/kg) each nostril 8H. SC: 0.5mg/dose (NOT/kg) 8H.

Buspirone. 0.1mg/kg/dose 8H oral, incr to max 0.4 mg/kg/dose (max 15mg) 8-12H.

Busulfan. Induction: 0.06mg/kg (max 4mg) daily oral if leucocytes $>$20,000/mm3 and platelets $>$100,000/mm3. Maintenance: 0.01-0.03mg/kg (max 2mg) daily.

Butabarbital. see secbutobarbitone.

Butalbital. 1-2mg/kg/dose (max 100mg) 8-24H oral.

Butobarbitone. 2-4mg/kg (max 200mg) at night oral.

Butorphanol. IM: 0.02-0.1mg/kg/dose (max 4mg) 3-4H.
IV: 0.01-0.05mg/kg (max 2mg) 3-4H.

Butriptyline. 0.5-1.0mg/kg/dose (max 50mg) 8H oral.

Caffeine. 1-5mg/kg/dose (max 250mg) 4-8H oral or PR.

Calamine, lotion. Usually applied 6-8H.

Calcitonin. Hypercalcaemia: 4iu/kg/dose 12-24H IM or SC, may incr up to 8iu/kg/dose 6-12H. Paget's: 1.5-3iu/kg (max 160mg) x3/wk IM or SC.

Calcitriol. see vitamin D.

Calcium (as carbonate, lactate or phosphate). NOT/kg: < 3yr: 100mg x2-5/day oral; 4-12yr: 300mg x2-3/day; > 12yr: 1000mg x1-2/day.

Calcium carbimide. 1-2mg/kg/dose (max 100mg) 12H oral.

Calcium carbonate. 840mg (NOT/kg) 8-12H oral.

Calcium chloride 10% (0.7mmol/ml Ca). 0.2ml/kg (max 10ml) slow IV stat. Requirement 2ml/kg/day. Inotrope: 0.5-2mmol/kg/day (0.03-0.12ml/kg/hr).

Calcium edetate (EDTA). see sodium calcium edetate.

Calcium gluconate 10% (0.22mmol/ml Ca). 0.5ml/kg (max 20ml) slow IV stat. Requirement 5ml/kg/day. Inotrope: 0.5-2mmol/kg/day (0.1-0.4ml/kg/hr).

Canrenoate. see potassium canrenoate.

Capreomycin. 20mg/kg (max 1g) IM on 2-7 days/wk.

Captopril. 0.1-1.0mg/kg/dose (max 50mg) 8H oral.

Carbachol. 0.01%: max 0.5ml in anterior chamber of eye.

Carbamazepine. 2mg/kg/dose 8H oral, may incr over 2wk to 5-10mg/kg/dose (max 500mg) 8H.
Level 20-50umol/l (x0.24 = μg/ml).

Carbenicillin. 25-100mg/kg/dose 4-6H IM or IV.

Carbenoxolone. Adult: 20-50mg (NOT/kg) 6H oral. Mouth gel 2%, or 2g granules in 40ml water, apply 6H.

Carbidopa. see levodopa and carbidopa.

Carbimazole. 0.25mg/kg/dose (max 15mg) 8H oral for 2wk, then 0.1mg/kg/dose 8-12H.

Carbinoxamine. NOT/kg: 2mg (1-3yr), 2-4mg (3-6yr), 4-8mg (> 6yr) 6-8H oral.

Carbocaine. see mepivacaine.

Carbocisteine. 10-15mg/kg/dose (max 750mg) 8H oral.

Carboplatin. 300-400mg/m^2 IV over 60min every 4wk.

Carboprost (15-Me-PGF2-alpha). Termination: 250-500 μg/dose (NOT/kg) 1-4H (max total 12mg) IM. Post partum haemorrhage: 250 μg/dose (NOT/kg) every 15-120min IM (max total 12mg).

Carisoprodol. 7mg/kg/dose (max 350mg) 6H oral.

Carmustine (BCNU). 200mg/m^2 IV over 2hr every 6wk (reduce dose if nadir in leucocytes < 3000/mm3 or platelets < 75,000).

Carnitine. 20-35mg/kg/dose (max 1g) 8H oral or IV.

Carob bean gum (Carobel Instant). NOT/kg: 1 scoop (1.8g) in 100ml water, give 10-20ml by spoon; or add ½ a scoop to every 100-200ml of milk.

Carteolol. 0.05-0.2mg/kg (max 10mg) daily oral.

Castor oil. Laxative: 1ml/kg (max 45ml) oral. Purgative: 2ml/kg (max 90ml) oral.

Cefaclor (Ceclor). 10-15mg/kg/dose (max 500mg) 8H oral.

Cefadroxil. 10-20mg/kg/dose (max 1g) 12H oral.

Cefamandole. 25mg/kg/dose 8H IV. Severe infection: 40 mg/kg/dose (max 2g) 6H or constant infusion.

Cefazolin. see cephazolin.

Cefixime. 4mg/kg/dose (max 200mg) 12H oral.

Cefmetazole. 40mg/kg/dose (max 2g) 6-12H IV.

Cefodizime. 20mg/kg/dose (max 1g) 12H IV or IM.
Cefonicid. 10-40mg/kg (max 2g) IV over 10min or IM daily.
Cefoperazone. 20-50mg/kg/dose (max 3g) 6-12H IV over 1hr or IM.
Ceforanide. 10-20mg/kg/dose (max 1g) 12H IM or IV.
Cefotaxime. 75mg/kg/dose 12H (<4wk), 8H (4+wk) IV. Severe infection: 50mg/kg/dose (max 3g) IV 12H (preterm), 8H (1st wk life), 6H (2-4 wk), 4-6H or constant infusion (4+ wk).
Cefotetan. 10-20mg/kg/dose (max 1g) 12H IM, IV. Severe infection: 40mg/kg/dose (max 3g) 12H or constant infusion.
Cefoxitin (Mefoxin). 20-40mg/kg/dose (max 3g) 12H (1st wk life), 8H (1-4wk), 6H (>4wk) IV.
Cefpodoxime. 2-4mg/kg/dose (max 200mg) 12H oral.
Cefprozil. 15mg/kg/dose (max 500mg) 12-24H oral.
Cefsulodin. 20-50mg/kg/dose (max 2g) 6H IV.
Ceftazidime. 30mg/kg/dose 8H IV or IM. Severe infection: 50 mg/kg/dose (max 2g) 12H (1st wk life), 8H (2-4 wk), 6H or constant infusion (4+ wk).
Ceftizoxime. 20-60mg/kg/dose (max 3g) 6-8H IV.
Ceftriaxone. 30mg/kg/dose 12-24H IV, or IM (in 1% lignocaine). Severe infection: 50-75mg/kg/dose (max 4g) daily (1st wk life), 12H (2+ wk). Epiglottitis: 100mg/kg stat, then 50mg/kg after 24hr. Haemophilus or meningococcus prophylaxis: 100mg/kg IM in 1% lignocaine once.
Cefuroxime. Oral: 5-10mg/kg/dose 12H. IV: 15-30mg/kg /dose 8H. Severe infection: 50mg/kg/dose (max 2g) IV 12H (1st wk life), 8H (2nd wk), 6H or constant infusion (>2wk).
Celiprolol. 4-8mg/kg (max 400mg) daily oral.
Cellulose phosphate (Calcisorb). Adult: 5g/dose (NOT/kg) 8H oral.
Celmoleukin (synthetic interleukin-2). see interleukin-2.
Cephalexin. 10-25mg/kg/dose (max 1g) 6-12H oral. Streptococcus: 10mg/kg/dose (max 500mg) 12H. Severe infection: 20mg/kg/dose (max 1g) IV 4H or constant infusion.
Cephalothin. 10-20mg/kg/dose 6H IV or IM. Severe infection: 50mg/kg/dose (max 2g) IV 4H or constant infusion. Irrigation fluid: 2g/l (2mg/ml).
Cephamandole. 15mg/kg/dose 6H IV over 10min or IM. Severe infection: 20-40mg/kg/dose (max 2g) IV over 20min 4H or constant infusion.
Cephazolin (Kefzol). 20mg/kg stat, then 10mg/kg/dose 6H IV or IM. Severe infection: 20-30 mg/kg /dose (max 2g) IV 4H or constant infusion.
Cephradine. Oral: 5-25mg/kg/dose (max 1g) 6H. IM or IV: 20-40mg/kg/dose (max 1-2g) 6H.
Cerumol. see dichlorobenzene + chlorbutol otic.
Cetirizine. 0.2mg/kg/dose (max 10mg) 12-24H oral.
Cetylpyridinium + benzocaine, mouth wash (Cepacaine). Apply 3H prn. Do not swallow.
Charcoal (Activated). Check bowel sounds present: 0.25 g/kg/dose hourly NG. Laxative: sorbitol 1g/kg (1.4ml/kg of 70%) once NG, may repeat once.
Chenodeoxycholic acid. 5-10mg/kg/dose 12H oral.
Chloral betaine. 1.7mg = 1mg chloral hydrate.
Chloral hydrate. Hypnotic: 50mg/kg (max 2g) stat (up to 100mg/kg, max 5g, in ICU). Sedative: 6mg/kg/dose 6H oral.

Chlorambucil. Typically 0.1-0.2mg/kg/day oral.

Chloramphenicol. Severe infection: 40mg/kg (max 2g) stat, then 25mg/kg/dose (max 1g) IV, IM or oral. 1st wk life: daily; 2-4wk: 12H; 5+ wk: 8H for 5 days, then 6H. Ensure serum level 20-30mg/l peak, < 15mg/l trough.

Chlordiazepoxide. 0.1mg/kg/dose 12H oral, may incr to max 0.5mg/kg/dose 6-8H.

Chlorhexidine. 0.1%: catheterisation prep, impetigo. 0.2%: mouthwash. 1%: skin disinfection. 2-4%: hand wash.

Chlorhexidine 0.5% + alcohol 70%, solution.
Skin disinfection.

Chlorhexidine 1.5% + cetrimide 15%.
1/30 in water: cleaning tissues or wounds, equipment before sterilisation. 140ml in 1 litre water: disinfecting skin, equipment (soak 2min, rinse in sterile water).

Chlorhexidine + cetrimide, 0.05%/0.5%, 0.1%/1%, 0.15%/0.15%.
Wound cleaning.

Chlorhexidine 1% + hexamidine 0.15%, powder.
Wound cleaning.

Chlormethiazole. IV (edisylate 0.8%): 1-2ml/kg (8-16 mg/kg) over 15min, then 0.5-1.0ml/kg/hr (4-8mg/kg/hr). Oral (capsule 192mg base): adult 2-4cap stat (may repeat in 1-2hr), then 1-2cap 8H.

Chlormezanone. 5mg/kg/dose (max 200mg) 6-8H, or 10mg/kg (max 400mg) at night oral.

Chlorophyllin copper complex. 2mg/kg/dose 8-24H oral.

Chloroprocaine. Max 11mg/kg (max 800mg). With adrenaline (1/200,000) max 14mg/kg (max 1000mg).

Chloroquine. Oral: 10mg/kg daily x3 days. IM: 4mg/kg /dose 12H for 3 days. Prophylaxis: 5mg/kg (max 300mg) oral x1/wk. Lupus, rheumatoid arthritis: 12mg/kg (max 600mg) daily, reducing to 4-8mg/kg (max 400mg) daily oral.

Chlorothiazide. 5-20mg/kg/dose (max 1g) 12-24H oral, IV.

Chlorotrianisene. 0.25-0.5mg/kg (max 25mg) daily oral.

Chloroxylenol, cream 0.3%, liquid 2.5-5%.
To clean skin or wounds.

Chlorphenasin, ointment 1%. Apply 12H.

Chlorpheniramine. 0.1mg/kg/dose (max 4mg) 6-8H oral.

Chlorpheniramine 1.25mg + phenylephrine 2.5mg in 5ml syrup (Demazin).
NOT/kg: 1.25-2.5ml (0-1yr) 2.5-5ml (2-5yr), 5-10ml (6-12yr), 10-15ml (> 12yr) 6-8H oral.

Chlorpromazine. Oral or PR: 0.5-2mg/kg/dose (max 100 mg) 6-8H; up to 20mg/kg/dose 8H for psychosis. Slow IV or IM: 0.25-1mg/kg/dose (usual max 50mg) 6-8H.

Chlorpropamide. Adult: initially 125-250mg (NOT/kg) daily oral, max 500mg daily.

Chlorprothixene. Usually 0.5-1mg/kg/dose 6-8H oral or IM.

Chlorquinaldol, paste 5%. Apply 12H.

Chlortetracycline, cream or ointment 3%.
Apply 8-24H.

Chlorthalidone. 2mg/kg (max 100mg) 3 times a wk oral.

Chlorzoxazone. 5-15mg/kg/dose (max 750mg) 6-8H oral.

Cholecalciferol (Vitamin D3). 1u = 1u ergocalciferol see vitamin D.

Cholera vaccine (CSL). Inactivated. 2 doses SC 7-28 days apart: 0.1ml then 0.3ml (< 5yr), 0.3ml then 0.5ml (5-9yr), 0.5ml then 1ml (> 9yr). Boost every 6mo (use 1st dose).

Cholestyramine. 50-150mg/kg/dose (max 9g) 6-8H oral.

Choline salicylate, mouth gel (Bonjela).
Apply 3H prn.

Choline theophyllinate (200mg = theophylline 127mg).
see theophylline.

Chorionic gonadotrophin. Usually 100iu/kg (max 5000iu) IM x3/wk for 2-8wk. After FSH: 10,000iu (NOT/kg) IM once. Men: 7000iu (NOT/kg) IM x2/wk, with 75iu FSH and 75iu LH IM x3/wk.

Chymopapain. Adult: 2000-4000 picokatal units per disc (NOT/kg), max 10,000 picokatal units per patient.

Cilazapril. Usually 0.02-0.1mg/kg (max 5mg) daily oral. Renal hypertension: 0.005-0.01mg/kg daily oral.

Cimetidine. 10-15mg/kg/dose (usual max 200mg/dose) 12H (newborn), 6H (> 4wk) IV or oral.

Cinnarizine. 0.3-0.6mg/kg/dose 8H oral. Peripheral vascular disease: 1.5mg/kg/dose (max 75mg) 8H oral.

Cinchocaine. Max dose 2mg/kg (0.4ml/kg of 0.5%).

Cinoxacin. 10mg/kg/dose (max 500mg) 12H oral.

Ciprofibrate. 2-4mg/kg (max 200mg) daily oral.

Ciprofloxacin. 5-10mg/kg/dose (max 750mg) 12H IV or oral. Reduce dose of theophylline.

Cisapride. 0.2-0.6mg/kg/dose (max 25mg) x4/day oral before meals and at bedtime.

Cisplatin. 60-100mg/m^2 IV over 6hr every 3-4wk x6 cycles.

Clarithromycin. 5-10mg/kg/dose (max 500mg) 12H oral.

Clavulanic acid with amoxycillin or ticarcillin.
Dose as for amoxycillin or ticarcillin.

Clemastine. 0.02-0.06mg/kg/dose (max 3mg) 12H oral.

Clidinium. 0.05-0.1mg/kg/dose (max 5mg) 6-8H oral.

Clindamycin. 5mg/kg/dose 6H oral, IM or IV over 30min. Severe infection: 10-20mg/kg/dose (max 1g) 6H IV over 1hr. Acne solution 1%: apply 12H.

Clioquinol, cream 10mg/g, powder 100%.
Apply 6-12H.

Clobazam. 0.1-0.4mg/kg/dose (max 20mg) 8-12H oral.

Clobetasone, 0.1% eye drops. 1-2drops/eye 1-6H.

Clofazimine. 2mg/kg (max 100mg) daily oral. Lepra reaction: up to 6mg/kg (max 300mg) daily for max 3mo.

Clofibrate. 10mg/kg/dose 8-12H oral.

Clomiphene citrate. Adult: 50mg (NOT/kg) daily for 5 days oral, incr to 100mg daily for 5 days if no ovulation.

Clomipramine. 0.5mg/kg/dose 8-12H oral.

Clonazepam. 0.02mg/kg/dose (max 0.5mg) 12H oral, slowly incr to 0.05mg/kg/dose (max 2mg) 6-12H oral. Status (may be repeated), NOT/kg: neonate 0.25mg, child 0.5mg, adult 1mg IV.

Clonidine. 3-5µg/kg slow IV, 1-6µg/kg/dose (max 300µg) 8-12H oral. Migraine: start with 0.5µg/kg /dose 12H oral.

Clorazepate. 0.3-2mg/kg (max 90mg) daily at night oral, or 0.1-0.5mg/kg/dose (max 30mg) 8H.

Clostridia antitoxin. See gas gangrene antitoxin.

Clotrimazole. Topical: 1% cream or solution 8-12H. Vaginal (NOT/kg): 1% cream or 100mg tab daily for 6 days, or 2% cream or 500mg tab daily for 3 days.

Cloxacillin. 15mg/kg/dose (max 500mg) 6H oral, IM or IV. Severe infection: 25-50 mg/kg/dose (max 2g) IV 12H (1st wk life), 8H (2-4 wk), 4-6H (>4 wk).

Clozapine. 0.5mg/kg/dose 12H oral, incr over 7-14 days to 2-5mg/kg/dose (max 300mg) 8-12H; later reducing to 2mg/kg/dose 8-12H.

Coal tar, topical. 0.5% incr to max 10%, applied 6-8H.

Cocaine. Topical: 1-3mg/kg.

Codeine. Analgesic: 0.5-1mg/kg/dose 4H oral. Antitussive: 0.25-0.5mg/kg/dose 6H.

Co-dergocrine mesylate. Adult: usually 3.0-4.5mg (NOT/kg) daily before meal oral or sublingual. 300μg (NOT/kg) daily IM, SC or IV infusion.

Colaspase. see asparaginase.

Colchicine. Acute gout: 0.02mg/kg/dose (max 1mg) 2H oral (max 3 doses/day). Chronic use (gout, FMF): 0.01-0.04mg/kg (max 2mg) daily oral.

Colestipol granules. 0.1-0.2g/kg/dose (max 10g) 8H oral.

Colfosceril palmitate. see surfactant, synthetic.

Colic mixture (RCH). Atropine 12μg/ml + phenobarbitone 3 mg/ml. Infant: 2.5-5ml/dose (NOT/kg) before feed, max 15ml/day.

Colistimethate sodium. see colistin.

Colistin (1mg = 200,000u approx).
Oral: 1.5-3mg/kg/dose 8H. IM or slow IV: 2mg/kg/dose (max 100mg) 8H.

Colistin 3mg/ml + neomycin 3.3mg/ml otic.
4 drops 8H.

Colonic lavage solution. Poisoning: if bowel sounds present, 30ml/kg/hr NG for 4-8hr (until rectal effluent clear).

Coloxyl. See dioctyl sodium sulphosuccinate, poloxalkol.

Corticotrophin (corticotropin). See ACTH.

Cortisone acetate. Physiological: 0.2mg/kg/dose 8H oral. Cortisone acetate 1mg = hydrocortisone 1.25mg in mineralocorticoid and glucocorticoid action.

Coryza vaccine (Neisseria, Klebsiella and Haemophilus; CSL).
Inactivated. 4 doses 1wk apart: 0.25ml, 0.5ml, 0.75ml, 1ml (<12yr half dose).

Cosyntropin. see tetracosactrin zinc injection.

Cotrimoxazole (trimethoprim 1mg + sulphamethoxazole 5mg). TMP 2.5mg/kg/dose 12H IV over 1hr or oral. Pneumocystis: TMP 250mg/m^2 stat, then 150mg/m^2 8H (<11yr) or 12H (>10yr) IV over 1hr, in renal failure dose interval = serum creatinine (mmol/l) x 135 (max 48hr); peak serum TMP 5-10μg/ml, SMX 100-200μg/ml. IV infusion: TMP max 1.6mg/ml in 5% dextrose.

Coumarin. Oral: 1-8mg/kg (max 400mg) daily. Cream 100mg/g: apply 8-12H.

Cromoglycate, sodium. Inhalation (Intal): 1 cap (20mg) 6-8H, 2ml solution (20mg) 6-8H, aerosol 1-10mg 6-8H. Eye drops (2%): 1-2 drops per eye 4-6H. Oral: 5-10mg/kg /dose (max 200mg) 6H oral. Nasal (Rynacrom): insufflator 5mg in each nostril 6H, spray 1 puff in each nostril 6H.

Cromolyn sodium. see cromoglycate.

Crotamiton, cream or lotion 10%.
Apply x2-3/day.

Cryoprecipitate (factor 8 about 5u/ml and 100u/bag, fibrinogen about 10mg/ml and 200mg/bag). Low factor 8: 1u/kg incr activity 2% (half life 12hr); usual dose 5ml/kg or 1 bag/4kg 12H IV for 1-2 infusions (muscle, joint), 3-6 infusions (hip, forearm, retroperitoneal, oropharynx), 7-14 infusions (intracranial). Low fibrinogen: usual dose 5ml/kg or 1bag/4kg IV. A bag is usually 20-30ml.

Cyanocobalamin. Use hydroxocobalamin.

Cyclizine. 1mg/kg/dose (max 50mg) 8H oral, IM or IV.

Cyclobenzaprine. 0.2-0.4mg/kg/dose (max 20mg) 8H oral.
Cyclofenil. Adult: 200mg/dose (NOT/kg) 12H oral, starting 3rd day of menstruation.
Cyclopenthiazide. 5-10μg/kg/dose (max 500μg) 12-24H oral.
Cyclopentolate, eye drops 0.5% or 1%.
1 drop per eye, repeat after 5min. Pilocarpine 1% speeds recovery.
Cyclophosphamide. A typical regimen is 600mg/m^2 IV over 30min daily for 3 days, then 600mg/m^2 IV wkly or 10mg/kg twice wkly (if leucocytes >3000/mm^3).
Cycloserine. 5-10mg/kg/dose (max 500mg) 12H oral. Keep plasma concentration <30μg/ml.
Cyclosporin. 1-3μg/kg/min IV for 24-48hr, then 5-8mg/kg/dose 12H reducing by 1mg/kg/dose each month to 3-4 mg/kg/dose oral. Trough level by Abbott TDx monoclonal specific assay (x 2.5 = non-specific assay level) on whole blood: 120-200ng/ml (marrow), 150-200ng/ml first 3mo then 100-150ng/ml (kidney), 100- 400ng/ml (heart, liver).
Cyclosporine. see cyclosporin.
Cyproheptadine. 0.1mg/kg/dose 8-12H oral.
Cyproterone acetate. 25-50mg/m^2/dose 8-12H oral.
Cyproterone acetate + ethinyloestradiol (2mg/35μg) x 21 tab, + 7 inert tab.
Contraception: 1 tab orally daily, starting 1st day of menstruation.
Cytarabine. Usually 100mg/m^2 daily for 10 days by IV injection or constant infusion. Intrathecal: 30mg/m^2 every 4 days until CSF normal (dissolve in saline not diluent).
Cytomegalovirus immunoglobulin.
see immunoglobulin, CMV.
Dacarbazine. 250mg/m^2 IV daily for 5 days every 3wk.
Dactinomycin. Usually 400-600μg/m^2 IV daily for 5 days, repeat after 3-4wk.
Danazol. 2-4mg/kg/dose (max 200mg) 6-12H oral.
Danthron. 1-6yr 25mg, 7-12yr 50mg, adult 100mg stat.
Dantrolene. Hyperpyrexia: 1mg/kg/min until improves (max 10mg/kg), then 1-2mg/kg/dose 6H for 1-3day IV or oral. Spasticity: 0.5-2mg/kg/dose (max 100mg) 6H oral.
Dapsone. 1-2mg/kg (max 100mg) daily oral.
Derm herpet. 1-6mg/kg (max 300mg) daily. See also pyrimethamine.
Daunorubicin. 30mg/m^2 wkly slow IV, or 60-90mg/m^2 every 3wk. Max total dose 500mg/m^2.
DDAVP. see desmopressin.
Debrisoquine. 0.2-1mg/kg/dose (max 60mg) 12-24H oral.
Deferoxamine. see desferrioxamine.
Demeclocycline. >8yr: 3mg/kg/dose (max 150mg) 6-12H oral.
Deserpidine. 0.005-0.02mg/kg (max 1mg) daily oral.
Desferrioxamine. Antidote: 10-15mg/kg/hr IV for 12-24hr (max 6g/24hr); some also give 5-10g (NOT/kg) once oral. Thalassaemia (NOT/kg): 500mg per unit blood, and 1-3g in 5ml SC over 10hr 5-6 nights per wk.
Desipramine. 0.5-1.0mg/kg/dose (max 50mg) 8-12H oral.
Desmopressin (DDAVP). 5-10μg (0.05-0.1ml) per dose (NOT/kg) 12-24H nasal. Low factor VIII: 0.3μg/kg in 1ml/kg saline IV over 1hr 12-24H.
Desogestrel + ethinyloestradiol (150μg/30μg) x21 tab, + 21 inert tab.
Contraception: 1 tab daily, starting 1st day of menstruation.
Dexamethasone. 0.1-0.25mg/kg/dose 6H oral or IV. BPD: 0.1mg/kg/dose 6H for 3 days, then 8H 3 days, 12H 3 days, 24H 3 days, 48H 7 days. Severe croup: 0.6mg/kg (max 12mg) IM stat, then prednisolone 1mg/kg/dose 8-12H oral. Eye drops 0.1%: 1-2 drops per eye 3-8H. Dexamethasone has no mineralocorticoid action, but 1mg = 25mg hydrocortisone in glucocorticoid action.

Dexamphetamine. 0.2mg/kg daily oral, incr to max 0.6 mg/kg/dose (max 30mg) 12H.
Dexchlorpheniramine. 0.04mg/kg/dose (max 2mg) 6-8H oral.
Dexfenfluramine. Adult: 15mg (NOT/kg) 12H oral.
Dextran 1 (Promit). 0.3ml/kg IV 1-2min before giving dextran 40 or dextran 70.
Dextran 40. 10% solution: 10ml/kg/dose (max 20ml/kg day 1, then 10ml/kg/day). Half life about 3hr.
Dextran 70. 6% solution: 10ml/kg/dose (max 20ml/kg day 1, then 10ml/kg/day). Half life about 12hr.
Dextroamphetamine. see dexamphetamine.
Dextromethorphan. 0.2-0.5mg/kg/dose 6-8H oral.
Dextromoramide. 0.1mg/kg/dose 8H, may incr to 0.5 mg/kg /dose (max 20mg) 8H.
Dextropropoxyphene. Hydrochloride 1.3mg/kg/dose (max 65mg) or napsylate 2mg/kg/dose (max 100mg) 6H oral.
Dextrose (glucose). Hypoglycaemia: 1ml/kg 50% dextrose IV, then incr infusion rate. Hyperkalaemia: 0.1u/kg insulin + 2ml/kg 50% dextrose IV. Neonates: 6g/kg/day (about 4mg/kg/min) day 1, incr to 12 g/kg/day (up to 18 g/kg/day with hypoglycaemia). Infusion rate (ml/hr) = (4.17 x Wt x g/kg/day)/%dextrose. Dose (g/kg/day) = (ml/hr x %dextrose)/(4.17 x Wt). mg/kg/min = g/kg/day/1.44.
Dezocine. IM: usually 0.2mg/kg/dose (max 10mg) 3-6H. IV: usually 0.1mg/kg/dose 2-4H.
Diazepam. 0.2mg/kg/dose IV. 0.2-0.5mg/kg/dose 8-12H oral or PR. Do not give by IV infusion (binds to PVC).
Diazoxide. Hypertension: 1-3mg/kg stat by rapid IV injection (severe hypotension may occur) repeat once prn, then 2-5mg/kg/dose IV 6H. Hyperinsulinism: 30-100 mg/m^2/dose 8H oral.
Dibromopropamidine, cream 0.15%. Apply on dressing prn.
Dibucaine. see cinchocaine.
Dichlorobenzene 2% + chlorbutol 5% otic (Cerumol). 5 drops to ear 15min before syringing.
Dichlorphenamide. 2-4mg/kg (max 200mg) stat, then 2mg/kg/dose (max 100mg) 12H until response, then 0.5-1mg/kg/dose (max 50mg) 8-24H oral.
Diclofenac. 1mg/kg/dose (max 50mg) 8-12H oral.
Dicloxacillin. 3-6mg/kg/dose 6H oral.
Dicobalt edetate. 6mg/kg (max 300mg) IV over 1-5min, repeat x2 if no response.
Dicyclomine. 0.5mg/kg/dose (max 15mg) 6H oral.
Didanosine. 50-150mg/m^2/dose 12H oral.
Dideoxycytidine (ddC). see zalcitabine.
Diethylcarbamazine. Filariasis, onchocerciasis, loiasis: 2mg/kg/dose 8H oral for 3-4wk. Ascariasis: 6-10mg/kg/dose 8H oral 7-10days. Tropical eosinophilia: 13mg/kg daily 4-7 days.
Diethylpropion. 6-12yr: 25mg (NOT/kg) 12H oral. >12yr: 25mg (NOT/kg) 6-8H oral.
Diethylstilboestrol. see stilboestrol.
Difenoxin 1mg and atropine 0.025mg. Adult: 1-2 tab (NOT/kg) 6-8H oral.
Diflunisal. 5-10mg/kg/dose (max 500mg) 12H oral.
Digoxin. 15µg/kg stat and 5µg/kg after 6H, then 5 µg/kg/dose (max 200µg IV, 250µg oral) 12H slow IV or oral. Level 0.5-2.5 nmol/l (x0.78 = ng/ml).
Digoxin FAB antibodies. IV over 30min. Dose (to nearest 40mg) = serum digoxin (nmol/l) x Wt (kg) x 0.3, or mg ingested x 55. Give if >0.3mg/kg ingested, or level >6.4 nmol/l.
Dihydrocodeine. 0.5-1mg/kg/dose 4-6H oral.

Dihydroergotamine mesylate. Adult: 1mg (NOT/kg) IM or IV, repeat hourly x2 if needed. Max 6mg/wk.
Dihydromorphinone. 0.02-0.1mg/kg/dose 3-6H SC, IM, slow IV, PR or oral.
Dihydrotachysterol. see vitamin D.
Diltiazem. 1mg/kg/dose 6H, incr to max 2mg/kg/dose (max 90mg) 6H oral.
Dimenhydrinate. 1.0-1.5mg/kg/dose (max 50mg) 4-6H oral, IM or IV.
Dimercaprol (BAL). 3mg/kg/dose (max 150mg) IM 4H for 2 days, then 6H for 1 day, then 12H for 10 days.
Dimethicone, cream 10%, 15%. Barrier cream, apply prn.
Dimethindene. 0.02-0.04mg/kg/dose (max 2mg) 8H oral.
Dimethyl sulfoxide, 50%. 50ml in bladder for 15min 2wkly.
Dinoprost (Prostaglandin F2 alpha). Extra-amniotic: 1ml of 250 μg/ml stat, then 3ml 2H. Intra-amniotic: 40mg stat, then 10-40mg after 24hr if required.
Dinoprostone (Prostaglandin E2). Labour induction: 1mg into posterior vagina, may repeat dose 1-2mg after 6hr (max 60μg/kg over 6hr). Maintain PDA: 25 μg/kg 1H (less often after 1wk) oral; or 0.003-0.01 μg/kg/min IV.
Dioctyl sodium sulphosuccinate. see docusate sodium.
Diphemanil, powder 20mg/g (2%). Apply 8-12H.
Diphenhydramine. 1-2mg/kg/dose (max 100mg) 6-8H oral.
Diphenidol. 0.5-1mg/kg/dose (max 50mg) 4H oral.
Diphenoxylate 2.5mg and atropine 25μg tab (Lomotil). Adult: 1-2 tab (NOT/kg) 6-8H oral.
Diphenylmethane. See bisacodyl.
Diphenylpyraline. 7-12yr: 2.5mg (NOT/kg) 8H oral. >12yr: 2.5-5mg (NOT/kg) 8H oral.
Diphtheria antitoxin (horse). IM or IV: 2500u (nasal), 10,000u (unilateral tonsillar), 20,000u (bilateral tonsillar), 30,000u (laryngeal), 50,000u (beyond tonsillar fossa) IM. Bullneck: 150,000u. Repeat dose may be needed. See also immunoglobulin, diphtheria.
Diphtheria vaccine, adult (CSL). Inactivated. 0.5ml IM stat, 6wk later, and 6mo later. Boost every 10yr.
Diphtheria vaccine, child (CSL). Inactivated. 0.5ml IM stat, 6wk later, and 6mo later. Boost with adult vaccine.
Diphtheria + pertussis + tetanus vaccine (Triple Antigen). 0.5ml IM at 2mo,4mo,6mo, 18mo and (not Australia) 5yr.
Diphtheria + tetanus vaccine, adult (ADT). Inactivated. 0.5 ml IM stat, 6wk later, and 6mo later. Boost every 10yr.
Diphtheria + tetanus vaccine, child Inactivated. 0.5ml IM stat, 6wk later, and 6mo later. Boost with ADT.
Dipivefrin, eye drops 0.1%. 1 drop per eye 12H.
Diprophylline. Usually 15mg/kg/dose 6H oral or IM.
Dipyridamole. 1-2mg/kg/dose (max 100mg) 6-8H oral.
Disodium edetate. see trisodium edetate.
Disodium pamidronate. 0.5-1.5mg/kg/dose (max 90mg) IV over 24hr, repeat every 2-3wk.
Disopyramide. Oral: 5mg/kg stat, then 2-5mg/kg/dose (max 200mg) 6H. IV: 2mg/kg (max 150mg) over 5min, then 0.4mg/kg/hr (max 800mg/day). Level 9-15umol/l (x0.3395 = μg/ml).
Distigmine. Neurogenic bladder, megacolon: 0.01mg/kg IM daily, 0.1mg/kg oral daily. Myasthenia gravis: 0.1-0.2mg/kg/dose 12-24H (max 20mg daily) oral.

Disulfiram. Adult: 500mg (NOT/kg) oral daily for 1-2wk, then 125-500mg daily.

Divalproex. 5-25mg/kg/dose (max 500mg) 8-12H oral.

Dobutamine. 1-20μg/kg/min IV.

Docusate sodium. NOT/kg: 100mg (3-10yr), 120-240mg (> 10yr) daily oral. Enema (5ml 18% + 155ml water): 30ml (newborn), 60ml (1-12mo), 60-120ml (> 12mo) PR.

Docusate sodium 100mg + bisacodyl 10mg, suppository. ½ suppository (< 12mo), 1 suppository (> 1yr) when required PR.

Docusate sodium 50mg + sennoside 8mg, tab. > 12yr: 1-4 tab at night oral.

Domperidone. Oral: 0.2-0.4mg/kg/dose (max 20mg) 4-8H. Rectal suppository: adult 30-60mg (NOT/kg) 4-8H.

Dopamine. 1-20μg/kg/min IV.

Dopexamine. 0.5-6μg/kg/min IV infusion.

Dothiepin. 0.5-1.0mg/kg/dose (max 50mg) 8-12H oral.

Doxacurium. 50-80μg/kg stat, then 5-10μg/kg/dose IV.

Doxapram. 5mg/kg IV over 1hr, then 0.5-1.0mg/kg/hr for 1hr (max total dose 400mg).

Doxazosin. Usually 0.02-0.1mg/kg (max 4mg) daily oral.

Doxepin. 0.2-2mg/kg/dose (max 100mg) 8H oral.

Doxorubicin. 30mg/m^2 IV over 15min wkly, or 30mg/m^2 daily for 2-3days every 3-4wk. Max total dose 480mg/m^2 (300mg/m^2 if mediastinal irradiation).

Doxycycline. Over 8yr: 2mg/kg/dose (max 100mg) 12H for 2 doses, then daily.

Doxylamine. 0.25-0.5mg/kg/dose (max 25mg) 8H oral. Hypnotic: 0.5-1mg/kg (max 50mg).

Dronabinol. Initially 5mg/m^2/dose 2-4H (max 4-6 doses per day) oral, slow incr by 2.5mg/m^2/dose to max 15mg/m^2/dose 4H.

Droperidol. Oral: 0.1-0.4mg/kg/dose (max 20mg) 4-8H. IM or slow IV: 0.1-0.15mg/kg/dose (max 15mg) 4-6H.

Dydrogesterone. 0.2mg/kg/dose (max 10mg) 12-24H oral.

Dyphylline. see diprophylline.

Econazole. Topical: 1% cream, powder or lotion 8-12H. Vaginal: 75mg cream or 150mg ovule twice daily.

Ecothiopate, eye drops 0.03%, 0.06%, 0.125%, 0.25%. Usually 1 drop 0.125% per eye every 1-2 days nocte.

Edrophonium. Test dose 20μg/kg, then 100μg/kg IV.

EDTA. see sodium calcium edetate.

Electrolyte solution. see glucose electrolyte solution.

EMLA cream. see lignocaine + prilocaine.

Emulsifying ointment. Soap substitute or emollient for dry skin.

Enalapril. 0.2-1.0mg/kg (max 40mg) daily oral.

Enalaprilat. Usually 0.025mg/kg/dose (max 1.25mg) 6H IV, max 0.1mg/kg/dose (max 5mg) 6H.

Enoxacin. 4-8mg/kg/dose (max 400mg) 12H oral.

Enoxaparin (1mg = 100u). Prevent DVT: 0.4-0.8mg/kg/dose (max 40mg) 2-12hr preoperatively, then daily SC. Haemodialysis: 1mg/kg into arterial line at start 4hr session.

Enoximone. IV: 5-20μg/kg/min. Oral: 1-3mg/kg/dose (max 150mg) 8H.

Ephedrine. 0.3-1mg/kg/dose (max 60mg) 6-8H oral. Nose drops (0.25%-1%): 1 drop each nostril 6-8H for 3-4 days.

Epinephrine. see adrenaline.

Epirubicin. Adult: 75-90mg/m^2 IV over 10min every 3wk.

Epoetin. see erythropoietin.

Epoprostenol (prostacyclin, PGI2). 0.01μg/kg/min IV. Pulmonary vasodilatation: 0.01μg/kg/min epoprost = 5μg/kg/min nitroglycerine = 2μg/kg/min nitroprusside = 0.1μg/kg/min PGE1.

Epsilon aminocaproic acid. see aminocaproic acid.

Ergocalciferol. see vitamin D.

Ergoloid mesylates. see co-dergocrine mesylate.

Ergometrine maleate. Adult: 500μg (NOT/kg) IM or IV; 500μg/dose (NOT/kg) 8H oral, sublingual

Ergonovine maleate. see ergometrine maleate.

Ergotamine tartrate. > 10yr (NOT/kg): 2mg sublingual stat, then 1mg/hr (max 6mg/episode, 10mg/wk). Suppository (1-2mg): 1 stat, may repeat once after 1hr.

Erythrityl tetranitrate. 0.1-0.2mg/kg/dose 6-8H sublingual, may incr to 0.5mg/kg/dose (max 25mg) 6H.

Erythromycin. 10-25mg/kg/dose (adult 0.25-1g) 6-8H oral or IV over 1hr.

Erythropoietin. 50u/kg x3/wk, incr to max 200u/kg x3/wk. Maintenance: 150u/kg x1-2/wk.

Esmolol. 0.5mg/kg over 1min, then 50μg/kg/min for 4min; if no response repeat 0.5mg/kg and give 50-200 μg/kg/min for up to 48hr.

Estazolam. 0.02-0.1mg/kg (max 4mg) at night oral.

Estradiol. see oestradiol.

Estramustine. 200mg/m^2/dose 8H oral (avoid milk).

Estrone. see oestrone.

Estropipate. Adult: 0.625-7.5mg (NOT/kg) daily starting 1st day of menstruation, for 3 of every 4wks. Intravaginal: 2-4g cream daily.

Ethacrynic acid. IV: 0.5-1mg/kg/dose (max 50mg) 12-24H. Oral: 1-4mg/kg/dose (max 200mg) 12-24H.

Ethambutol. 25mg/kg once daily for 8wk, then 15mg/kg daily oral. Intermittent: 35mg/kg x3/wk.

Ethamsylate. 12.5mg/kg/dose (max 500mg) 6H oral, IM, IV.

Ethchlorvynol. 10-20mg/kg (max 1g) at night oral.

Ethinyloestradiol. see desogestrel, ethynodiol, levonorgestrel, norethisterone and oestradiol.

Ethionamide. TB: 15-20mg/kg (max 1g) at night oral. Leprosy: 5-8mg/kg (max 375mg) daily.

Ethosuximide. 2.5mg/kg/dose 6H oral, incr by 50% each wk to max 10mg/kg/dose (max 500mg) 6H.

Ethotoin. 5mg/kg/dose 6H oral after meal, incr to max 15mg/kg/dose (max 750mg) 6H.

Ethylnoradrenaline. 0.02-0.04mg/kg IM or SC.

Ethylnorepinephrine. see ethylnoradrenaline.

Ethyloestrenol. 0.1mg/kg (max 4mg) daily oral.

Ethynodiol diacetate + ethinyloestradiol (0.5mg/50μg or 1mg/50μg) x 21 tab, + 7 inert tab. Contraception: 1 tab daily, starting 1st day of menstruation.

Etidocaine, 0.5%-1.5%. Max 6mg/kg (0.6ml/kg of 1%) parenteral, or 8mg/kg (0.8ml/kg of 1%) with adrenaline.

Etidronate. see sodium etidronate.

Etodolac. 4-8mg/kg/dose (max 400mg) 6-8H oral.

Etomidate. 0.3mg/kg slow IV.

Etoposide. 50-60mg/m^2 IV over 1hr daily for 5 days, repeat after 2-4wk. Oral dose 2-3 times IV dose.

Etretinate. 0.4mg/kg/dose 8-12H oral for 2-4wk, then 0.5-1mg/kg (max 75mg) daily for 6-8wk, then reducing to 0.25-0.5mg/kg daily. Teratogenic.

Factor 8 concentrate (vial 200-250u). Joint 20u/kg, psoas 30u/kg, cerebral 50u/kg.

Factor 9 complex (factor 2, 9, 10, and some 7). 40-60iu/kg, then 5-10iu/kg/dose 12H IV. Prophylaxis: 10-20iu/kg x1-2/wk. Factor 8 antibodies: 75iu/kg, repeat in 12hr prn.

Famotidine. 0.5-1.0mg/kg/dose (max 40mg) 12-24H oral. 0.5mg/kg/dose (max 20mg)12H slow IV.

Fat emulsion 20%. 1-3g/kg/day IV (ml/hr = g/kg/day x Wt x 0.21).

Fatty acids (Nandicelle). Adult: 1-2cap (NOT/kg) 8-12H.

Felodipine. 0.05mg/kg/dose (max 2.5mg), incr to 0.2 mg/kg/dose (max 10mg) 12H oral.

Fenbufen. 10mg/kg/dose (max 450mg) 12H oral.

Fenfluramine. Adult: 60mg (NOT/kg) daily oral.

Fenofibrate. 2mg/kg/dose (max 100mg) 6-12H oral.

Fenoprofen. 4mg/kg/dose (max 200mg) 6-8H oral, may incr gradually to 12mg/kg/dose (max 800mg).

Fenoterol. Oral: 0.1mg/kg/dose 6H. Respiratory solution 1mg/ml: 0.5ml/dose diluted to 2ml 3-6H (mild), 1.0ml/dose diluted to 2ml 1-2H (moderate), undiluted continuous (severe, in ICU). Aerosol (200µg/puff): 1-2 puffs 4-8H.

Fentanyl. 1-4µg/kg/dose (max 200µg) IM or IV; infuse 2-4µg/kg/hr. Ventilated: 5-10µg/kg stat or 50µg/kg IV over 1hr; infuse 5-10µg/kg/hr (amp 50µg/ml at 0.1-0.2ml/kg/hr).

Ferrous salts. Prophylaxis 2mg/kg/day elemental iron oral, treatment 6mg/kg/day elemental iron oral. Fumarate 1mg = 0.33mg iron. Gluconate 1mg = 0.12mg iron; so Fergon (60mg/ml gluconate) prophylaxis 0.3ml/kg daily, treatment 1ml/kg daily oral. Sulphate (dried) 1mg = 0.3mg iron; so Ferro-Gradumet (350mg dried sulphate) prophylaxis 7mg/kg (max 350mg) daily, treatment 20mg/kg (max 1050mg) daily oral.

Fibrinolysin 8-10u/ml and desoxyribonuclease 500-667 u/ml, ointment or solution. Apply topically 6-24H.

Filgrastim (granulocyte CSF). Idiopathic or cyclic neutropenia: 5µg/kg daily SC or IV over 30min. Congenital neutropenia: 12µg/kg daily SC or IV over 1hr. Marrow transplant: 20-30µg/kg daily IV over 4-24hr, reducing if neutrophils $>1x10^9$/l.

Finasteride. Adult: 5mg (NOT/kg) daily oral.

Flavoxate. 2-4mg/kg/dose (max 400mg) 6-8H oral.

Flecainide. 2mg/kg/dose (max 100mg) 12H oral or IV over 30min, may incr over 2wk to 5mg/kg/dose (max 200mg) 12H.

Flosequinan. 1-3mg/kg (max 150mg) daily oral.

Floxuridine (FUDR). 100-300µg/kg/day by constant intra-arterial infusion (400-600µg/kg/day in hepatic artery). Stop if WCC $<3500/mm^3$ or platelets $<100,000/mm^3$.

Fluclorolone, cream 0.025%. Apply sparingly 12H.

Flucloxacillin. 10mg/kg/dose (max 250mg) 6H oral, IM or IV. Severe infection: 25-50mg/kg/dose (max 2g) IV 12H (1st wk life), 8H (2-4 wk), 4-6H or constant infusion (>4 wk).

Fluconazole. 4mg/kg (max 200mg) stat, then 2mg/kg (max 100mg) daily oral or IV. Severe infection: 8mg/kg (max 400mg) stat, then 4-8mg/kg (max 200-400mg) daily IV.

Flucytosine (5-fluorocytosine). 400-1200mg/m^2/dose (max 2g) 6H IV over 30 min, or oral. Peak level 25-100 µg/ml, trough<20µg/ml (x7.75=umol/l).

Fludarabine. 25mg/m^2 daily x5 IV over 30min.

Fludrocortisone. 0.05-0.2mg (NOT/kg) daily oral. Fludrocortisone 1mg = hydrocortisone 125mg in mineralocorticoid activity, 10mg in glucocorticoid.

Flumazenil. 5µg/kg stat IV, repeat every 60sec to max total 40µg/kg (max 2mg), then 2-10µg/kg/hr IV.

Flunarizine. Migraine: 0.1-0.2mg/kg (max 10mg) oral daily at night. Epilepsy: 0.4mg/kg (max 20mg) daily at night.

Flunisolide. Asthma (250μg/puff): 1-2 puffs 12H. Nasal (25μg/puff): 1-2 puffs/nostril 8-24H.

Flunitrazepam. Adult: 0.5-2mg (NOT/kg) at night, oral.

Fluocinolone, cream or ointment 0.025%. Apply 8-12H.

Fluocortolone, cream or ointment 0.25%. Apply 8-12H.

Fluorescein, eye drops 1%, 2%. 1-2 drops per eye.

5-Fluorocytosine. see 5-flucytosine.

9-alpha-fluorohydrocortisone. see fludrocortisone.

Fluorometholone, eye drops 0.1%. 1-2drops/eye 6-12H.

Fluorothiocarbanilide, powder 1%. Apply daily.

5-Fluorouracil. 15mg/kg (max 1g) IV over 4hr daily until side effects, then 5-10mg/kg wkly. see folinic acid.

Fluoxetine. 0.5mg/kg (max 20mg) daily, incr to max 1.0 mg/kg/dose (max 40mg) 12H oral.

Fluoxymesterone. 0.1-0.2mg/kg (max 10mg) daily oral.

Flupenthixol. Oral: 0.05-0.2mg/kg/dose (max 9mg) 12H. Depot IM: usually 0.4-0.8mg/kg (up to 5mg/kg, max 300 mg) every 2-4wk (1mg flupenthixol deconate = 0.625mg fluphenazine decanoate = 1.25mg haloperidol).

Fluphenazine. 0.02-0.2mg/kg/dose (max 10mg) 8-12H oral.

Flurazepam. Adult: 15-30mg (NOT/kg) at night, oral.

Flurbiprofen. 1-2mg/kg/dose (max 100mg) 8H oral or PR. Eye drops 0.03%: 1 drop/eye every 30min.

Fluspirilene. Wkly IM: 0.02mg/kg, incr to 0.05-0.2mg/kg; occasionally 0.4mg/kg (max 20mg) wkly.

Flutamide. Adult: 250mg (NOT/kg) 8H oral.

Fluticasone. Inhaled (NOT/kg): 50-100μg/dose (child), 100-1000μg/dose (adult) 12H. 0.05% solution: 1-4 sprays /nostril daily.

Fluvoxamine. 2mg/kg/dose (max 100mg) 8-24H oral.

Folic acid. Treatment: 0.1-0.3mg/kg (max 15mg) daily IV, IM or oral. Pregnancy: 0.2-0.5mg (NOT/kg) daily.

Folinic acid. 5-15mg (NOT/kg) oral or 1mg IM or IV daily. Rescue starting up to 24hr after methotrexate: 10-15 mg/m^2/dose 6H for 36-48hr IV. Methotrexate toxicity: 100-1000mg/m^2/dose 6H IV. Before a fluorouracil dose of 370 mg/m^2: 200mg/m^2 IV daily x5, repeat every 3-4wk.

Follicle stimulating hormone (FSH). Initially 75iu (NOT/kg) IM daily for 9-12 days (monitor urinary oestrogen and adjust dose).

Fomepizole. 10mg/kg stat IV over 1hr, then 5mg/kg/dose 12H IV over 30min for 4 doses.

Formestane. Adult: 250mg (NOT/kg) 2wkly deep IM.

Foscarnet. 20mg/kg IV over 30min, then 200mg/kg/day by constant IV infusion (less if creatinine >0.11mmol/l).

Fosfestrol. Adult. Initial: 0.5g (NOT/kg) IV over 1hr day 1, then 1.0g x5 days. Maintenance: 120-240mg/dose (NOT/kg) 8H oral, later reducing to 120-240mg daily.

Fosinopril. 0.2-0.8mg/kg (max 40mg) daily oral.

Framycetin (Soframycin). Subconjunctival: 500mg in 0.5-1ml water daily x3 days. Bladder: 500mg in 50ml saline 8hrly for 10 days. Eye/ear 0.5%: 2-3 drops 8H, ointment 8H.

Framycetin 15mg/g + gramicidin 0.05mg/g, cream or ointment (Soframycin topical). Apply 8-12H.

Framycetin 5mg + gramicidin 0.05mg + dexamethasone 0.5mg/ml eye/ear (Sofradex). 2-3 drops 6-8H, ointment 8-12H.

Fresh frozen plasma. Contains all clotting factors. 10-20 ml/kg IV. 1 bag is about 230ml.

Frusemide. Usually 0.5-1.0mg/kg/dose 6-12H (daily if preterm) IM, IV or oral. Up to 5mg/kg/dose in resistant cases. IV infusion: 0.1-1.0mg/kg/hr.

Furazolidone. 2mg/kg/dose (max 100mg) 6H oral 7-10day.

Furosemide. see frusemide.

Fusidic acid. 10mg/kg/dose (max 500mg) 8H oral or IV over 2-8hr. Peak level 30-200μmol/l (x 0.52 = μg/ml).

Gabapentin. 5-15mg/kg/dose (max 800mg) 8-24H oral.

Galactosidase. see tilactase.

Gallamine. 1-2mg/kg/dose (max 100mg) IV.

Gallium nitrate. 100-200mg/m^2/day for 5 days by constant IV infusion.

Gamma benzene hexachloride. see lindane.

Gamma globulin. see immunoglobulin.

Gammahydroxybutyrate. 40-100mg/kg IV stat (use the high dose for long anaesthetic or children).

Gamolenic acid. 2-5mg/kg/dose (max 240mg) 12H oral.

Ganciclovir. 2.5-5mg/kg/dose 8-12H IV over 1hr.

Gas gangrene (Clostridia) antitoxin. Prophylaxis: 25,000u IM or IV. Treatment: 75,000-150,000u IV over 1hr, repeat x1-2 after 8-12hr. Give 100,000u IM as well for severe infection.

Gaviscon. see alginic acid.

Gemeprost (PGE1 analogue). Cervical dilatation: 1 pessary (1mg) into posterior vagina 3hr before surgery. Termination: 1 pessary (1mg) into posterior vagina 3H (max 5 pessaries).

Gemfibrozil. 10mg/kg/dose (max 600mg) 12H oral.

Gentamicin. Single daily dose IV or IM: 2.5mg/kg (< 30wk gestation), 3.5mg/kg (30-35wk gestation), 5mg/kg (1st wk life), 7.5mg/kg (2+ wk), 6mg/kg (> 10yr). Trough level < 1.0 mg/l.

Gestrinone. Adult: 2.5mg (NOT/kg) x2/wk on day 1 and 4 of menstrual cycle, then on same days each wk.

Gestronol. Adult: 200-400mg (NOT/kg) every 5-7 days IM.

Glibenclamide. Adult: initially 2.5mg (NOT/kg) daily oral, max 20mg daily.

Gliclazide. Adult: initially 40mg (NOT/kg) daily oral, max 160mg 12H.

Glipizide. Adult: initially 5mg (NOT/kg) daily oral, max 20mg 12H.

Gliquidone. 0.25-1mg/kg/dose (max 60mg) 8-12H oral.

Glucagon. 1u = 1mg. 0.2u/kg (max 2mg) IV or IM stat, then 0.005-0.01 u/kg/hr IV.

Glucose. see dextrose.

Glucose electrolyte solution. Not dehydrated: 1 heaped teaspoon sucrose in a large cup of water (4% sucrose = 2% glucose); do NOT add salt. Dehydrated: 1 sachet of Gastrolyte in 200ml water; give frequent small sips, or infuse through a nasogastric tube.

Glutamic acid. 10-20mg/kg (max 1g) oral with meals.

Glyburide. see glibenclamide.

Glyceryl trinitrate. Adult (NOT/kg): sublingual tab 0.3-0.9 mg/dose (lasts 30-60min); sublingual aerosol 0.4-0.8 mg/dose; slow-release buccal tab 1-10mg 8-12H; transdermal 0.5-5cm of 2% ointment, or 5-15mg patch 8-12H. IV: see nitroglycerine.

Glycopyrrolate. see glycopyrronium.

Glycopyrronium. To reduce secretions or treat bradycardia: 4-8µg/kg/dose (max 400µg) 6-8H IV or IM. With 0.05mg/kg neostigmine: 10-15µg/kg IV. Anticholinergic: 0.02-0.04mg/kg/dose (max 2mg) 8H oral.

GM-CSF. see sargramostim.

Gold sodium thiomalate. see sodium aurothiomalate.

Gonadorelin (GnRH or LHRH). 100µg/dose (NOT/kg) IV. See also leuprorelin.

Gonadotrophin. see chorionic g., and menotrophin.

Goserelin. Adult: 3.6mg (NOT/kg) SC every 28 days.

Gramicidin 25µg/ml + neomycin 2.5mg/ml + polymyxin B 5000u/ml (Neosporin). Eye drops: 1-2 drops/eye every 15-30min, reducing to 6-12H.

Granisetron. 0.05mg/kg (max 3mg) IV over 10min; up to 3 doses/day, with at least 10min between doses.

Granulocyte-macrophage colony stimulating factor (GM-CSF). see sargramostim.

Griseofulvin. 10-20mg/kg (max 1g) daily oral.

Griseofulvin (ultramicrosize) 5.5mg/kg (max 330mg) daily oral.

Growth hormone. see somatropin.

Guanabenz. 0.1mg/kg/dose (max 4mg) 12H oral, incr to max 0.6mg/kg/dose (max 32mg) 12H.

Guanadrel. 0.1mg/kg/dose (max 5mg) 12H oral, incr to max 0.5mg/kg/dose (max 25mg) 8-12H.

Guanethidine. 0.2mg/kg (max 10mg) daily oral, incr to 0.5-6mg/kg (max 300mg) daily. Regional sympathetic block (adult): cuff 55mmHg > systolic BP, 10-20mg in 10-25ml saline (arm) or 15-30mg in 15-50ml (leg) IV, wait 10-20min, release cuff over 5min; > = 7 days between injections (max 12/yr).

Guanfacine. 0.02mg/kg (max 1mg) daily oral, incr over several weeks to max 0.06mg/kg (max 3mg) daily.

Haemaccel. 10-20ml/kg (may be repeated). Half life 2hr.

Haemophilus influenzae type b, vaccines. Inactivated. < 12mo: give diphtheria protein conjugate (HibTITER), or tetanus protein conjugate (Act-HIB) 0.5ml IM at 2mo, 4mo, 6mo and 15mo; meningococcal conjugate (Pedvax HIB) 0.5ml IM at 2mo, 4mo and 15mo. If 1st dose > 18mo: give diphtheria toxoid conjugate (Prohibit) 0.5ml IM x1.

Halcinonide, cream 0.1%. Apply sparingly 8-12H.

Halofantrine. 10mg/kg/dose (max 500mg) 6H for 3 doses oral, repeat after 1wk if nonimmune.

Haloperidol. 0.01mg/kg (max 0.5mg) daily, incr up to 0.1 mg/kg/dose 12H IV or oral; up to 2mg/kg/dose (max 100mg) 12H used rarely. Long-acting decanoate ester: 1-6mg/kg IM every 4wk.

Hemin. 1-3mg/kg/dose 12-24H IV over 30min.

Heparin. 1mg = 100u. Low dose: 75u/kg IV stat, then 10-15u/kg/hr IV (500u/kg in 50ml at 1ml/hr = 10u/kg/hr). Full dose: 200u/kg stat, then 15-30u/kg/hr. Extracorporeal circuits: 10-20u/kg/hr prefilter, 2-5u/kg/hr postfilter.

Heparin calcium. Low dose: 75u/kg/dose SC 12H.

Heparin, low molecular weight. Venous thrombosis: 100u/kg/dose 12H SC, or 100u/kg IV over 12hr. Haemodialysis: 5-10u/kg stat, then 4-5u/kg/hr IV (acute renal failure, anti-Xa 0.2-0.4u/ml); 30-40u/kg stat, then 10-15u/kg/hr (chronic renal failure, anti-Xa 0.5-1.0u/ml).

Hepatitis A vaccine (Havrix). Inactivated. 1ml IM stat, after 1mo, and after 12mo (3 doses).

Hepatitis B vaccine (Engerix-B, HB Vax II). Inactivated. Engerix-B 10µg/dose (< 10yr), 20µg (> 9yr); HBVax II 2.5µg/dose (< 10yr), 5µg (10-19yr), 10µg (> 19yr), 40µg (dialysis) IM stat, after 1mo, and after 6mo (3 doses). Boost every 5yr approx.

Hetastarch, 6%. 10-20ml/kg IV.

Hexamine mandelate. 15mg/kg/dose (max 1g) 6H oral.

Hexetidine. 0.1% solution: rinse/gargle 15ml (NOT/kg) 8-12H.

Histrelin. Usually 10µg/kg daily SC.

Homatropine, eye drops 2%. 1-2 drops 4H.

Human chorionic gonadotrophin (HCG). see chorionic gonadotrophin.

Hyaluronidase. Hypodermoclysis: add 1-1.5u/ml fluid. Local anaesthesia: add 50u/ml solution.

Hydralazine. 0.1-0.2mg/kg (max 10mg) stat IV or IM, then 4-6µg/kg/min (max 300µg/min) IV. Oral: 0.2mg/kg /dose 12H, slow incr to 1mg/kg/dose (usual max 50mg).

Hydrochloric acid. Use solution of 150mmol/l, give IV by central line only. Dose(ml) = BE x Wt x 2.2 (give ½ this). Maximum rate = 1.33ml/kg/hr.

Hydrochlorothiazide. 1mg/kg/dose (max 50mg) 12-24H oral.

Hydrocodone. 0.1-0.2mg/kg/dose (max 10mg) 4-6H oral.

Hydrocortisone. Cream or ointment 0.1%, 0.5%, 1%: apply 8-24H. Eye drops 0.5%, 1%: 1-2 drops/eye 2-4H.

Hydrocortisone acetate. Cream or ointment 0.5%: apply 6-12H. Rectal foam 10%: 125mg/dose (Colifoam). Usually 125mg 12-24H for 2-3wk, then 48H.

Hydrocortisone 1% + clioquinol 3%, cream. Apply 8-24H.

Hydrocortisone sodium succinate. 2-4mg/kg/dose 3-6H IM or IV. Physiological: 0.2 mg/kg/dose 8H IM or IV.

Hydroflumethiazide. 0.5-2mg/kg/dose (max 100mg) 12-48H oral.

Hydrogen peroxide 10 volume (3%). Mouthwash 1:2 parts water. Skin or ear disinfectant 1:1 part water.

Hydromorphone. See dihydromorphinone.

Hydrotalcite. 20mg/kg/dose 6H oral.

Hydroxocobalamin (Vitamin B12) 20µg/kg/dose IM daily for 7 days then wkly (treatment), monthly (prophylaxis). IV dangerous in megaloblastic anaemia.

Hydroxyapatite. 20-40mg/kg/dose 8H oral before meals.

Hydroxychloroquine. 10mg/kg daily for 3 days oral. Prophylaxis: 5mg/kg (max 300mg) once a wk oral.

Hydroxyethylcellulose, eye drops 0.44%. 1-2 drops per eye 6-8H.

Hydroxyprogesterone. Adult: 250-500mg/wk (NOT/kg) IM.

Hydroxyurea. 20-30mg/kg daily oral.

Hydroxyzine. 0.5-2.0mg/kg/dose (max 100mg) 6-8H oral.

Hyoscine. 0.01mg/kg/dose (max 0.6mg) 6H, IM or IV.

Hyoscine hydrobromide. NOT/kg: 0.25 tab (2-7yr), 0.5 tab (7-12yr), 1-2 tab (> 12yr) 6-24H oral.

Hyoscine N-butylbromide. 0.5mg/kg/dose (max 40mg) 6-8H IV, IM or oral.

Hyoscine transdermal 1.5 mg. > 10yr: 1 patch every 72hr.

Hyoscyamine (L-atropine). 2-5µg/kg/dose (max 300µg) 4-6H oral, sublingual, IM or IV.

Hypromellose, eye drops 0.5% 2-3 drops per eye prn.

Hypromellose 0.3% + dextran 70 0.1%, eye drops. 1-2 drops per eye prn.

Ibuprofen. 2.5-10mg/kg/dose (max 600mg) 6-8H oral.

Idarubicin. 12 mg/m^2 IV over 15min daily for 3 days.

Idoxuridine. Eye drops 0.1%: 1-2 drops every 15min for 2hr, then hourly by day and 2H at night. 0.1% solution or 0.5% ointment: apply hourly first 24hr, then 4H.

Ifosfamide. Usually 1.2-2.0g/m^2 IV over 4hr daily x5, or 5-6g/m^2 (max 10g) IV over 24hr once. Repeat every 2-4wk.

Imipenem/cilastatin. 10mg/kg/dose 6H IV over 30min. Severe infection: 25mg/kg/dose IV over 1hr (max 1g) 12H (1st wk life), 8H (2-4 wk), 6H or constant infusion (4+ wk).

Imipramine. 0.5-1.5mg/kg/dose (max 75mg) 8H oral. Enuresis: 5-6yr 25mg, 7-10yr 50mg, >10yr 50-75mg nocte.

Immunoglobulin. See also antivenoms.

Immunoglobulin, CMV. 100-200mg/kg IV over 2hr. Transplant: daily for first 3 days, wkly x6, monthly x 6.

Immunoglobulin, diphtheria. 250u IM once.

Immunoglobulin, hepatitis B. 400u IM within 5 days of needle stick, repeat in 30 days; 100u IM within 24hr birth to baby of Hepatitis B carrier.

Immunoglobulin, lymphocyte (anti-thymocyte immunoglobulin, equine; Atgam).
10mg/kg daily for 3-5 days IV over 4hr in saline.

Immunoglobulin, normal, human.
Hypogammaglobulinaemia: 10-15ml/kg of 6% solution (600-900mg/kg) IV over 4hr, then 5-7.5 ml/kg (300-450mg/kg) monthly; or 0.6ml/kg of 16% solution (100mg/kg) every 2-4wk IM. Kawasaki, Guillain-Barre, ITP, myasthenia gravis, Still's disease: 35ml/kg of 6% solution (2g/kg) IV over 10hr stat, then if required 15 ml/kg (900mg/kg) IV over 4hr each month. Prevention hepatitis A: 0.1ml/kg (16mg/kg) IM. Prevention measles: 0.2ml/kg (32mg/kg) IM (repeat next day if immunocompromised).

Immunoglobulin, rabies (Hyperab, Imogam).
20iu (0.133ml)/kg IM once (½ infiltrated around wound), with rabies vaccine.

Immunoglobulin, Rh. 1ml (625iu, 125μg) IM within 72hr of exposure. Large transfusion: 0.16ml (100iu, 20μg) per ml RH positive red cells (maternal serum should be anti-D positive 24-48hr after injection).

Immunoglobulin, tetanus (intramuscular, TIG).
250-500iu (1-2amp) IM.

Immunoglobulin, tetanus (intravenous).
4000iu (100ml) given IV at 0.04ml/kg/min for 30min, then 0.075 ml/kg/min.

Immunoglobulin, vaccinia (16%).
To prevent vaccine complications (NOT/kg): 4ml (<6mo), 8ml (6mo-14yr), 12ml (>14yr); double dose to treat complications.

Immunoglobulin, Zoster. Prevention of chickenpox in immunocompromised, 0.4-1.2ml/kg IM.

Indapamide. Adult: 2.5mg (NOT/kg) daily oral.

Indomethacin. PDA: 0.1mg/kg daily for 6 days oral or IV in saline over 1hr (0.13mg/kg daily if >14 days old). Arthritis: 0.25-1mg/kg/dose (max 50mg) 6-8H oral or PR.

Indoramin. 0.5-1.5mg/kg/dose (max 75mg) 8-12H oral.

Influenza A and B vaccine (Fluvax, Vaxigrip).
Inactivated. 0.125ml (<2yr), 0.25ml (2-6yr), 0.5ml (>6yr) SC stat and 4wk later (2 doses). Boost annually (1 dose).

Inosine pranobex. Herpes 20mg/kg/dose (max 1g) 6-8H oral. SSPE: 10-15mg/kg/dose 4H oral.

Inosiplex. See inosine pranobex.

Inositol nicotinate. 20mg/kg/dose (max 1g) 6-8H oral.

Insulin. Regular insulin: 0.05-0.2u/kg prn, or 0.1u/kg/hr; later 1u/10g dextrose IV. For hyperkalaemia: 0.1u/kg insulin and 2ml/kg 50% dextrose IV. In TPN: 5-25u/250g dextrose. SC: regular insulin onset 30-60min, peak 4hr, duration 6-8hr; isophane (NPH) insulin onset 2-4hr, peak 4-12hr, duration 18-24hr; zinc (Lente) insulin onset 2-3hr, peak 7-15hr, duration 24hr; crystalline zinc (Ultralente) insulin onset 4-6hr, peak 10-30hr, duration 24-36hr; protamine zinc insulin onset 4-8hr, peak 15-20hr, duration 24-36hr.

Interferon alfa-2a, recombinant. 1,700,000u/m^2 (max 3,000,000u) SC or IM daily for 16-24wk, then x3/wk.

Interferon alfa-2b, recombinant. Leukaemia: 2,000,000 u/m^2 SC x3/wk. Condylomata: 1,000,000u into each lesion (max 5) x3/wk for 5wk.

Interferon alpha-n3. Adult: 250,000u injected into base of wart (max 10 doses per session) x2/wk for max 8wk.

Interferon gamma-1b. 1.5μg/kg/dose (body area $<=0.5m^2$) or 50μg/m^2 (area $>0.5m^2$) x3/wk SC.

Interleukin-2. Malignancy: constant IV infusion less toxic than bolus injection: 3,000,000 – 5,000,000u/m^2/day for 5 days, repeat x1-2 if tolerated (5 days between courses).

Ipecacuanha syrup. 1-2ml/kg (max 30ml) stat oral, NG.

Ipratropium. Respiratory solution (250μg/ml): 0.25-1.0ml diluted to 4ml 4-6H. Aerosol 20μg/puff: 2-4 puffs 6-8H.

Iprindole. 0.3-1mg/kg/dose (max 60mg) 8H oral.

Iron. See ferrous gluconate, ferrous sulphate.

Iron dextran. Fe 50mg/ml: dose (ml) = 0.05 x Wt in kg x (15 – Hb in g%) IM. IV infusion dangerous.

Isocarboxazid. Adult: 30mg (NOT/kg) daily oral (may incr to 60mg/day after 4wk), reducing to 10-40mg daily.

Isoconazole. Topical: 1% cream 12H. Vaginal: 600mg (2 tab) once.

Isoetharine. Inhalation solution (1%): 0.5ml diluted to 4ml 3-6H (mild), 1.0ml diluted to 4ml 1-2H (moderate), undiluted constant (severe, in ICU). Aerosol 340μg/puff: 1-puff 4-6H.

Isoniazid. 10-15mg/kg (max 300mg) daily oral. TB meningitis: 15-20mg/kg (max 500mg) daily oral.

Isoprenaline. 0.1-2.0μg/kg/min. <33kg: 0.3mg/kg in 50ml at 1ml/hr = 0.1μg/kg/min. >33kg: 0.1μg/kg/min using 1/5000 (0.2 mg/ml) solution = 0.03 x Wt ml/hr. Aerosol 80-400μg/puff: 1-3puffs 4-8H.

Isoproterenol. see isoprenaline.

Isosorbide dinitrate. Sublingual: 0.1-0.2mg/kg/dose (max 10mg) 2H or as needed. Oral: 0.5-1.0 mg/kg/dose (max 40mg) 6H or as needed. Sustained release tab: adults 1-2 tab (NOT/kg) daily.

Isotretinoin. Adult: 0.5-1.0mg/kg daily oral for 2-4wk, reducing if possible to 0.1-0.2mg/kg daily for 15-20wk.

Isoxsuprine. 0.2-0.5mg/kg/dose (max 20mg) 6-12H oral.

Ispaghula husk. Adult: 1-2 teaspoonfuls (NOT/kg) 6-12H oral. Half this dose in child.

Isradipine. 0.05mg/kg/dose 12H oral, may incr after 2-4wk gradually to 0.1-0.2mg/kg/dose (max 10mg) 12H.

Itraconazole. 2-4mg/kg/dose (max 200mg) 12-24H oral after food.

Ivermectin. 0.15-0.2mg/kg (max 12mg) oral every 6-12mo.

Josamycin. 10-15mg/kg/dose (max 750mg) 8-12H oral.

Kanamycin. Single daily dose IV or IM: 7.5mg/kg (< 30wk gestation), 10mg/kg (30-35wk gestation), 15mg/kg (1st wk life), 22.5mg/kg (2+ wk), 18mg/kg (> 10yr). Trough < 5mg/l.

Ketamine. 1-2mg/kg IV, 5-10mg/kg IM. Infusion: anaesthesia 10-20μg/kg/min, analgesia 4μg/kg/min.

Ketoconazole. 3-5mg/kg/dose (max 400mg) 12-24H oral. Cream 2%: apply 12-24H.

Ketoprofen. 0.5-2mg/kg/dose (max 50-100mg) 8-12H oral, PR. Slow release (adults): 200mg (NOT/kg) daily.

Ketorolac. Oral: 0.2mg/kg/dose (max 10mg) 4-6H (max 0.8mg/kg/day or 40mg/day). IM: 0.6mg/kg (max 30mg) stat, then 0.2-0.4mg/kg/dose (max 20mg) 4-6H for 5 days, then 0.2mg/kg/dose (max10mg) 6H.

Ketotifen. Child > 2yr: 1mg/dose (NOT/kg) 12H oral with food. Adult: 1-2mg/dose (NOT/kg) 12H oral with food.

Labetalol. 1-2mg/kg/dose (max 100mg) 12H oral, may incr wkly to max 10mg/kg/dose (max 600mg) 6H.

Lacidipine. 0.04-0.12mg/kg (max 6mg) daily oral with food.

Lactulose 50% (Duphalac). Laxative: 0.5ml/kg/dose 12-24H oral. Hepatic coma: 1ml/kg/dose hourly until bowel cleared, then 6-8H.

Lamotrigine. 0.5mg/kg oral daily for 2wk, then 1mg/kg daily 2wk, then 1-4mg/kg/dose (max 200mg) 12H (double dose if taking carbamazepine, phenobarbitone, phenytoin or primidone; halve dose if taking valproate).

L-asparaginase. see colaspase.

Latamoxef (Moxalactam). 25-50mg/kg/dose (max 2g) 4-6H IV, IM.

Lenograstim (rHuG-CSF, Granocyte).
150μg/m^2 daily SC or IV over 30min. Keep WCC 5,000-10,000/mm3.

Leucovorin. see folinic acid.

Leuprolide. see leuprorelin.

Leuprorelin (GnRH or LHRH) Adult: 7.5 mg (NOT/kg) depot injection monthly IM.

Levamisole. Anthelmintic: 3mg/kg (max 150mg) oral once (ascaris), repeat in 1wk (hookworm). Adenocarcinoma colon (with 5-fluorouracil 450mg/m^2 IV wkly): mg/kg (max 50mg) 8H oral for 3 days every 2wk.

Levobunolol. 0.5% solution: 1drop/eye 12-24H.

Levocarnitine. see carnitine.

Levodopa and benserazide (4:1)
Adult: initially levodopa 100mg/dose (NOT/kg) 8H oral; if not controlled, incr wkly by 100mg/day to max 250mg/dose (NOT/kg) 6H.

Levodopa and carbidopa (250mg/25mg and 100mg/10mg tabs).
Adult (NOT/kg): initially one 100/10 tab 8H oral; if not controlled, substitute one 250/25 tab for one 100/25 tab every 2nd day; if not controlled on 250/25 8H, incr by one 250/25 tab every 2nd day to max 6-8 tab/day.

Levonorgestrel. Contraception: 30μg daily oral, starting 1st day of menstruation.

Levonorgestrel + ethinyloestradiol (150μg/30μg or 125μg/50μg) x 21 tab, + 7 inert tab.
Contraception: tab daily, starting 1st day of menstruation.

Levorphanol. 0.03-0.1mg/kg/dose 12-24H oral or SC.

Levothyroxine sodium. see thyroxine.

Lidocaine. see lignocaine.

Lignocaine. IV: 1mg/kg stat (0.1ml/kg of 1%), then 15-50μg/kg/min (see p.35). Nerve block: without adrenaline max 4mg/kg, with adrenaline 7mg/kg. Topical spray: max 3-4mg/kg (Xylocaine 10% spray pack: about 10mg/puff). Topical gel 2%, solution 2% and 4%, ointment 5%, dental ointment 10%: apply prn.

Lignocaine 2.5% compound, mouth paint/gel (SM-33). Apply 3H prn.

Lignocaine 2.5% + prilocaine 2.5%, cream (EMLA). $1.5g/10cm^2$ under occlusive dressing for 1-3hr.

Lincomycin. 10mg/kg/dose (max 600mg) 8H oral, IM or IV over 1hr. Severe infection: up to 20mg/kg/dose (max 1.2g) IV over 2hr 6H.

Lindane, cream or lotion 1% Scabies: apply from neck down, wash off after 8-12hr. Lice: rub into hair for 4min, then wash off; repeat after 24hr (max x2/wk).

Linoleic acid. see fatty acids.

Liothyronine (T3). Oral: 0.2μg/kg/dose (max 10μg) 8H, may incr to 0.4μg/kg/dose (max 20μg) 8H. IV: 0.1-0.4μg/kg/dose (max 20μg) 8-12H.

Liotrix. Liothyronine (T3) plus thyroxine (T4) mixture.

Lipid emulsion 20%. 1-3g/kg/day IV (ml/hr = g/kg/day x Wt x 0.21).

Lipolytic enzymes. see pancreatic enzymes.

Lisinopril. 0.1mg/kg daily oral, may incr over 4-6wk to 0.2-0.4mg/kg (max 20mg) daily.

Lithium carbonate. 5-20mg/kg/dose 12-24H to maintain trough serum level 0.8-1.6mmol/l (> 2mmol/l toxic).

Lodoxamide. 0.1% solution: 1-2drops/eye 6H.

Lofepramide. Adult (NOT/kg): 70mg morning, 70-140mg night oral.

Lofexidine. 2-8μg/kg/dose (max 400μg) 6-12H oral.

Lomefloxacin. 8mg/kg (max 400mg) daily oral.

Lomustine (CCNU). $100\text{-}130mg/m^2$ oral every 6 wk.

Loperamide. 0.05-0.1mg/kg/dose (max 2mg) 8-12H oral.

Loracarbef. 4-8mg/kg (max 400mg) 12H oral.

Loratadine. 0.2mg/kg (max 10mg) daily oral.

Lorazepam. Acute: 0.05-0.2mg/kg (max 10mg) IV over 2min. Chronic: 0.02-0.06mg/kg/dose 8-24H oral.

Lovastatin. 0.4-0.8mg/kg/dose (max 40mg) 12-24H oral.

Loxapine. 0.2-1mg/kg/dose (max 60mg) 6-12H oral or IM.

Lymecycline. 408mg = 300mg tetracycline base.

Lymphocyte immune globulin see immunoglobulin, lymphocyte immune.

Lypressin (lysine-8-vasopressin) 1 spray (2.5iu) into 1 nostril 4-8H, may incr to 1 spray both nostrils 4-8H.

Lysuride. Migraine: 0.5μg/kg/dose (max 25μg) 8H oral. Parkinson's, adults (NOT/kg): 0.2mg daily, incr by 0.2 mg daily each wk to max 1.6mg/dose 8H oral.

Magaldrate. 5-30mg/kg/dose (max 1.6g) 6H oral.

Magnesium chloride. 0.48g/5ml (1mmol/ml Mg). 0.4mmol (0.4ml)/kg/dose 12H slow IV. Myocardial infarct (NOT/kg): 5mmol/hr IV for 6hr, then 1mmol/hr for 24-48hr.

Magnesium hydroxide. Antacid: 10-40mg/kg/dose (max 2g) 6H oral. Laxative: 50-100mg/kg (max 5g) oral.

Magnesium sulphate. Deficiency: 50% magnesium sulphate (2 mmol/ml) 0.2ml/kg/dose (max 10ml) 12H IM, slow IV.
Myocardial infarction: (NOT/kg): 5mmol/hr IV for 6hr, then 1.0 mmol/hr for 24-48hr.
Digoxin tachyarrhythmia: 50% magnesium sulphate 0.1 ml/kg (max 5ml) IV over 10min, then infuse 0.4ml/kg (max 20ml) over 6hr, then 0.8ml/kg (max 40ml) over 18hr (keep serum Mg 1.5-2.0 mmol/l).
Pulmonary hypertension newborn: aim for 3-4mmol/l.
Laxative: 0.5g/kg/dose (max 15g) as 10% solution 8H for 2 days oral.
Asthma: 25mg/kg (max 1.2g) IV over 30min once.

Malathion. see maldison.

Maldison, liquid 0.5%. 20ml to hair, wash off after 12hr.

Mannitol. 0.25-0.5g/kg/dose IV (2-4ml/kg of 12.5%, 1.25-2.5ml/kg of 20%, 1-2ml/kg of 25%) 2H prn, provided serum osmolality < 330mmol/l.

Maprotiline. 0.15-1mg/kg/dose (max 50mg) 8-24H oral.

Mazindol. Adult: 0.5mg (NOT/kg) daily oral, may incr to 1-3mg daily.

Measles vaccine (Attenuvax). Live. > 12mo: 0.5ml SC once.

Measles + mumps vaccine (Rimparix).
Live. > 12mo: 0.5ml SC once.

Measles + mumps + rubella vaccine (MMRII).
Live. > 12mo: 0.5ml SC.

Mebendazole. 100mg/dose (NOT/kg) 12H x3 days. Enterobiasis: 100mg once (NOT/kg), repeat after 2-4wks.

Mebeverine (135mg tab). Adult: 1-3 tab (NOT/kg) daily oral.

Mebhydrolin. 1-2mg/kg/dose (max 100mg) 8-12H oral.

Mecamylamine. 0.05mg/kg/dose (max 2.5mg) 12H oral; may incr to max 0.5mg/kg/dose (max 25mg) 6H oral.

Mechlorethamine. see mustine HCl.

Meclizine. see meclozine.

Meclocycline sulfosalicylate, 1% cream.
Apply 12H.

Meclofenamate. 1-2mg/kg/dose (max 100mg) 6-8H oral.

Meclozine. 0.5-1.0mg/kg/dose (max 50mg) 12-24H oral.

Medazepam. 0.05-0.2mg/kg/dose (max 10mg) 6-8H oral.

Medroxyprogesterone. Adult (NOT/kg): 5mg daily for 5-10 days per month oral; malignancy 0.5g daily IM or oral for 4wk, then 1g wkly.

Medroxyprogesterone (MP) + conjugated oestrogens (CO).
MP (NOT/kg): 10mg (up to 20mg) daily oral for last 10-14 days of 28 day cycle. CO (NOT/kg): 0.625mg (0.3-1.25mg) daily continuously.

Medroxyprogesterone 10mg tab + oestradiol 4mg patch.
NOT/kg: 10mg tab daily oral for first 10-14 days of each 28 day cycle, and 4mg patch x2/wk continuously.

Medrysone, eye drops 1%. 1 drop/eye 6-12H.

Mefenamic acid. 10mg/kg/dose (max 500mg) 8H oral.

Mefloquine. 15mg/kg (max 750mg) stat, then 10mg/kg (max 500mg) after 6-8hr.
Prophylaxis: 5mg/kg (max 250mg) once a wk.

Mefruside. 0.5-1mg/kg (up to 2mg/kg for 3 days) daily for 10-14 days, then 0.5-1mg/kg (max 50mg) every 2-3 days.

Megestrol acetate. 80mg per dose (NOT/kg) 12H oral.

Melphalan. Typically 6mg/m^2 daily for 4-6days, repeat every 6wk.

Menadione, menadiol. see menaphthone sod. bisulphate.

Menaphthone sodium bisulphate. 0.6mg/kg (max 30mg) daily oral.

Meningococcus groups A and C vaccine (Mencevax AC). Inactivated. >2yr: 0.5ml SC. Boost every 2-3yr.

Menotrophin (FSH + LH activity). Females: 75 + 75iu or 150 + 150iu (NOT/kg) IM daily for 9-12 days until oestrogen levels rise, then give HCG. Males: 75 + 75iu (NOT/kg) IM x2-3/wk with HCG 7000iu IM x2/wk.

Mepacrine. Giardia: 2mg/kg/dose (max 100mg) 8H oral 5-7 days.

Mepenzolate. 0.5-1mg/kg/dose (max 50mg) 6-8H oral.

Meperidine. see pethidine.

Mephenytoin. see methoin.

Mephobarbital. see methylphenobarbitone.

Mepivacaine. Max dose 5-7mg/kg.

Meprobamate. 5-10mg/kg/dose (max 800mg) 8-12H oral.

Meptazinol. 4mg/kg/dose (max 200mg) 3-6H oral.

Mepyramine. 2-4mg/kg/dose (max 200mg) 8H oral.

Mequitazine. 0.1mg/kg/dose (max 5mg) 12H oral.

Mercaptopurine (6MP). 75-100mg/m^2 daily oral

Mesalamine. see mesalazine.

Mesalazine. Initially 15-30mg/kg/dose (max 1.6g) 8H oral, reducing to 10-15mg/kg/dose (max 750mg) 8H. Suppository: 5-10mg/kg (max 500mg) 8H. Enema: 20mg/kg (max 1g) nocte.

Mesna. 20% (up to 40%) of the cyclophosphamide or ifosfamide dose IV over 30min 4H for 3 doses (at 0, 4 and 8 hr). Nebuliser: 0.6-1.2g/dose (NOT/kg) 4-6H.

Mesoridazine. 0.25-3mg/kg/dose (max 150mg) 8H oral. 0.5mg/kg/dose (max 75mg) 8H IM.

Mesterolone. 0.5mg/kg/dose (max 25mg) 6-12H oral.

Mestranol. see norethisterone.

Metaproterenol. see orciprenaline.

Metaraminol. IV: 0.01mg/kg stat (repeat prn), then 0.1-1.0μg/kg/min and titrate dose against BP. SC: 0.1mg/kg.

Metaxalone. 15mg/kg/dose (max 800mg) 6-8H oral.

Metformin. Adult: initially 500mg (NOT/kg) 8-24H oral, max 1g per dose 8H.

Methacycline. Over 8yr: 150mg (NOT/kg) 12H oral. Adult: 300mg (NOT/kg) 12H oral.

Methadone. Usually 0.1-0.2mg/kg/dose (max 10mg) 6-12H oral, SC or IM.

Methamphetamine. see methylamphetamine.

Methazolamide. 1-2mg/kg/dose (max 100mg) 8-12H oral.

Methdilazine. 0.1-0.3mg/kg/dose (max 16mg) 12-24H oral.

Methenamine mandelate. see hexamine mandelate.

Methicillin. 20-50mg/kg/dose (max 2g) 4-6H IV or IM.

Methimazole. 0.3-1mg/kg (max 60mg) daily oral, reducing when euthyroid to 0.1-0.5mg/kg (max 30mg) daily.

Methionine. 50mg/kg/dose (max 2.5g) oral 4H for 4 doses.

Methixene. 0.05-0.4mg/kg/dose (max 20mg) 8H oral.

Methocarbamol. Oral: 30mg/kg/dose (max 1.5g) 6H for 3 days, then 15-20mg/kg/dose (max 1g) 6-8H. IV over 5-10 min or IM: 15mg/kg/dose (max 750mg) 6H.

Methohexital. see methohexitone.

Methohexitone. 1.5-2.0mg/kg/dose (max 120mg) slow IV.

Methoin. 1mg/kg daily oral, may incr by 1mg/kg each wk to max 10mg/kg (max 600mg) daily.

Methoserpidine. 0.2-0.4mg/kg/dose (max 20mg) 8H oral.

Methotrexate. Leukaemia: typically $3.3 mg/m^2$ IV daily for 4-6wk; then 2.5mg/kg IV every 2wk, or $30 mg/m^2$ oral or IM x2/wk; much higher doses with folinic acid rescue. Intrathecal: $12 mg/m^2$ wkly for 2wk, then monthly. Adult psoriasis: 0.2-0.5mg/kg wkly oral, IV or IM until response, then reduce.

Methotrimeprazine. Psychosis: 0.5-4mg/kg (max 200mg) daily oral. Pain: 0.25-1mg/kg/dose (max 50mg) 4-8H.

Methoxamine. 0.1-0.4mg/kg (max 20mg) IM, or 0.1-0.2 mg/kg (max 10mg) IV over 5-10min (at least 15min between doses). Nose drop 0.25%: 1-3drop/nostril 6-12H.

Methoxsalen. Adult: 20mg (NOT/kg) 2hr before UV exposure. Lotion 1%: wkly before 1min of UV light.

Methscopolamine. see hyoscine.

Methsuximide. 5mg/kg daily, may incr to max 10mg/kg /dose (max 400mg) 8-12H oral.

Methyclothiazide. 0.05-0.2mg/kg (max 10mg) daily oral.

Methylamphetamine. >5yr (NOT/kg): 2.5-5.0mg/dose 12-24H oral, incr to about 10-15mg/dose 12H.

Methylcellulose. Constipation: 30-60mg/kg/dose (max 3g) with at least 300ml fluid 12H oral.

Methylcysteine. 4mg/kg/dose (max 200mg) 6-12H oral.

Methyldopa. 3mg/kg/dose 8H oral, may incr to max 15 mg/kg/dose (max 750mg).

Methyldopate. 5-20mg/kg/dose (max 1g) 6H IV over 1hr.

Methylene blue. 1-4mg/kg/dose IV.

Methylergometrine. Adult: 200μg (NOT/kg) IM, IV over 5min, or oral; may repeat in 2hr, then 4-6H.

Methylergonovine. see methylergometrine.

Methylphenidate. Hyperactivity: 0.25mg/kg daily oral, may incr to max 2mg/kg daily. Narcolepsy: 0.1-0.4mg/kg per dose (max 20mg) 8H oral.

Methylphenobarbitone. 4-12mg/kg (max 600mg) daily.

Methylphenylsuccinimide. see phensuximide.

Methylprednisolone. Asthma: 0.5-1.0mg/kg/dose 6H oral, IV or IM day 1, 12H day 2, then 1.0 mg/kg daily, reducing to minimum effective dose. Severe croup: 4mg/kg IV stat, then 1mg/kg/dose 12H. Spinal cord injury (within 8hr): 30mg/kg stat, then 5mg/kg/hr 2 days. Lotion 0.25%: apply sparingly 12-24H. Methylprednisolone 1mg = hydrocortisone 5mg in glucocorticoid activity, 0.5mg in mineralocorticoid.

4-Methylpyrazole. see fomepizole.

Methyltestosterone. 2.5-12.5mg/day (NOT/kg) buccal.

Methysergide. 0.02mg/kg/dose (max 1mg) 12H oral, incr to max 0.04mg/kg/dose (max 2mg) 8H oral for 3-6mo.

Metirosine. 5-20mg/kg/dose (max 1g) 6H oral.

Metoclopramide. 0.12mg/kg/dose (max 15mg) 6H IV, IM or oral. 0.2-0.4mg/kg/dose (max 20mg) 8H PR.

Metocurine iodide. ICU: 0.4mg/kg IV prn. Theatre: 0.1-0.4mg/kg stat, then 0.01-0.02 mg/kg/dose.

Metolazone. 0.1-0.2mg/kg (max 10mg) daily oral. Up to 0.5mg/kg (max 30mg) daily short term.

Metoprolol. IV: 0.1mg/kg (max 5mg) over 5 min, repeat every 5 min to max 3 doses, then 1-5μg/kg/min. Oral: 1-2mg/kg/dose (max 100mg) 6-12H.

Metronidazole. 15mg/kg stat, then 7.5mg/kg/dose (max 800mg) 12H in neonate (1st maintenance dose 48hr after load in preterm, 24hr in term baby), 8H (4+ wk) IV, PR or oral. Topical gel 0.5%: apply daily. Level 60-300umol/ml (x0.17μg/ml).

Metyrapone.	Diagnosis: 15mg/kg/dose (minimum 250mg) 4H x6 dose oral. Cushing: 1-20 mg/kg/dose (max 1g) 4H.
Metyrosine.	see metirosine.
Mexiletine.	IV infusion: 2-5mg/kg (max 250mg) over 15 min, then 5-20µg/kg/min (max 250mg/hr). Oral: 8mg/kg (max 400mg) stat, then 4-8mg/kg/dose (max 400mg) 8H starting 2hr after loading dose.
Mezlocillin.	50mg/kg/dose 6-8H (1st wk life), 4-6H (2+ wk) IM or IV. Serious infection: 60mg/kg/dose (max 3g) 4H.
Mianserin.	0.2-0.5mg/kg/dose (max 40mg) 8H oral.
Miconazole.	7.5-15mg/kg/dose (max 1.2g) 8H IV over 1hr. Topical: 2% cream, powder, lotion, tincture or gel 12-24H. Vaginal: 2% cream or 100mg ovule daily.
Microlax enema.	<12mo 1.25ml, 1-2yr 2.5ml, >2yr 5ml.
Midazolam.	Sedation: usually 0.1-0.2mg/kg IV or IM; up to 0.5mg/kg used safely in children. Anaesthesia: 0.5 mg/kg, then 2µg/kg/min (3mg/kg in 50ml at 2ml/hr) IV.
Mifepristone.	Termination: 600mg (NOT/kg) oral once, then gemeprost 1mg PV in 36-48hr if abortion incomplete.
Milrinone.	50µg/kg IV over 10min, then 0.375-0.75µg/kg/min (max 1.13mg/kg/day).
Mineral mixture (Aminogram).	<5.5kg: 1.5g/kg daily oral, mixed with feed. >5.5kg: 8g daily (NOT/kg).
Mineral oil.	see paraffin liquid.
Minocycline.	Over 8yr: 4mg/kg (max 200mg) stat, then 2mg/kg/dose (max 100mg) 12H oral or IV over 1hr.
Minoxidil.	0.1mg/kg (max 5mg) daily, incr to max 0.5mg/kg /dose (max 25mg) 12-24H oral. Male baldness: 2% solution 1ml 12H to dry scalp.
Misoprostol (PGE1 analogue)	5µg/kg/dose (max 200µg) 4-6H oral.
Mitomycin C, crystalline.	2mg/m^2 IV daily x10 days, repeat only if leucocytes >3000/mm3 + platelets >75,000/mm3.
Mitotane.	10-80mg/kg/dose (max 4g) 6H oral.
Mitoxanthrone.	see mitozanthrone.
Mitozantrone.	Breast cancer or lymphoma: 10-14mg/m^2 IV over 10min every 3wk. Leukaemia: 10-12mg/m^2 IV over 10min daily for 3-5 days.
Mivacurium.	150µg/kg stat, then 100µg/kg/dose IV. Infusion: 5-15µg/kg/min.
Moclobemide.	2-3mg/kg/dose (max 150mg) 6-12H oral.
Molgramostim.	see sargramostim.
Molidone.	0.1-1.5mg/kg/dose (max 75mg) 8H oral.
Mometasone furoate.	0.1% cream or ointment: apply daily.
Moracizine.	4-6mg/kg/dose (max 300mg) 8H oral.
Moricizine.	see moracizine.
Morphine.	0.1-0.2mg/kg/dose IV, 0.2mg/kg/dose IM (half life 2-4hr). Infusion: 0.5mg/kg in 50ml 5%D at 1-5ml/hr (10-50µg/kg/hr).
Morrhuate sodium.	Adult: 50-250mg per injection (NOT/kg).
Moxalactam.	see latamoxef.
Mumps vaccine (Mumpsvax)	Live. >12mo: 0.5ml SC once. See also measles + mumps + rubella vaccine.
Mupirocin, ointment 2%.	Apply 8-12H.
Muromonab-CD3 (Orthoclone OKT3).	0.1mg/kg (max 5mg) daily for 10-14 days IV over 1min.
Mustine HCl (nitrogen mustard).	0.1mg/kg IV daily for 3-4 days. Hodgkins: 6mg/m^2 IV.
Nabilone.	0.02-0.04mg/kg/dose (max 2mg) 12H oral.
Nabumentone.	10-20mg/kg/dose (max 1g) 12-24H oral.

Nadolol. 1-5mg/kg (max 240mg) daily oral.

Nafarelin. Adult: 200µg (NOT/kg) spray to 1 nostril 12H.

Nafcillin. Oral: 15-30mg/kg/dose 6H. Severe infection (slow IV, IM): 40mg/kg/dose (max 2g) 12H (1st wk life), 8H (2nd wk), 6H or constant infusion (>2wk).

Naftidrofuryl. 2-4mg/kg/dose (max 200mg) 8H (oral) or 12H (IM, or IV or IA infusion over 2hr).

Nalbuphine. 0.2-0.5mg/kg/dose (max 20-30mg) 3-6H SC, IM or IV. Anaesthesia: 0.3-1.0mg/kg IV over 15min, then 0.2-0.5mg/kg every 30min.

Nalidixic acid. 15mg/kg/dose (max 1g) 6H oral, reducing to 7.5mg/kg/dose 6H after 2wk.

Nalorphine. 0.1-0.2mg/kg stat, repeat every 10-15min to max 0.8mg/kg (max 40mg).

Naloxone. Opiate intoxication (including newborn): 0.1 mg/kg (max 2mg) stat IV or intratracheal, then 0.01 mg/kg/hr IV. Postoperative sedation: 0.002mg/kg/dose repeat every 2min, then 0.01 mg/kg/hr (0.2µg/kg/min) IV.

Naltrexone. 1mg/kg (max 50mg) daily oral.

Nandrolone in oil. 0.5-4mg/kg (max 0.4g) each 1-3wk IM.

Naphazoline. 0.025-0.1%: 1-2drops each nostril or eye 3H.

Naproxen. 5-7.5mg/kg/dose (max 500mg) 12-24H oral.

Nedocromil. Inhalation: 4mg/dose (NOT/kg) 6-12H.

Nefopam. Oral: 0.5-2mg/kg/dose (max 90mg) 8H. IM: 0.4 mg/kg (max 20mg) stat, may repeat in 6hr.

Neomycin. 12.5-25mg/kg/dose (max 1g) 6H oral. Bladder washout: 40-2000mg/l.

Neostigmine. Oral: 0.3-0.6mg/kg/dose 3-4H (max 400mg /day). IV, IM: 0.01-0.05mg/kg/dose 3-4H (max 20mg /day). Reverse relaxants: 0.05-0.07 mg/kg/dose IV; suggested dilution: neostigmine (2.5mg/ml) 0.5ml + atropine (0.6mg/ml) 0.5ml + saline 0.5ml, give 0.1ml/kg IV.

Netilmicin. Single daily dose IV or IM: 2.5mg/kg (<30wk gestation), 3.5mg/kg (30-35wk gestation), 5mg/kg (1st wk life), 7.5mg/kg (2+ wk), 6mg/kg (>10yr). Trough<1.0mg/l.

Nicardipine. 0.4-0.8mg/kg/dose (max 40mg) 8H oral.

Niclosamide. 40mg/kg (max 2g) oral.

Nicofuranose. 10-20mg/kg/dose (max 1g) 8H oral.

Nicotine resin chewing gum. NOT/kg: 2-4mg chewed over 30min when inclined to smoke; usually need 16-24 mg/day, max 60mg/day.

Nicotine transdermal patches (Nicabate 7mg, 14mg, 21mg; Nicotinell 10 = 17.5mg, 20 = 35mg, 30 = 52.5mg). Adult: if smoked >20cig/day apply strongest patch daily 3-4wk, then medium patch daily 3-4wk (initial dose if smoked< =20cig/day), then weakest patch daily 3-4wk.

Nicotinic acid. Hypercholesterolaemia and hypertriglyceridaemia: 5mg/kg/dose (max 200mg) 8H, gradually incr to 20-30 mg/kg/dose (max 2g) 8H oral.

Nicoumalone. 0.1-0.25mg/kg (max 12mg) daily oral. INR usually 2-2.5 for prophylaxis, 2-3 for treatment.

Nifedipine. Caps 0.25-0.5mg/kg (max 20mg) 6-8H, tabs 0.5-1.0mg/kg/dose (max 40mg) 12H oral or sublingual.

Nimodipine. 10-15µg/kg/hr (max 1mg/hr) IV for 2hr, then 10-45µg/kg/hr.

Nitrazepam. NOT/kg: 1-5mg/dose 12H. Hypnotic: 2-5mg.

Nitric oxide. 5-10ppm (up to 80ppm used occasionally). [NO] = Cylinder [NO] x (1 – (Patient FIO2 / Supply FIO2)).

Nitrofurantoin. 1.5mg/kg/dose (max 100mg) 6H oral. Prophylaxis: 1-2.5mg/kg at night.

Nitrofurazone. 0.2% cream, solution: apply every 1-3 days.

Nitrogen mustard. see mustine HCl.

Nitroglycerine. 1-10μg/kg/min IV. Use polyethylene-lined syringe and tubing (not PVC). Pulmonary vasodilator: 5μg/kg/min nitroglycerine = 2μg/kg/min nitroprusside = 0.1μg/kg/min PGE1.

Nitroprusside. 0.5-10μg/kg/min; used for > 24hr, max 4μg/kg/min. Max total 70mg/kg with normal renal function (or sodium thiocyanate < 1725 mol/l, x 0.058 = mg/l). Pulmonary vasodilator: 5μg/kg/min nitroglycerine = 2 μg/kg/min nitroprusside = 0.1 μg/kg/min PGE1 approx.

Nizatidine. 3mg/kg/dose (max 150mg) 12H oral for max 8wk, then 3mg/kg (max 150mg) daily.

Nonoxynol. Cream 2% (Ortho) or 5% (Delfen): 1 applicator full just before intercourse. Foam 12.5% (Delfen): 1 applicator full < 60min before intercourse.

Noradrenaline. IV infusion: 0.05-0.5μg/kg/min. See p.35.

Norepinephrine. see noradrenaline.

Norethindrone. see norethisterone.

Norethisterone. Contraception: 350μg daily, starting 1st day of menstruation. Menorrhagia: 10mg 3H until bleeding stops, then 5mg 6H for 1wk, then 5mg 8H for 2wk.

Norethisterone + ethinyloestradiol (0.5mg/35μg or 1mg/35μg) x 21 tab, + 7 inert tab.
Contraception: 1 tab daily, starting 1st day of menstruation.

Norethisterone 1mg + mestranol 50μg.
Contraception: 1 tab daily from 5th to 25th day of menstrual cycle.

Norfloxacin. 7.5mg/kg/dose (max 400mg) 12H oral.

Norgestrel. see levonorgestrel.

Normacol granules. 6mo-5yr ½ teaspoon 12H, 6-10yr 1 teaspoon 12H, over 10yr 1 teaspoon 8H.

Nortriptyline. 0.5-1.5mg/kg/dose (max 75mg) 8H oral.

Noxythiolin. 1-2.5% solution into body cavity 12-24H, left at least 30min. Max daily dose 200mg/kg (max 10g).

Nystatin. 500,000u (1 tab) 6-8H NG or oral. Neonates: 100,000u (1ml) 8H, prophylaxis 50,000u (0.5ml) 12H. Topical: 100,000u/g gel, cream or ointment 12H. Vaginal: 100,000u 12-24H.

Octoxinol (octoxynol). Jelly 1% (Ortho-Gynol): 1 teaspoonful on diaphragm before intercourse.

Octreotide. 1μg/kg/dose 12-24H SC, may incr to 4μg/kg/dose (max 250μg) 8H. IV: 3-5μg/kg/hr.

Oestradiol, vaginal tab 25μg.
1 tab daily for 2wk, then 1 tab x2/wk.

Oestradiol 2mg or 4mg (x12 tab), oestradiol 1mg (x6 tab), oestradiol 2mg or 4mg + norethisterone 1mg (x10 tab).
1 tab daily, starting 5th day of menstruation.

Oestriol. Vaginal: 0.5mg daily, reducing to twice a wk.

Oestrogen. see ethinyloestradiol.

Oestrone. Vaginal: 0.1-1mg daily, decrease to 1mg x2-3/wk.

Ofloxacin. 4-8mg/kg/dose (max 400mg) 12-24H oral or IV over 1hr.

OKT3. see muromonab-CD3.

Olsalazine. 250mg cap: 1-3 cap (NOT/kg) 6-12H oral.

Omeprazole. Usually 0.4-0.8mg/kg (max 40mg) daily oral. ZE syndrome: 0.4-1.0mg/kg (max 60mg) 12-24H oral. IV: 2 mg/kg (max 80mg) stat, then 1mg/kg (max 40mg) 8-12H. H. pylori: 0.4 mg/kg/dose (max 20mg) 12H with amoxycillin 10mg/kg/dose 6H oral for 2wk.

Ondansetron. IV: 0.1-0.2mg/kg (usual max 8mg) over 15 min, then 0.25-0.5μg/kg/min. Oral: 0.1-0.2 mg/kg/dose (usual max 8mg) 8-12H.

IV. Drug dose compendium

Oral rehydration solution (ORS).
see glucose electrolyte solution.

Orciprenaline. Oral: 0.25-0.5mg/kg/dose (max 20mg) 6H. Respiratory solution (2%): 0.5ml/dose diluted to 4ml 3-6H (mild), 1.0 ml/dose diluted to 4ml (moderate), undiluted continuously (severe, in ICU). Aerosol 750μg/dose: 2 puffs 4-6H.

Ornipressin (POR 8). IV: 0.1u/kg/hr (max 6u/hr) for max 4hr, then 0.03u/kg/hr (max 1.5u/hr). SC: 5u in 30ml saline, max total dose 0.1u/kg.

Orphenadrine. 2-5mg/kg/dose (max 150mg) 8-12H oral.

Oxacillin. Oral: 15-30mg/kg/dose 6H. Severe infection (IV,IM): 40mg/kg/dose (max 2g) 12H (1st wk life), 8H (2nd wk), 6H or constant infusion (> 2wk).

Oxandrolone. 0.1mg/kg daily oral.

Oxatomide. 0.6-1.2mg/kg/dose (max 60mg) 12-24H oral.

Oxazepam. 0.2-0.5mg/kg/dose 6-8H oral.

Oxerutin. 10mg/kg/dose (max 500mg) 12H oral.

Oxitropium. Inhalation: 200μg/dose (NOT/kg) 8-12H.

Oxpentifylline. Sustained release tab: 8mg/kg/dose (max 400mg) 8-12H oral.

Oxprenolol. 0.5-2mg/kg/dose (max 120mg) 8-12H oral.

Oxtriphylline. see choline theophyllinate.

Oxybutynin. NOT/kg: 5-12yr 5mg/dose 8-12H oral, > 12yr 5mg/dose 6-8H.

Oxycodone. 0.1-0.2mg/kg/dose (max 10mg) 4-6H oral.

Oxymetazoline, nasal. 0.25mg/ml (6yr): 2-3 drops or sprays in each nostril 8-12H.

Oxymetholone. 1-2mg/kg/dose 12-24H oral.

Oxymorphone. Usually 0.02-0.03mg/kg/dose (max 1.5mg) 4-6H IM or SC. Slow IV: 0.01mg/kg/dose (max 0.5mg) 4-6H. PR: 0.1mg/kg (max 5mg) 4-6H.

Oxypentifylline. 8mg/kg/dose (max 400mg) 8-12H oral.

Oxyphenbutazone, 10% ointment.
Apply x2-5 times/day.

Oxytetracycline. > 8yr: 250-500mg/dose (NOT/kg) 6H oral, or 250-500mg/dose (NOT/kg) 6-12H slow IV.

Oxytocin. Labour: 1-4mU/min (NOT/kg) IV, may incr to 20 mU/min max. Lactation: 1 spray (4iu) into each nostril 5min before infant feeds.

Packed cells. 4ml/kg raises Hb 1g%. 1 bag is about 300ml.

Paclitaxel. 100-250mg/m^2 IV over 24hr each 3wk, total of 3-6 doses.

Pamidronate. see disodium pamidronate.

Pancreatic enzymes. With meals (NOT/kg): 1-3 Cotazyme-S Forte cap, 1-5 Pancrease cap oral.

Pancuronium. ICU: 0.1-0.15mg/kg IV prn. Theatre: 0.1mg /kg IV, then 0.02mg/kg prn. Infusion: 0.25-0.75μg/kg/min.

Papaveretum (Omnopon). 0.2mg/kg/dose IV, 0.4 mg/ kg/dose IM (half life 2-4hr). ICU: 0.3mg/kg/dose IV, 0.6 mg/kg/dose IM.

Papaveretum (20mg/ml) and hyoscine (0.4mg/ml).
0.4 mg/kg (P) + 0.008mg/kg (H) = 0.02ml/kg/dose IM.

Papaverine. Adult (NOT/kg): 150-300mg 12H oral, 12-40 mg x1-2/wk intracavernosal. IA lines: 0.12mg/ml.

Paracetamol. 20mg/kg stat, then max 15mg/kg/dose 4H (max 4g/day) oral or PR. Overdose: see acetylcysteine.

Paraffin. Liquid: 1ml/kg (max 45ml) daily oral. Liquid 50% + white soft 50%, ointment: apply 6-12H.

Paraffin 65% + agar. NOT/kg: 6mo-2yr 5ml, 3-5yr 5-10ml, > 5yr 10ml 8-24H oral.

Paraffin, phenolphthalein and agar (Agarol).
NOT/kg: 6mo-2yr 2.5ml, 3-5yr 2.5-5ml, > 5yr 5ml 8-24H oral.

Paramethadione. 5-10mg/kg/dose (max 600mg) 6-8H oral.

Paraldehyde. IM: 0.2ml/kg (max 10ml) stat, then 0.1 ml/kg/dose 4-6H. IV: 0.2ml/kg (max 10ml) over 15 min, then 0.02ml/kg/hr (max 1.5ml/hr). Rectal or NG: 0.3 ml/kg/dose diluted 1:10.

Paromomycin. 10mg/kg/dose 8H for 5-10 days oral.

Paroxetine. 0.4-1.0mg/kg (max 50mg) daily oral.

Pegademase. 10u/kg IM wkly, incr to 20u/kg wkly.

Pemoline. >6yr: 20-120mg (NOT/kg) daily oral.

Penbutolol. 0.5-1.5mg/kg (max 80mg) daily oral.

Penicillamine. 5-7.5mg/kg/dose 8H (max 2g/day) oral.

Penicillin, benzathine. 25,000-50,000u(20-40mg)/kg (max 1.8g) IM once. Streptococcal prophylaxis: 25,000u(20mg)/kg (max 900mg) IM 3-4wkly, or 12,500(10mg)/kg IM 2 wkly.

Penicillin, benzathine co (Bicillin 1,200,000u). 0-2yr ½ vial, 3-6yr 3/4 vial, >6yr 1 vial IM once.

Penicillin G (benzyl). 50,000u(30mg)/kg/dose 4-6H. Severe infection: 100,000u (60mg)/kg/dose (max 3g) IV 12H (1st wk life), 6H (2-4 wk), 4H or constant infusion (>4 wk).

Penicillin, procaine. 25,000-50,000u(25-50mg)/kg (max 1.2-2.4g) 12-24H IM. Single dose: 100mg/kg (max 4.8g).

Penicillin V (phenoxymethylpenicillin). 7.5-15mg/kg/dose (max 500mg) 6H oral. Prophylaxis: 12.5mg/kg/dose 12H oral.

Penicilloyl polylysine (Prepen, 0.00006 molar). Scratch: 1 drop. Intradermal: 0.01-0.02ml (NOT/kg).

Pentaerythritol tetranitrate. 0.2-1.0mg/kg/dose (max 60mg) 6-8H oral.

Pentagastrin. 6μg/kg SC, or 0.6μg/kg/hr IV.

Pentastarch. 10% solution: 10-40mg/kg IV.

Pentamidine isethionate. 4mg/kg of base IV over 2hr or IM daily for 10-14 days (1mg base = 1.5mg mesylate = 1.74 mg isethionate).

Pentazocine. Oral: 0.5-2.0mg/kg/dose (max 100mg) 3-4H. SC, IM or slow IV: 0.5-1.0mg/kg/dose (max 60mg) 3-4H. PR: 1.0 mg/kg/dose (max 50mg) 6-12H.

Pentobarbital. see pentobarbitone.

Pentobarbitone. 0.5-1.0mg/kg/dose (max 60mg) 6-8H oral, IM, slow IV. Hypnotic: 2-4mg/kg (max 200mg).

Pentostatin. 4 mg/m^2 IV wkly.

Pentoxifylline. see oxypentifylline.

Pergolide. Parkinson's: 1μg/kg (max 0.5mg) daily, incr to max 25μg/kg/dose (max 2mg) 8H oral. Hyperprolactinaemia: 0.5-3μg/kg daily.

Pericyazine. 0.15-1mg/kg/dose (max 150mg) 12H oral.

Perindopril. 0.05-0.15mg/kg (max 8mg) daily oral.

Permethrin. Creme rinse 1% (head lice): wash hair, apply creme for 10min, wash off; may repeat in 2wk. Cream 5% (scabies): apply to whole body except face, wash off after 12-24hr.

Perphenazine. 0.1-0.3mg/kg/dose (max 20mg) 8-12H oral.

Pertussis. see diphtheria + tetanus + pertussis vaccine.

Pethidine. 0.5-1.0mg/kg/dose IV, 1-1.5mg/kg/dose IM (half life 2-4hr). Infusion: 5mg/kg in 50ml heparin-5%D at 1-3ml/hr (100-300μg/kg/hr).

Phenacemide. 10-20mg/kg/dose (max 1g) 8H oral.

Phenazone 5.4% + benzocaine 1.4% otic (Auralgin). 3 drops 6-8H.

Phenazocine. 0.1-0.4mg/kg/dose (max 20mg) 4-6H oral or sublingual.

Phenazopyridine. 4mg/kg/dose (max 200mg) 6H oral for 2 days.

Phendimetrazine. 0.4-1.4mg/kg/dose (max 70mg) 8H oral.

Phenelzine. 0.3-2mg/kg/dose (max 90mg) 8H oral.

Phenethicillin. 5-10mg/kg/dose (max 500mg) 6H oral.

Phenindamine. 0.5-1.0mg/kg/dose (max 50mg) 8-12H oral.

Phenindione. Usually 0.25-1.0mg/kg/dose (max 50mg) 12H oral.

Pheniramine. 0.5-1mg/kg/dose (max 50mg) 6H oral.

Phenobarbital. see phenobarbitone.

Phenobarbitone. see also Colic Mixture. Loading dose in emergency: 20-30mg/kg IM or IV over 30min stat. Ventilated: repeat doses of 10-15mg/kg up to 100mg/kg in 24hr (beware hypotension). Usual maintenance: 5mg/kg (max 300mg) daily IV, IM or oral. Level 80-120umol/l (x0.23 = μg/ml).

Phenolphthalein. 0.5-5mg/kg (max 270mg) at night oral.

Phenoperidine. 0.03-0.05mg/kg/dose (max 1mg) every 40-60min. Ventilated: 0.1-0.15 mg/kg/dose (max 5mg) every 40-60min.

Phenoxybenzamine. 0.2-1mg/kg 12-24H oral. Cardiac surgery: 1mg/kg IV over 1hr stat, then 0.5mg/kg/dose 6-12H IV over 1hr or oral.

Phenoxymethylpenicillin. see penicillin V.

Phensuximide. 10-20mg/kg/dose (max 1g) 8-12H oral.

Phentermine. Adult (NOT/kg): 30-40mg daily oral, reducing to 15-40mg daily.

Phentolamine. 0.1mg/kg stat, then 5-50μg/kg/min IV.

Phenylacetate. see sodium phenylacetate.

Phenylbutazone. Initially 2mg/kg/dose (max 100mg) 4H, reducing to 1-2mg/kg/dose (max 100mg) 6-8H oral.

Phenylephrine. IV: 2-10μg/kg stat (max 500μg), then 1-5μg/kg/min. SC or IM: 0.1-0.2mg/kg (max 10mg). Eye drops (0.12%, 10%): 1-2 drops/eye 6-8H. Nose drops (0.25%, 0.5%): 1-3 drops/sprays per nostril 6-8H.

Phenylpropanolamine. 0.5mg/kg/dose (max 25mg) 6-8H oral.

Phenyltoloxamine. 1mg/kg/dose (max 50mg) 8H oral.

Phenytoin. Loading dose in emergency: 15-20mg/kg (max1.5g) IV over 1 hr. Maintenance: oral or IV 4mg/kg/dose 12H (1st wk life; ½ dose if preterm), 8H (2nd wk), 6H (3wk-5yr), 8H (5-9yr); 2 mg/kg/dose (usual max 100mg) 6-12H > 12 yr. Level 40-80 mol/l (x0.25 = μg/ml).

Pholcodine. 0.1-0.2mg/kg/dose (max 10mg) 6-12H oral.

Phosphate, potassium (1mmol/ml). 0.1-1mmol/kg/day (max 20mmol/day) IV infusion.

Phosphate, sodium (500mg tab). 0.5-1g (NOT/kg) 8H oral.

Physostigmine. 0.02mg/kg (max 1mg) IV every 5 min till response (max 0.1mg/kg), then 5-2.0μg/kg/min.

Phytomenadione. 0.3mg/kg (max 10mg), IM or IV over 1hr. Prophylaxis in neonates (NOT/kg): 1mg IM at birth; or 1mg oral or 0.1mg IM at birth, at 4-7 days, and 3-4 weeks (give ½ se if weight < 1500g).

Phytonadione. see phytomenadione.

Pilocarpine, eye drops 0.5%, 1%, 2%, 3%, 4%. 1-2 drops 2-4 times a day.

Pimozide. 0.04-0.4mg/kg (max 20mg) daily oral.

Pindolol. 0.3mg/kg/dose (max 15mg) 8-24H oral.

Pine tar, gel, solution. 5ml to baby bath, 15-30ml to adult bath; soak for 10min.

Pipenzolate. 0.1mg/kg/dose (max 5mg) 6H oral.

Piperacillin. 50mg/kg/dose (max 4g) IV 4-8H (1st wk life), 4-6H or constant infusion (2+ wk).

Piperazine. 75mg/kg (max 4g) oral daily for 2 days (ascaris), 7 days (pinworm).

Pipothiazine. Oily injection: initially 0.5mg/kg (max 25mg), then 1-4mg/kg (max 200mg) every 4wk IM.

Piracetam. 15mg/kg/dose (max 800mg) 8H oral, IM or IV.

Pirbuterol. Oral: 0.2-0.3mg/kg/dose (max 15mg) 6-8H. Inhalation: 0.2-0.4mg/dose (NOT/kg) 4-6H (max 2.4mg/day).

Pirenzepine. 1mg/kg/dose (max 50mg) 12H oral.

Piretanide. Sustained release tab: 0.1-0.2mg/kg (max 12mg) daily.

Piroxicam. 0.2-0.4mg/kg (max 20mg) daily oral.

Pivampicillin. 20mg/kg/dose (max 500mg) 8-12H oral.

Pivampicillin 1.25 mg + pivmecillinam 1mg. 5-10mg/kg per dose (max 250mg) of pivampicillin 12H oral.

Pizotifen. NOT/kg: 1-3mg daily oral, usually 0.5mg morning, 1mg night.

Plague vaccine (CSL). Inactivated. Adult (>11yr): 0.5ml SC stat, and 1-4wk later (2 doses); boost every 6mo. Child: 0.1ml (6mo-2yr), 0.2ml (3-6yr), 0.3ml (7-11yr) SC stat, 1-4wk later, and 1-4wk later (3 doses); boost every 6mo.

Platelets. 10ml/kg IV stat, then daily if necessary. 1 unit is about 60ml.

Plicamycin. Testicular tumours: 25-30µg/kg daily for 8-10 days IV over 6hr, repeat monthly if response. Hypercalcaemia: 25µg/kg daily for 3-4 days, then x1-3/wk.

Pneumococcus vaccine (Pneumovax 23). Inactivated. >2yr: 0.5ml SC or IM once.

Podofilox. see podophyllotoxin.

Podophyllotoxin, paint 0.5% Apply 12H for 3 days, then none for 4 days; 4wk course.

Podophyllum, solution or ointment 15%-25%. Apply to wart x2/day.

Poldine. 0.1mg/kg/dose (max 4mg) 6H oral.

Polio vaccine, oral (Sabin). Live. 2 drops oral at 2mo, 4mo and 6mo. Boost at 5yr, and if going to epidemic area.

Polio vaccine, SC (Enpovax HDC). Inactivated. 0.5ml SC stat, 8wk later, and 8wk later (3 doses). Boost 12mo later, and at school entry.

Poloxalkol. 10% solution: 1 drop per month of age (max 25 drops) 8H oral.

Polyestradiol. Adult: 40-80mg (NOT/kg) IM every 2-4wk.

Polyethylene glycol. see colonic lavage solution.

Polymyxin B. see bacitracin + neomycin + polymyxin.

Polynoxylin, gel 10%. Apply 12H.

Polycarbophil Ca. 20mg/kg/dose (max 1g) 4-24H oral.

Polystyrene sulphonate (Resonium). 0.3-0.6g/kg/dose (max 30g) 6H NG (give lactulose) or PR.

Polythiazide. 0.02-0.1mg/kg/dose (max 4mg) daily oral.

Polyvinyl alcohol, eye drops 1.4%, 3%. 1-2 drops per eye prn.

POR 8. see ornipressin.

Potassium. Max IV 0.4mmol/kg/hr. Need 2-4 mmol/kg/day. 1g KCl = 13.3mmol K, 7.5% KCl = 1mmol/ml.

Potassium canrenoate. 3-8mg/kg (max 400mg) daily IV.

Potassium guaiacolsulfonate. 1-3mg/kg/dose (max 160 mg) 4-6H oral.

Povidone-iodine, cream, ointment, paint, solution. Apply 6-12H.

Pralidoxime. 25-50mg/kg (max 2g) over 30min, then up to 10mg/kg/hr (max 12g/day).

Pravastatin. 0.2-0.4mg/kg (max 20mg) at bedtime oral.

Prazepam. 0.2-1mg/kg (max 60mg) at night oral.

Praziquantel. 20mg/kg/dose 4H for 3 doses oral.

Prazosin. 0.005mg/kg (max 0.25mg) test dose, then 0.025-0.1 mg/kg/dose (max 5mg) 6H oral.

Prednisolone. Asthma: 0.5-1.0mg/kg/dose 6H for 24hr, 12H for the next 24hr, then 1.0mg/kg daily. Severe croup: 4mg/kg stat, then 1mg/kg/dose 8-12H oral. Prednisolone 1mg = hydrocortisone 0.8mg in mineralocorticoid action, 4mg in glucocorticoid. see also methylprednisolone.

Prednisolone acetate 1% + phenylephrine 0.12%, eye drops. 1-2 drops per eye 6-12H.

Prednisolone sodium phosphate, ear/eye drops 0.5%. 1-3 drops per eye 2-6H.

Prednisone. Action equivalent to prednisolone.

Prilocaine. Max dose 6mg/kg (0.6ml/kg of 1%). With adrenaline max dose 9mg/kg (0.9ml/kg of 1%).

Primaquine. Usually 0.3mg/kg (max 15mg) daily for 14-21 days oral. Gameteocyte: 0.7mg/kg (max 45mg) once.

Primidone. 5-15mg/kg/dose (max 750mg) 12H oral.

Probenicid. 25mg/kg (max 1g) stat, then 10mg/kg/dose (max 500mg) 6H oral.

Probucol. 10mg/kg/dose (max 500mg) 12H oral.

Procainamide. 3-6mg/kg (max 100mg) IV over 15 min, then 20-80µg/kg/min (max 80mg/hr). 2.5-7.5mg/kg 4H oral.

Procaine. Max dose 20mg/kg (1ml/kg of 2%).

Procarbazine. 1mg/kg daily oral, incr over 4-6 days to 4-6mg/kg (max 300mg) daily until remission, then 1-2mg/kg daily. Suspend if leucocytes < 3000/mm3 or platelets < 80,000/mm^3.

Prochlorperazine (1mg base = approx 1.5mg edisylate, maleate or mesylate). Only use if > 10kg. IM or slow IV: 0.1-0.2mg/kg (max 15mg salt) 6-8H. Oral or PR: 0.1-0.4mg/kg/dose (max 25mg salt) 6-8H, slow incr to max 0.6mg/kg/dose (max 35mg) 6H in psychosis. Buccal: 0.05-0.1mg/kg (max 6mg salt) 12-24H.

Procyclidine. 0.05-0.2mg/kg/dose (max 10mg) 6-8H oral.

Progesterone. Adult. Premenstrual syndrome: 200-400mg/dose (NOT/kg) PV or PR 12-24H (last ½ cycle). Dysfunctional uterine haemorrhage: 5-10mg/day (NOT/kg) IM for 5-10 days before menses. Prevent abortion: 25-100mg (NOT/kg) IM every 2-4 days.

Proguanil. 4mg/kg (max 200mg) daily oral after food.

Promazine. Oral: 2-4mg/kg/dose (max 200mg) 6H. IM 0.7 mg/kg/dose (max 50mg) 6-8H.

Promethazine. Antihistamine, antiemetic: 0.2-0.5mg/kg/dose (max 25mg) 6-8H IV, IM or oral. Sedative, hypnotic: 0.5-1.5mg/kg/dose (max 100mg).

Propafenone. Oral: 3-5mg/kg/dose (max 300mg) 8H. IV: 1-2mg/kg over 15min, then 10-20µg/kg/min.

Propantheline bromide. 0.3-0.6mg/kg/dose (max 30mg) 6H oral.

Propofol. 1-3mg/kg stat, then 4-12mg/kg/hr IV. Beware acidosis and myocardial depression.

Propoxyphene. See dextropropoxyphene.

Propranolol. IV: 0.02mg/kg test dose then 0.1mg/kg (max 5 mg) over 10 min (repeat x1-3 prn), then 0.1-0.3mg/kg /dose 3H. Oral: 0.2-0.5mg/kg/dose 6-12H, slow incr to max 1.5 mg/kg/dose (max 80mg) 6-12H if required.

Propylthiouracil. 50mg/m^2/dose 8H oral, reduce according to response.

Prostaglandin. see alprostadil (PGE1), carboprost (15-Me-PGF2-alpha), dinoprost (PGF2-alpha), dinoprostone (PGE2), epoprostenol (PGI2), gemeprost (PGE1 analogue), and misoprostol (PGE1 analogue).

Protamine. IV 1mg/100u heparin (or 1mg per 25ml pump blood) IV stat; subsequent doses of protamine 1 mg/kg (max 50mg). Heparin 1mg = 100u (half life 1-2hr).

Prothionamide. TB: 15-20mg/kg (max 1g) at night oral. Leprosy: 5-8mg/kg (max 375mg) daily.

Prothrombinex (factors 2, 9 and 10; 250u/10ml). 1ml/kg slow IV daily. Risk of thrombosis in acute liver failure.

Protionamide. see prothionamide.

Protirelin. 200µg (NOT/kg) IV stat.

Protriptyline. 0.1-0.2mg/kg/dose (max 20mg) 6-8H oral.

Proxymetacaine, eye drops 0.5%. 1-2 drops stat, then 1 drop every 10min.

Pseudoephedrine. 1mg/kg/dose (max 60mg) 6H oral.

Psyllium. Usually 0.1-0.2g/kg (max 10g) at night oral.

Pyrantel embonate. 10mg/kg once oral. Necator: 20mg/kg daily x2 doses. Enterobius: 10mg/kg each 2wk x3 doses.

Pyrazinamide. 20-35mg/kg/dose (max 3g) daily oral.

Pyridostigmine. 1-3mg/kg/dose (usual max 200mg) 4-12H oral. 180mg slow release tab (Timespan): adult 1-3 tab (NOT/kg) 12-24H. 1mg IV, IM or SC = 30mg oral.

Pyridoxine. With isoniazid: 5-10mg daily (NOT/kg) IV or oral. Neonatal fitting: 50-100mg daily (NOT/kg) IV or oral. Sideroblastic anaemia: 2-8mg/kg (max 400mg) daily IV or oral.

Pyrilamine. See mepyramine.

Pyrimethamine 12.5mg and dapsone 100mg (Maloprim). 1-4yr quarter tab wkly, 5-10yr ½ tab, > 10yr 1tab.

Pyrimethamine 25mg and sulphadoxine 500mg (Fansidar). < 4yr ½ tab once, 4-8yr 1 tab, 9-14yr 2 tab, > 14yr 3 tab. Prophylaxis: < 4yr ¼ tab wkly, 4-8yr ½ tab, 9-14yr 3/4 tab, > 14yr 1 tab.

Q fever vaccine (Q-Vax). Inactivated. 0.5ml SC once.

Quazepam. 0.15-0.6mg/kg (max 30mg) at night oral.

Quinacrine. see mepacrine.

Quinalbarbitone. Sedative 5mg/kg. Premed 10mg/kg.

Quinapril. 0.2-0.8mg/kg (max 40mg) daily oral.

Quinestrol. Adult (NOT/kg): 100µg daily for 7 days, then 100-200µg wkly oral.

Quinethazone. 1-3mg/kg (max 200mg) daily oral.

Quinidine sulphate. 12mg/kg stat, then 6mg/kg/dose (max 400mg) 4-6H oral. IV: 7.5mg/kg IV over 2hr, then 15µg/kg/min. IM: 15mg/kg stat, then 7.5mg/kg/dose (max 400mg) 8H.

Quinine sulphate. Oral: 10mg/kg/dose (max 600mg) 8H for 7-10 days. Parenteral: 20mg/kg IV over 4hr or IM, then 7.5 mg/kg/dose 8H IV over 1hr or IM for 2-3 days, then 10mg/kg/dose 8H oral for 5 days.

Rabies vaccine, inactivated (HDCV, Merieux).	
	1ml IM stat, 7 days later, and 28 days later (3 doses). Boost every 2yr. Post exposure: if immune, 1ml IM day 0 and day 3; if non-immune, give 1ml IM on days 0,3,7,14,30 and 90, with immunoglobulin.
Ramipril.	0.05mg/kg (max 2.5mg) oral daily, may incr over 4-6wk to 0.1-0.2mg/kg (max 10mg) daily.
Ranitidine.	IV: 1mg/kg/dose slowly 6-8H, or 2μg/kg/min. Oral: 2-4mg/kg/dose (max 300mg) 12H.
Razoxone.	2mg/kg/dose (max 125mg) 8-24H oral; or 7.5-15mg/kg (max 750mg) daily for 2-3 days every 1-4wk. Kaposi sarcoma, leukaemia: max 0.33g/m^2/dose 8H oral.
Remoxipride.	1.5-6mg/kg/dose (max 300mg) 12H oral.
Renatonium, solution 2mg/ml.	Apply 8H and after washing hands.
Reproterol.	Aerosol 0.5mg/puff: 1-2 puffs 3-8H.
Reserpine.	0.005-0.01mg/kg/dose (max 0.5mg) 12-24H oral.
Resonium.	see polystyrene sulphonate.
Retinol A.	see vitamin A.
Ribavirin.	Inhalation (Viratek nebulizer): 20mg/ml at 25ml/hr (190μg/l of gas) for 12-18 hr/day for 3-7 days.
Riboflavine.	5-10mg daily (NOT/kg) oral.
Rifabutin.	3-12mg/kg (max 600mg) daily oral.
Rifampicin.	10-15mg/kg (max 600mg) daily oral fasting, or IV over 3hr (monitor AST). Prophylaxis (meningococcus 2 days, haemophilus 4 days): 10 mg/kg/dose (max 600mg) daily (newborn), 12H (>4wk old) oral.
Rifampin.	see rifampicin.
Rimipril.	Initially 0.05mg/kg (max 2.5mg) oral daily, incr over 4-6wk to max 0.2mg/kg (max 10mg) daily if needed.
Rimiterol.	Aerosol 0.2mg/puff: 1-3puffs 3-8H.
Risperidone.	0.02-0.15mg/kg/dose (max 8mg) 12H oral.
Ritodrine.	Premature labour: 0.05-0.45mg/min (NOT/kg) IV; 10-20mg/dose (NOT/kg) 4-6H oral.
Rolitetracyline (Reverin).	>8yr: 10mg/kg/dose (max 275 mg) daily slow IV.
Roxithromycin.	2.5mg/kg/dose (max 150mg) 12H oral before meals.
Rubella vaccine (Ervevax, Meruvax II)	
	Live. >12mo: 0.5ml SC once. See also measles + mumps + rubella vaccine.
Salbutamol.	0.1-0.15 mg/kg/dose (max 8mg) 6H oral. Inhalation – mild: respiratory solution (5mg/ml, 0.5%) 0.5 ml/dose diluted to 4ml, or nebulise 2.5mg/2.5ml 3-6H; moderate: 0.5% solution 1ml/dose diluted to 4ml, or nebulise 5mg/2.5ml 1-2H; severe (in ICU): 0.5% solution undiluted continuous. Aerosol 100μg/puff: 1-2 puff 4-6H. Rotahaler: 200-400μg 6-8H. IM or SC: 8μg/kg. IV: child 5μg/kg over 10 min, then 1-5μg/kg/min (1μg/kg/min using 1mg/ml solution = 0.06 x Wt ml/hr); adult 4μg/kg over 10min, then (NOT/kg) 10-50μg/min (0.6ml/hr of 1mg/ml solution = 10μg/min).
Salcatonin.	Hypercalcaemia: 4u/kg/dose 12H IM or SC, may incr to 8u/kg/dose 6-12H.
Salicylic acid.	Cradle cap: 6% solution (Egocappol) 12H 3-5 days. Plantar warts: 15% solution x 1-2 /day, 40% medicated disc 24-48H.
Salicylsalicylic acid.	See salsalate.
Salmeterol.	Aerosol or diskhaler (NOT/kg): 50-100mg 12H.
Salmonella typhi vaccine.	see typhoid vaccine.
Salsalate.	10-20mg/kg/dose (max 1g) 6H oral.

Sargramostim (GM-CSF, Leucomax). 3-5μg/kg daily SC, or IV over 6hr. Keep WCC 5,000-10,000/mm3.

Scopolamine. see hyoscine.

Secbutobarbitone. 0.3-0.6mg/kg/dose (max 30mg) 6-8H, or 1-4mg/kg (max 200mg) nocte oral.

Secobarbital sodium. see quinalbarbitone.

Secretin (1cu = 4chr units). 1-2cu/kg slow IV.

Selegiline. Adult (NOT/kg): 10mg each morning, oral.

Selenium sulphide, 2.5%. Shampoo x2/wk for 2wk.

Sennoside. Tab 7.5mg daily (NOT/kg): 6mo-2yr ½-1 tab, 3-10yr 1-2 tab, >10yr 2-4 tab. Granules 22.5mg/teasp, 12-24H (NOT/kg): <6mo ¼-½teasp, 6mo-2yr ½-1teasp, 3-10yr 1-2teasp.

Sermorelin (GHRH). 1μg/kg fasting in morning IV.

Sertraline. 1-2mg/kg (max 100mg) daily oral; may give 3-4mg/kg (max 200mg) daily for up to 8wk.

Silver nitrate, stick. Apply daily to affected area only.

Silver sulfadiazine 1% + chlorhexidine 0.2%, cream. Apply in 3-5mm layer.

Simethicone. see aluminium hydroxide compound.

Simvastatin. Initially 0.2mg/kg (max 10mg) daily, may incr every 4wk to max 1mg/kg (max 40mg) daily oral.

Sodium. Deficit: ml of 20% NaCl = weight x 0.2 x (140 – serum Na); do not increase serum Na faster than 2 mmol/l/hr. Need 2-6 mmol/kg/day. NaCl MW = 58.45, 1g NaCl = 17.1mmol Na, NaCl 20% = 3.4mmol/ml.

Sodium alginate. see alginic acid.

Sodium aurothiomalate. 0.25mg/kg wkly IM, incr to 1 mg/kg (max 50mg) weekly for 10wk, then every 2-6wk. IM, then every 1-4wk.

Sodium benzoate. Neonate: 250mg/kg over 2hr stat, then 10-20mg/kg/hr IV.

Sodium bicarbonate. see bicarbonate.

Sodium calcium edetate (EDTA). 30-40mg/kg/dose 12H IM or IV over 1hr for 5 days.

Sodium chloride. see sodium.

Sodium citrotartrate. 40-80mg/kg/dose (max 4g) in 50ml water 8-12H oral.

Sodium clodronate. 6mg/kg (max 300mg) IV over 2hr daily for 7 days, then 15-30/mg/kg/dose (max 1.6g) 12H oral.

Sodium cromoglycate (Intal). see cromoglycate.

Sodium etidronate. 5-20mg/kg daily oral (no food for 2hr before and after dose) for max 6mo.

Sodium fluoride. NOT/kg: <2yr 0.55mg oral daily, 2-4yr 1.1 mg, >4yr 2.2mg. Osteoporosis, Paget's, bone secondaries in adult: 20-40mg/dose (NOT/kg) 8-12H.

Sodium nitrite. 3% solution: 0.2ml/kg (max 10ml) IV over 5min.

Sodium nitroprusside. see nitroprusside.

Sodium phenylacetate. Neonate: 250mg/kg IV over 2hr, then 10mg/kg/hr.

Sodium picosulphate. 0.1-0.3mg/kg (max 15ml) at night oral.

Sodium tetradecyl sulphate. 0.25-1ml per vein (NOT/kg) as 1% (max 10 small veins) or 3% (max 4 large veins).

Sodium thiosulphate. 1ml/kg (max 50ml) 25% solution IV over 10min.

Sofradex, Soframycin. see framycetin.

Somatostatin. see octreotide.

Somatrem. 4u/m^2 3 days a wk IM.

Somatropin. Usually 2-3iu/m^2 on 5-7 days a wk SC, or 4-6iu/m^2 on 3 days a wk IM.

Sorbitol 70%. 0.2-0.5ml/kg/dose (max 30ml) 8H oral. With activated charcoal: 1g/kg (1.4ml/kg) NG, may repeat x1.

Sorbolene cream; pure, with 10% glycerin, or with 5% or 10% olive oil or peanut oil. Skin moisturiser, apply prn.

Sotalol. IV: 0.5-2mg/kg/dose (max 100mg) over 10min 6H. Oral: 1-4 mg/kg/dose (max 200mg) 8H.

Spectinomycin. 40-80mg/kg (max 4g) IM once.

Spironolactone. Oral: 0-10kg 6.25mg/dose (NOT/kg) 12H, 11-20kg 12.5 mg/dose (NOT/kg) 12H, 21-40kg 25 mg/dose (NOT/kg) 12H, over 40kg 25mg/dose (NOT/kg) 8H. IV: see potassium canrenoate.

Stanozolol. 0.05-0.2mg/kg oral (max 10mg) daily at first, then every 2-3 days.

Sterculia. 3.5-7g/dose (NOT/kg) 12-24H oral.

Stilboestrol. Ca breast: 10-20mg (NOT/kg) daily oral. Ca prostate: 1-3mg (NOT/kg) daily oral or IV.

Streptokinase (SK). Short term (myocardial infarct): 30,000u/kg (max 1,500,000u) IV over 60min, repeat if occlusion recurs < 5 days. Long term (DVT, pulmonary embolism, art thrombosis): 5,000 u/kg (max 250,000u) IV over 30min, then 2000 u/kg/hr (max 100,000u/hr); stop heparin and aspirin, if PTT < x2 normal at 4hr give extra 10,000u/kg (max 500,000u) IV over 30min, stop SK if PTT > x5 normal then give 1000u/kg/hr. Local infusion: 50 u/kg/hr (continue heparin 10-15u/kg/hr). Blocked IV cannula: 5000u/kg in 2ml in cannula for 2hr then remove, repeat x1.

Streptomycin. 20-30mg/kg (max 1g) IM daily.

Streptozocin. 1.0-1.5g/m^2 wkly IV.

Succinyl choline. see suxamethonium.

Sucralfate 1g tab. NOT/kg: 0-2yr quarter tab 6H, 3-12 yr ½ tab 6H, > 12yr 1 tab 6H oral.

Sufentanil. 2-50μg/kg slow IV; may then infuse so that total dose is 1μg/kg/hr of expected surgical time.

Sulbactam. see ampicillin + sulbactam.

Sulfacetamide. see sulphacetamide.

Sulfadiazine. 50mg/kg/dose (max 2g) 6H slow IV.

Sulfadoxine. see pyrimethamine and sulfadoxine.

Sulfamethizole. see sulphamethizole.

Sulfamethoxazole. see cotrimoxazole.

Sulfametopyrazine. 40mg/kg (max 2g) wkly oral.

Sulfasalazine. see sulphasalazine.

Sulfinpyrazone. see sulphinpyrazone.

Sulfisoxazole. see sulphafurazole.

Sulindac. 4mg/kg/dose (max 200mg) 12H oral.

Sulphacetamide 10% + prednisolone 0.2% + phenyl-ephrine 0.12%, eye drops. 1 drop per eye 6-12H.

Sulphafurazole. 5mg/kg (max 4g) stat, then 35mg/kg /dose (max 1.5g) 4-6H oral.

Sulphamethizole. 15mg/kg/dose (max 1g) 8H oral.

Sulphamethoxazole. see cotrimoxazole.

Sulphasalazine. Active disease: 10-15mg/kg/dose (max 1g) 6H oral. Remission: 5-7.5mg/kg/dose (max 0.5g) 6H.

Sulphinpyrazone. 2-3mg/kg/dose (max 200mg) 6-12H oral.

Sulpiride. 4mg/kg/dose (max 200mg) 12H, slow increase to 4-24mg/kg/dose (max 1.2g) 12H oral.

Sulthiame. 1mg/kg/dose 8-12H oral, may incr to 5mg/kg /dose (max 200mg) 8H.

Sumatriptan. Oral: 2mg/kg (max 100mg) stat, may repeat twice. SC: 0.12mg/kg (max 6mg) stat, may repeat once after 1hr.

Surfactant, bovine (Survanta) see beractant.

Surfactant, synthetic (Exosurf Neonatal). Prophylaxis: 5 ml/kg intratracheal over 5min immediately after birth, and at 12hr and 24hr if still ventilated. Rescue: 5ml/kg intratracheal over 5min, repeat in 12hr if still ventilated.

Suxamethonium. IV: neonate 3mg/kg/dose, child 2mg/kg /dose, adult 1mg/kg/dose. IM: double IV dose.

Tacrine (THA). 0.5-2mg/kg/dose (max 120mg) 3H IV.

Talampicillin. 5-10mg/kg/dose (max 500mg) 8H oral.

Tamoxifen. Adult: 20mg daily (NOT/kg), incr to 40mg daily if no response after 1mo.

Tar. See coal tar.

Teceleukin (synthetic interleukin-2). see interleukin-2.

Teicoplanin. 250mg/m^2 IV over 30min stat, then 125 mg/m^2 IV or IM daily. Severe infection: 250mg/m^2 12H x3 doses, then 250mg/m^2 IV or IM daily.

Temazepam. Adult: 10-30mg (NOT/kg) at night, oral.

Temocillin. 20-50mg/kg/dose (max 2g) 12H IV or IM.

Teniposide. 100-150mg/m^2 IV over 1hr wkly.

Tenoxicam. 0.2-0.4mg/kg (max 20mg) daily oral.

Terazosin. 0.02mg/kg test, then 0.04-0.4mg/kg (max 20 mg) daily oral.

Terbinafine. 5mg/kg (max 250mg) daily oral.

Terbutaline. Oral: 0.05-0.1mg/kg/dose (max 5mg) 6H. SC: 5-10µg/kg/dose (max 500µg). IV: 5µg/kg stat over 10min, then 1-10µg/kg/hr. Inhalation – mild: respiratory solution (1%, 10mg/ml) 0.25ml/dose diluted to 4ml 3-6H; moderate: 0.5ml of 1% diluted to 4ml, or respule 5mg/2ml 1-2H; severe (in ICU): undiluted continuous. Aerosol 250µg /puff: 1-2 puffs 4-6H.

Terfenadine. 1mg/kg/dose (max 60mg) 12H oral.

Testolactone. 5-10mg/kg/dose (max 250mg) 6H oral.

Testosterone. Esters: 100-500mg (NOT/kg) IM every 2-4wk. Implant: 8mg/kg (to nearest 100mg). Undecanoate: 40-120mg (NOT/kg) daily oral. Testosterone level: < 16yr 5-10nmol/L, > 16yr 10-30nmol/l.

Tetanus toxoid (CSL). 0.5ml IM stat, 6wk later, and 6mo later. Boost every 10yr, or if contaminated wound. See also diphtheria (+ pertussis) + tetanus vaccines.

Tetrabenazine. 0.5-2mg/kg/dose (max 100mg) 12H oral.

Tetracaine. see amethocaine.

Tetracosactrin zinc injection (Synacthen Depot). 600µg/m^2 (max 1mg) IM every 1-7 days.

Tetracycline. Over 8yr: 250-500mg/dose (NOT/kg) 6H oral. see also rolitetracycline.

Tetrahydrozoline, eye drops 0.05%. 1-2 drops/eye 8-12H.

Tetrahydrozoline 0.05% + macrogol 400 (polyethylene glycol) 1%, eye drops. 1-2 drops/eye 8-12H.

THAM. see tromethamine.

Theophylline (80mg theophylline = 100mg aminophylline). Loading dose: 8mg/kg (max 500mg) oral. Maintenance: 1st wk life 2mg/kg/dose 12H; 2nd wk life 3mg/kg/dose 12H; 3wk-12mo (0.1 x age in wk) + 3mg/kg/dose 8H; 1-9yr 4mg/kg/dose 4-6H, or 10mg/kg/dose slow release 12H; 10-16yr or adult smoker 3mg/kg/dose 4-6H, or 7mg/kg /dose 12H slow release; adult non-smoker 3 mg/kg/dose 6-8H; elderly 2mg/kg/dose 6-8H. Monitor serum level: neonate 60-80 mol/l, asthma 60-110 (x0.18 =μg/ml).

Thiabendazole. 25mg/kg/dose (max 1.5g) 12H oral for 3 days.

Thiamine. Beriberi: 1-2mg/kg IV, IM or oral daily.

Thiamylal. 0.05-0.1ml/kg of 2.5% solution IV over 1min; may then infuse 0.3% solution.

Thiethylperazine maleate. >10kg: 0.2mg/kg/dose (max 10mg) 8-24H oral, IM, or PR.

Thioguanine. 100mg/m^2 daily oral; or 100mg/m^2/dose 12H for 5-7 days.

Thiopentone. 3-5mg/kg slowly stat (beware hypotension), then 1-5mg/kg/hr IV. Level 150-200umol/l (x 0.24 =μg/ml).

Thioridazine. 0.5-3mg/kg/dose (max 150mg) 6-8H oral, IM.

Thiosulphate. see sodium thiosulphate.

Thiotepa. 10-14mg/m^2 IV every 1-4wk.

Thiotepa, eye drops 1 in 2000. 2 drops/eye 4-6H for 6wk.

Thiothixene. >12yr: initially 2mg/dose (NOT/kg) 8H oral, slow incr to 2-20mg per dose.

Thrombin, topical. 100-2000u/ml onto bleeding surface.

Thymoxamine. Adult: 40-80mg/dose (NOT/kg) 6H oral.

Thyroxine. Infants: 25μg daily (NOT/kg), gradually incr to 3-5μg/kg/day oral. Adult: 100-200μg daily (NOT/kg).

Tiaprofenic acid. 2-4mg/kg/dose (max 200mg) 8H oral.

Tibolone. Adult: 2.5mg (NOT/kg) daily oral.

Ticarcillin. 50mg/kg/dose (max 3g) IV 6-8H (1st wk life), 4-6H or constant infusion (2+ wk).

Ticarcillin and clavulanic acid. Dose as for ticarcillin.

Ticlopidine. 5 mg/kg/dose (max 250mg) 12H oral.

Tilactase. 200u/drop: 5-15 drops/l milk 24hr before use. 3300u/tab: 1-3tabs with meals.

Timolol. 0.1mg/kg/dose (max 5mg) 8-12H, incr to max 0.3 mg/kg/dose (max 15mg) 8H. Eye drops (0.25%, 0.5%): 1 drop/eye 12H.

Tinidazole. Giardia: 50mg/kg (max 2g) stat, repeat after 48hr. Amoebic Dys: 50mg/kg (max 2g) daily for 3 days.

Tinzaparin (1mg = 75 anti-Xa IU) 50u/kg SC 2hr before surgery, then daily for 7-10 days.

Tioconazole, 280mg/ml. Apply to nails 12H for 6-12mo.

Tissue plasminogen activator. see alteplase.

Tobramycin. Single daily dose IV or IM: 2.5mg/kg (<30wk gestation), 3.5mg/kg (30-35wk gestation), 5mg/kg (1st wk life), 7.5mg/kg (2+ wk), 6mg/kg (>10yr). Trough level<1.0 mg/l.

Tocainide. 5-10mg/kg/dose (max 400-800mg) 8-12H IV over 30min or oral.

Tocopherol. see vitamin E.

Tolazamide. 2-5mg/kg/dose (max 250mg) 6-24H oral.

Tolazoline. Newborn: 1-2mg/kg slowly stat (beware hypotension), then 2-6μg/kg/min (0.12-0.36mg/kg/hr) IV. Note: 1-2mg/kg/hr too much (*Pediatrics* 1986;77:307).

Tolbutamide. Adult: initially 1g (NOT/kg) 12H oral, often reducing to 0.5-1g daily.

Tolmetin. 5-10mg/kg/dose (max 400-600mg) 8H oral.

Tolnaftate, cream, ointment, powder, solution 1%. Apply 8-12H.

Tramazoline 120µg + dexamethasone 20µg per dose, nasal.
Aerosol: 1 puff in each nostril 4-8H.
Trandolapril. 0.01-0.1mg/kg (max 4mg) daily oral.
Tranexamic acid. 15-20mg/kg/dose (max 1g) 8H oral.
Tranylcypromine. 0.2mg/kg/dose (max 10mg) 8-12H oral.
Trazodone. 1-4mg/kg/dose (max 200mg) 8H oral.
Tretinoin, cream or lotion 0.05%, gel 0.01%.
Apply daily.
Triacetyloleandomycin. 6-12mg/kg/dose (max 250-500 mg) 6H oral.
Triamcinolone. Joint, tendon: 2.5-15mg (NOT/kg) stat. IM: 0.05-0.2mg/kg every 1-7 days. Cream or ointment 0.02%, 0.05%: apply sparingly 6-8H. Triamcinolone has no mineralocorticoid action, 1mg = 5mg hydrocortisone in glucocorticoid action.
Triamcinolone 0.1% + neomycin 0.25% + gramicidin 0.025% + nystatin 100,000u/g.
Kenacomb cream, ointment: apply 8-12H. Kenacomb otic cream, ointment, drops: apply 8-12H (2-3 drops).
Triamterene. 2mg/kg/dose (max 100mg) 8-24H oral.
Triazolam. Adult: 0.125-0.5mg (NOT/kg) at night, oral.
Tribavirin. see ribavirin.
Triclosan, emulsion 2%. 2ml to wet skin for 20sec, rinse and repeat.
Trientine. 10mg/kg/dose (max 500mg) 6-12H oral.
Triethylenethiophosphoramide.
see thiotepa.
Trifluoperazine. 0.02-0.2mg/kg/dose (max 10mg, occasionally 20mg) 12H oral.
Trifluridine. 1% solution: 1 drop/eye 2H (max 9 drops/day) until epithelialised, then 4H (max 5 drops/day) for 7 days.
Trihexyphenidyl. see benzhexol.
Triiodothyronine (T3). see liothyronine.
Trilostane. 0.5-4mg/kg/dose (max 240mg) 6H oral.
Trimeprazine (Vallergan). Antihistamine: 0.1-0.5mg/kg/dose (max 25mg) 6H oral. Sedation: 0.5-1mg/kg/dose IM, 2-4 mg/kg/dose oral.
Trimetaphan. 0.04-0.1mg/kg/min (max 4mg/min) IV.
Trimethadione. see troxidone.
Trimethobenzamide. 5mg/kg/dose (max 250mg) 6-8H oral, IM or PR.
Trimethoprim. 3-4mg/kg/dose (usual max 150mg) 12H, or 6-8mg/kg (usual max 300mg) daily oral or IV.
Trimethoprim-sulphamethoxazole.
see cotrimoxazole.
Trimipramine. 1-2mg/kg/dose (max 100mg) 8-24H oral.
Trioxsalen. see trioxysalen.
Trioxysalen. Adult: 5-10mg (NOT/kg) daily 2hr before UV exposure.
Tripelennamine. 1.25mg/kg/dose (max 75mg) 6H oral.
Tripotassium dicitratobismuthate (bismuth subcitrate).
50 mg/kg/dose (max 240mg) 12H oral 30min before meal. H. pylori (> 5yr old): 25mg/kg/dose 6H oral for 2-4wk, with metronidazole and (if > 7yr) tetracycline. Avoid milk.
Triprolidine 2.5mg + pseudoephedrine 60mg (Actifed).
10ml elixir = 1tab. NOT/kg: 2.5ml (< 2yr), 2.5-5ml (2-5yr), 0.5tab (6-12yr), 1tab (> 12yr) 6-8H oral.

Trisodium edetate. 40-70mg/kg (max 3g) IV over 6hr daily for 5 days; max 3 courses each 2 days apart.

Troleandomycin. see triacetyloleandomycin.

Tromethamine (THAM). ml of 0.3 molar (18g/500ml) solution = Wt x BE (give ½ this) IV over 30-60min.

Tropicamide, eye drops 0.5%, 1%.
1-2 drops/eye, repeat after 5min.

Tropisetron. 0.1mg/kg (max 5mg) slow IV just before chemotherapy, then oral 1hr before breakfast for 5 days.

Troxidone. 10-15mg/kg/dose (max 800mg) 8H oral.

Tubocurarine. ICU: 0.6mg/kg IV prn. Theatre: 0.3-0.6mg/kg IV stat, then 0.15mg/kg/dose.

Tulobuterol. 0.04mg/kg/dose (max 2mg) 8-12H oral.

Typhoid vaccine, oral (Typh-Vax).
Live. 1 cap oral days 1, 3, 5 and (for better immunity) 7. Boost yearly.

Typhoid vaccine, parenteral (CSL).
Inactivated. 0.1ml (<6yr), 0.25ml (6-12yr), 0.5ml (>12yr) SC stat, and 4wk later. Boost every 3yr.

Typhoid vaccine, parenteral, polysaccharide (Typhim Vi).
Inactivated. >5yr: 0.5ml IM once. Protects 3yr or more.

Urea, cream 10%. Apply 8-12H.

Urofollitrophin. As for menotrophin.

Urokinase. 4000u/kg IV over 10min, then 4000u/kg/hr for 12hr (start heparin 3-4hr later). Blocked cannula: instil 5000-25000u (NOT/kg) in 2-3ml saline for 2-4hr.

Ursodeoxycholic acid. 4-8mg/kg/dose 12H oral.

Ursodiol. see ursodeoxycholic acid.

Valproate. 5-25mg/kg/dose (max 500mg) 8-12H oral. Level 0.3-0.7mmol/l (x144=μg/ml),

Vancomycin. 20mg/kg/dose (max 500mg) IV over 2hr: daily (preterm), 12H (1st wk life), 8H (2+ wk). Oral: 5-10mg/kg/dose 6H. Intraventricular: 10mg per dose (NOT/kg) 48H. Peak level 25-40mg/l, trough<10mg/l.

Vasopressin. Aqueous: put 1-2u in 1l fluid, and replace urine output + 10% IV; or 2-10u IM or SC 8H. Brain death: 0.0003u/kg/min (1u/kg in 50ml at 1ml/hr) + adrenaline 0.1-0.2μg/kg/min. Oily: 2.5-5u (NOT/kg) IM every 2-4 days. GI haemorrhage (aqueous solution): 0.4u/min IV in adult; 0.1 u/min local IA in adult. See desmopressin and lypressin.

Vecuronium. ICU: 0.1mg/kg prn. Theatre: 0.1mg/kg stat, then 1-10μg/kg/min IV.

Verapamil. IV: 0.1-0.2mg/kg (max 10mg) over 10min, then 5μg/kg/min. Oral: 1-3 mg /kg /dose (max 120mg) 8-12H.

Vidarabine. Eye ointment: x5/day until epithelialised, then 12H 7 days. IV infusion: 10mg/kg/day 5-10 days (varicella-zoster), 15mg/kg/day 10 days (herpes encephalitis).

Vigabatrin. Initially 40mg/kg (max 2g) daily oral, may incr to 80-100mg/kg (max 4g) daily (given in 1-2 doses).

Viloxazine. 1-4mg/kg (max 250mg) morning, and 1-2mg/kg (max 150mg) noon oral.

Vinblastine. 6.5mg/m^2 IV over 1 min every 1-4wk.

Vincristine. 1.5mg/m^2 wkly IV over 1 min.

Vindesine. 3-4mg/m^2 IV every 7-10day if WCC >2500/mm^3.

Vitamin A. High risk: 200,000iu (NOT/kg) oral every 4-6mo.

Vitamin A, B, C, D compound (Pentavite).
Neonate 12drop, 0-6yr 2.5-5ml, >6yr 5ml (NOT/kg) daily oral.

Vitamin A+D (RCH 12,000u A, 2,000u D/ml).
1ml/day.

Vitamin B group. Amp: IV over 30 min. Tab: 1-2/day.

Vitamin B1. see thiamine.

Vitamin B12. see hydroxycobalamin.

Vitamin C. see ascorbic acid.

Vitamin D. Nutritional rickets: ergocalciferol (D2) 10,000u daily (NOT/kg) for 30 days, oral. Renal rickets or hypoparathyroidism: calcitriol (1,25-OH D3) start 0.01μg/kg daily; dihydrotachysterol (1-OH D2) 20μg/kg/day; ergocalciferol (D2): 50,000-300,000u/day (NOT/kg).

Vitamin E (Copherol E). Preterm babies: 40u (2 drops) daily (NOT/kg) oral. 1u = 1mg.

Vitamin K1. see phytomenadione.

Vitamins, parenteral. MVI-12 (for adult): 5ml in 1 litre IV fluid. MVI Paediatric, added to IV fluid: 65% of a vial (< 3kg), 1 vial (3kg to 11yr).

Vitaprem (RCH) (Pentavite, folate, B12, C). 1ml daily oral.

Warfarin. Usually 0.2mg/kg (max 10mg) stat, 0.2mg/kg (max 10mg) next day providing INR < 1.3, then 0.05-0.2mg/kg (max 10mg) daily oral. INR usually 2-2.5 for prophylaxis, 2-3 for treatment. Beware of drug interactions.

Whole blood. 8ml/kg incr Hb 1g%. 1bag = 400ml approx.

Xamoterol. 4mg/kg/dose (max 200mg) 12-24H oral.

Xipamide. 0.5-1.5mg/kg (max 80mg) every morning oral.

Xylometazoline. < 6yr: 0.05% 1 drop or spray 8-12H. 6-12yr: 0.05% 2-3 drops or sprays 8-12H. > 12yr: 0.1% 2-3 drops or sprays 6-12H.

Yellow fever vaccine (CSL). > 12mo: 0.5ml SC once. Boost every 10yr.

Yohimbine. 0.05-0.1mg/kg/dose (max 5.4mg) 8H oral.

Zalcitabine. 0.01mg/kg/dose 8H oral.

Zidovudine (AZT). 10mg/kg/dose (max 250mg) 4H oral.

Zinc sulphate. Adult: 50-220mg (NOT/kg) 8-24H oral.

Zopiclone. 0.1-0.3mg/kg (max 15mg) at bedtime oral.

Zuclopenthixol. 0.4-3mg/kg (max 150mg) daily oral.

Appendix 5

Drug infusion nomogram

multiplier	0.15	0.3	0.6	1.5	3.0	6	15	30	60
mg/kg/hr	ml/hr								
0.05	1	ml/hr							
0.1	2	1	ml/hr						
0.2	4	2	1						
0.3	6	3	1.5						
0.4	8	4	2	ml/hr					
0.5	10	5		1					
0.6	12	6	3						
0.7	14	7							
0.8	16	8	4						
0.9	18	9			ml/hr				
1.0	20	10	5	2	1				
1.5		15		3	1.5	ml/hr			
2.0		20	10	4	2	1			
3.0				6	3	1.5	ml/hr		
4.0			20	8	4	2	1		
5.0				10	5				
6.0				12	6	3			
7.0				14	7				
8.0				16	8	4			
9.0				18	9			ml/hr	
10				20	10	5	2	1	
12					12	6			
14					14	7			
15					15		3	1.5	ml/hr
20					20	10	4	2	1
25							5		
30						15	6	3	1.5
40						20	8	4	2
50							10	5	
100							20	10	5
150								15	
200								20	10

1. select drug dosage to be delivered in µg/kg/min
2. select infusion rate of syringe pump in ml/hour (from centre of the table)
3. calculate the number of milligrams of drug to be mixed in the 50 ml syringe

e.g. **10 kg child**
drug dosage range:
0.1 - 2 µg/kg/min
drug infusion rate:
1 - 20 ml/hr
put
0.3 mg/kg (i.e. 3 mg)
in 50 ml solution

multiplier x body weight (kg) = no. of mg to be made up to 50 ml

- 0.05–1.0: MORPHINE; NOR ADR ENA LINE; ISOPRENALINE; ADRENALINE; MAX IHRS
- 0.05–10: NITROPRUSSIDE (MAX INFUSION HRS: 10, 8, 7, 7, 6 beside rows 6.0–10)
- 0.6–10: NITROGLYCERINE
- 1.5–25: SALBUTAMOL; DOBUTAMINE; DOPAMINE
- 1.5–10: TOLAZOLINE
- 1.5–25: KETAMINE
- 12–200: LIGNOCAINE; THIOPENTONE

A nonogram for the calculation of the composition of drug infusions for a 50 ml syringe pump

Index

Q

U

V